CAROL DEALEY PhD MA BSc (Hons) RGN RCNT

Research Fellow
University Hospital Birmingham NHS Trust, and
School of Health Sciences
University of Birmingham

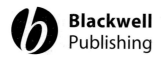

Blackwell
Publishing

© 2005 Blackwell Publishing Ltd

Editorial offices:
Blackwell Publishing Ltd, 9600 Garsington Road,
Oxford OX4 2DQ, UK
 Tel: +44 (0)1865 776868
Blackwell Publishing Inc., 350 Main Street, Malden,
MA 02148-5020, USA
 Tel: +1 781 388 8250
Blackwell Publishing Asia Pty Ltd, 550 Swanston
Street, Carlton, Victoria 3053, Australia
 Tel: +61 (0)3 8359 1011

First published 2005 by Blackwell Publishing Ltd

Library of Congress Cataloging-in-Publication Data

Dealey, Carol.
 The care of wounds : a guide for nurses / Carol
Dealey. – 3rd ed.
   p. ; cm.
 Includes bibliographical references and index.
 ISBN-13: 978-1-4051-1863-7 (pbk. : alk. paper)
 ISBN-10: 1-4051-1863-6 (pbk. : alk. paper)
 1. Wounds and injuries – Nursing.
 [DNLM 1. Wounds and Injuries – nursing.
2. Wound Healing – physiology. WO 700 D279c
2005] I. Title.
 RD93.95.D43   2005
 617.1 – dc22

                        2005001740

ISBN 10: 1-4051-1863-6
ISBN 13: 978-14051-1863-7

A catalogue record for this title is available from the
British Library

Set in 10/12pt Palatino
by SNP Best-set Typesetter Ltd., Hong Kong
Printed and bound in Spain
by GraphyCems, Navarra

The publisher's policy is to use permanent paper
from mills that operate a sustainable forestry policy,
and which has been manufactured from pulp
processed using acid-free and elementary chlorine-
free practices. Furthermore, the publisher ensures
that the text paper and cover board used have met
acceptable environmental accreditation standards.

For further information on Blackwell Publishing,
visit our website:
www.blackwellpublishing.com

Contents

Preface

This is an exciting time in wound care and there have been many new developments in the last few years, including new approaches as well as systematic reviews and guidelines. Much of this is reflected in this third edition of *The Care of Wounds* and as a result, several of the chapters have been rewritten rather than updated. I also believe that many of those involved in caring for patients with wounds are more sophisticated in their approach to the subject. I hope that I have managed to reflect this in the text.

I would like to thank all those people who have encouraged me to produce this new edition and for their kind remarks about the usefulness of the last edition. I hope they find it to be relevant to their clinical practice and that nurses especially will find it useful when caring for patients with wounds.

Carol Dealey

Dedication

To my husband for his endless patience

Chapter 1
The Physiology of Wound Healing

1.1 INTRODUCTION

Wound healing is a highly complex process. It is important that the nurse has an understanding of the physiological processes involved for several reasons.

- Understanding the physiology of skin assists in understanding the healing process.
- An understanding of the physiology of wound healing makes it possible to recognise the abnormal.
- Recognition of the stages of healing allows the selection of appropriate dressings.
- Understanding of the requirements of the healing process means that appropriate nutrition can, as far as is possible, be given to the patient.

1.2 DEFINITIONS ASSOCIATED WITH WOUNDS

Any damage leading to a break in the continuity of the skin can be called a wound. There are several causes of wounding.

- Traumatic – mechanical, chemical, physical
- Intentional – surgery
- Ischaemia – e.g. arterial leg ulcer
- Pressure – e.g. pressure ulcer

In both traumatic and intentional injury there is rupture of the blood vessels, which results in bleeding, followed by clot formation. In wounds caused by ischaemia or pressure, the blood supply is disrupted by local occlusion of the microcirculation. Tissue necrosis follows and results in ulcer formation, possibly with a necrotic eschar or scab.

Wounds in the skin or deeper have been labelled in various ways. Some of them can be described as follows.

Partial- and full-thickness wounds

- A partial-thickness wound is one where some of the dermis remains and there are shafts of hair follicles or sweat glands.
- In a full-thickness wound all the dermis is destroyed and deeper layers may also be involved.

Healing by first and second intention

These definitions were first described by Hippocrates around 350 BC.

- Healing by first intention is when there is no tissue loss and the skin edges are held in apposition to each other, such as a sutured wound.
- Healing by second intention means a wound where there has been tissue loss and the skin edges are far apart, such as a leg ulcer.

Open and closed wounds

These are the same as healing by second and first intention respectively.

1.3 THE STRUCTURE OF THE SKIN

The skin is the largest and one of the most active organs of the body. It is composed of two layers – the epidermis and dermis – with the epidermis forming the outer surface of the body and the dermis forming the deeper layer of the skin. The main structures of the skin can be found in the dermis. Figure 1.1 shows a cross-section of the skin.

1.3.1 Dermis

Dermis is composed of connective tissue, both collagen and elastic fibres, which is both elastic and resilient and provides support for the structures in the dermis. Within the dermis can be found blood vessels, lymph vessels, sensory nerve endings, sweat and sebaceous glands and hair follicles. The ducts of the glands and hair shafts pass through the epidermis to the skin surface. Sweat glands have their own ducts opening on the skin surface but sebaceous glands open onto the hair follicles. The base or bulb of hair follicles is sited deep into the dermis. They are lined with epithelial cells and can play a role in the healing of partial-thickness wounds.

The surface of the dermis where it interlocks with the epidermis is irregular, with projections of cells called papillae. The base of the dermis is less clearly defined as it blends into subcutaneous tissue, which contains both connective tissue and adipose tissue and helps to anchor the skin to muscle and bone.

1.3.2 Epidermis

The epidermis comprises several layers of cells. The deepest layer is the stratum basale and it is constantly producing new cells by cell division. These cells are gradually pushed towards the skin surface, taking about seven weeks to reach the surface. The stratum spinosum contains bundles of keratin filaments, which hold the skin together. The top three layers of epidermis are the stratum granulosum, which produces the precursor to keratin, the stratum lucidum and the stratum corneum. As they move through the strata, the cells gradually flatten

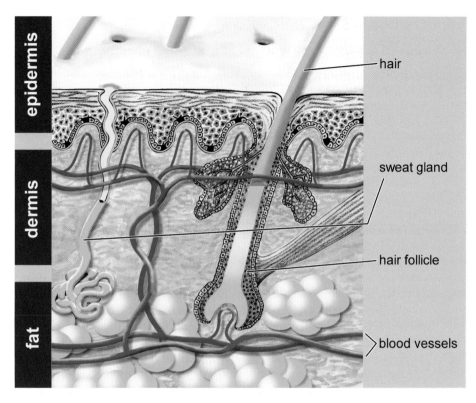

Fig. 1.1   A cross-section of the skin. Reproduced from www.nurseminerva.co.uk with permission.

and the protoplasm becomes replaced with keratin. The cells in the stratum corneum are flat with no nucleus and are essentially dead cells. They are constantly worn away and replaced by new cells moving to the surface.

In addition, the epidermis has cells called melanocytes containing melanin, which gives skin its colour. A high concentration of melanin produces a dark skin colour. Ultraviolet light increases melanin production. This may occur naturally by sunlight, resulting in a sun tan, or artificially such as a treatment in dermatology.

1.4 WOUND HEALING

The wound-healing process consists of a series of highly complex interdependent and overlapping stages. These stages have been given a variety of names but are described here as:

- inflammation
- reconstruction
- epithelialisation
- maturation.

The stages last for variable lengths of time. Any stage may be prolonged because of local factors such as ischaemia or lack of nutrients. The factors that can delay healing are discussed in more detail in Chapter 2.

1.4.1 Inflammation

The inflammatory response is a non-specific local reaction to tissue damage and/or bacterial invasion. It is an important part of the body's defence mechanisms and is an essential stage of the healing process. The signs of inflammation were first described by Celsus, in the first century AD, as redness, heat, pain and swelling. The factors causing them are shown in Table 1.1.

When there is traumatic or intentional injury that causes damage to the blood vessels, the first response is to stop the bleeding. This is achieved by a combination of factors: first by vasoconstriction, which reduces the blood flow, and second, by the release of a plasma protein called von Willebrand factor from both endothelial cells and platelets, resulting in platelet aggregation and formation of a platelet plug. The third factor is the initiation of the clotting cascade and the development of a fibrin clot to reinforce the platelet plug.

Hageman factor (factor XII in the clotting cascade) triggers both the complement and kinin systems. The complement system consists of plasma proteins which are inactive precursors. When activated, there is a cascade effect that leads to the release of histamine and serotonin from the mast cells and results in vasodilation and increased capillary permeability. The complement system also assists in attracting neutrophils to the wound. The complement molecule, C3b, acts as an opsonin. That is, it assists in binding neutrophils to bacteria. Five of the proteins activated during the cascade process form the membrane attack complex, which has the ability to directly destroy bacteria.

The effect of the complement system is enhanced by the kinin system which, through a series of steps, activates kininogen to bradykinin. Kinins attract neutrophils to the wound, enhance phagocytosis and stimulate the sensory nerve endings. The apparent delay in feeling pain after injury is explained by the short time lag taken for the kinin system to be activated.

Table 1.1 The signs of inflammation.

Signs and symptoms	Physiological rationale
Redness	Vasodilation results in large amount of blood in the area
Heat	Large amount of warm blood and heat energy produced by metabolic reactions
Swelling	Vasodilation and leakage of fluid into the wound area
Pain	May be caused by damage to nerve ends, activation of the kinin system, pressure of fluid in the tissues or the presence of enzymes, such as prostaglandins, which cause chemical irritation

As the capillaries dilate and become more permeable, there is a flow of fluid into the injured tissues. This fluid becomes the 'inflammatory exudate' and contains plasma proteins, antibodies, erythrocytes, leucocytes and platelets. As well as being involved in clot formation, platelets also release fibronectin and growth factors called platelet-derived growth factor (PDGF) and transforming growth factor alpha and beta (TGFα and TGFβ). Their role is to promote cell migration and growth at the wound site.

Growth factors are a subclass of cytokines, proteins that are used for cellular communication (Greenhalgh, 1996). The particular role of growth factors is to stimulate cell proliferation. There are a number of growth factors involved in the healing process and they are listed in Table 1.2. Some growth factors have been isolated and used as a treatment for chronic wounds. This will be discussed in more detail in Chapter 4.

The first leucocyte to arrive at the wound is the neutrophil. Wagner (1985) has described the role of fibronectin in relation to neutrophils. It attracts neutrophils to the wound site, a process known as chemotaxis. Neutrophils squeeze through the capillary walls into the tissues by diapedesis; again this ability is enhanced by fibronectin. Within about an hour of the inflammatory response being initiated, neutrophils can be found at the wound site. They arrive in large numbers, their role being to phagocytose bacteria by engulfing and destroying them. Neutrophils decay after phagocytosis as they are unable to regenerate the enzymes required for this process. As the numbers of bacteria decline, so too do the numbers of neutrophils.

Table 1.2   Growth factors involved in the healing process.

Growth factor	Abbreviation	Action
Platelet-derived growth factor	PDGF	Chemotactic for neutrophils, fibroblasts and, possibly, monocytes Encourages proliferation of fibroblasts
Transforming growth factor alpha	TGFα	Stimulates angiogenesis
Transforming growth factor beta	TGFβ	Chemotactic for monocytes (macrophages) Encourages angiogenesis. Regulates inflammation
Fibroblast growth factor	FGF	Stimulates fibroblast proliferation and angiogenesis
Epidermal growth factor	EGF	Stimulates the proliferation and migration of epithelial cells
Insulin-like growth factors	IGF-I, IGF-II	Promote protein synthesis and fibroblast proliferation. Work in combination with other growth factors

TGFβ attracts monocytes to the wound where they differentiate into macrophages. Fibronectin binds onto the surface receptors on the cells, promoting diapedesis and phagocytosis. Oxygen is vital to this process and macrophages can be inactivated and their ability to undertake phagocytosis reduced if the partial oxygen pressure falls below 30 mmHg (Cherry *et al.*, 2000). Macrophages are larger than neutrophils and so are able to phagocytose larger particles, such as necrotic debris, as well as bacteria. The lifespan of the neutrophil can be a few hours or a few days. When they die, they are also phagocytosed by the macrophages.

T lymphocytes also migrate into the wound, although in smaller numbers than macrophages (Martin & Muir, 1990). They influence macrophage phagocytic activity by the production of several macrophage-regulating factors. They also produce colony-stimulating factors that encourage the macrophage to produce a range of enzymes and cytokines. These include prostaglandins which maintain vasodilation and capilliary permeability and can be produced on demand to prolong the inflammatory response if required. A study by Martin and Muir (1990) found that both macrophages and lymphocytes are present in wounds from day 1, with macrophages peaking between days 3 and 6 and lymphocytes between days 8 and 14.

Inflammation lasts about 4–5 days. It requires both energy and nutritional resources. In large wounds the requirements may be considerable. If this stage is prolonged by irritation to the wound, such as infection, foreign body or damage caused by the dressing, it can be debilitating to the patient as well as delaying healing.

1.4.2 Reconstruction

The reconstruction phase is characterised by the development of granulation tissue. This consists of a loose matrix of fibrin, fibronectin, collagen and hyaluronic acid and other glycosaminoglycans. Within this matrix can be found macrophages and fibroblasts and the newly formed blood vessels. Macrophages play a major role in this phase of healing. They produce PDGF and fibroblast growth factor (FGF), which are chemotactic to fibroblasts, attracting them to the wound and stimulating them to divide and later to produce collagen fibres. Fibronectin also seems to play a role in enhancing fibroblast activity (Orgill & Demling, 1988). Collagen has been seen in a new wound as early as the second day. Collagen fibres are made up of chains of amino acids in a triple helix formation. There are a number of different types of collagen characterised by different formations of amino acids. Type III is present in the healing wound in greater proportions than would normally be found in skin. Over time, this proportion reduces in favour of higher levels of type I collagen.

Fibroblasts are key cells in this phase of healing (Harding *et al.*, 2002). As well as being responsible for the production of collagen, they also produce the extracellular matrix, which is seen visually as granulation tissue. As new extracellular matrix is synthesised, the existing matrix is degraded by enzyme systems such as matrix metalloproteinases (MMPs). There are a number of MMPs, in particular MMP1, MMP2 and MMP9, involved in the healing process, although their role is imperfectly understood at present.

The activity of fibroblasts depends on the local oxygen supply. If the tissues are poorly vascularised the wound will not heal well. The wound surface has a relatively low oxygen tension, encouraging the macrophages to produce TGFβ and FGF, which instigate the process of angiogenesis, the growth of new blood vessels. Undamaged capillaries beneath the wound, sprout buds, which grow towards the surface and loop over and back to the capillary. The loops form a network within the wound, supplying oxygen and nutrients. At this stage, a high oxygen tension promotes the continued growth of the capillary loops because collagen is required in their formation (Cherry et al., 2000).

Some fibroblasts have a further role as they are involved in the process of contraction. The exact mechanism is not clearly understood and there are currently two theories postulated: cell contraction and cell traction. The theory of cell contraction is based on specialised fibroblasts known as myofibroblasts (Gabbiani et al., 1973), which have a contractile apparatus, similar to that in smooth muscle cells. In in vitro models, they have been shown to cause contraction of the wound. Tomasek et al. (1989) found a higher level of contractile forces when a high level of myofibroblasts was present. The concept of cell traction was put forward by Stopak and Harris (1982), who demonstrated that fibroblasts could contract collagen gels by a physical pull, resulting in a rearrangement of the extracellular matrix. It must be noted that all these studies were undertaken in vitro and there is no certainty that they could be repeated in vivo.

Whatever the actual process, contraction may start at around the fifth or sixth day. It considerably reduces the surface area of open wounds. Irvin (1987) suggests that contraction could be responsible for as much as 40–80% of the closure. It is certainly of considerable importance in large cavity wounds. However, in shallower wounds with a large surface area such as burns, contraction may lead to contractures. Myofibroblasts disappear after healing is completed.

In wounds healing by first intention, little can be seen of this stage of healing but in those healing by second intention, the granulation tissue can be seen as it gradually fills the wound cavity. Figure 1.2 summarises cellular activity during reconstruction as the macrophage completes clearance of cellular debris and produces growth factors that will instigate angiogenesis and also attract fibroblasts to the wound site.

As the wound fills with new tissue and a capillary network is formed, the numbers of macrophages and fibroblasts gradually reduce. This stage may have started before the inflammation stage is completed and prolonged inflammation can result in excessive granulation with hypertrophic scarring. The length of time needed for reconstruction depends on the type and size of wound but may be about 24 days for wounds healing by first intention.

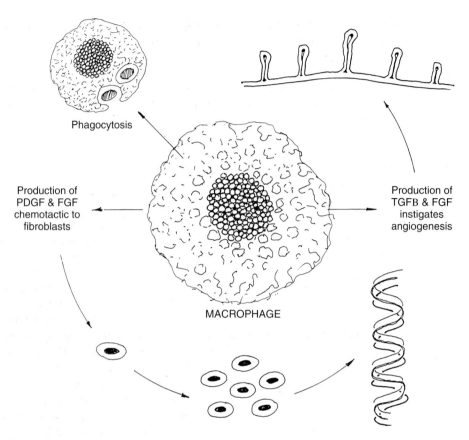

Fig. 1.2   The process of reconstruction.

1.4.3 Epithelialisation

This is the phase in which the wound is covered with epithelial cells. Macrophages release epidermal growth factor (EGF), which stimulates both the proliferation and migration of epithelial cells. Keratinocytes at the wound margins and around hair follicle remnants synthesise fibronectin, which forms a temporary matrix along which the cells migrate. The cells move over the wound surface in a leapfrog fashion, the first cell remaining on the wound surface and forming a new basement membrane. When cells meet, either in the centre of the wound, forming islets of cells, or at the margin, they stop. This is known as contact inhibition. Epithelial cells only move over viable tissue and require a moist environment (Winter, 1962). In sutured wounds, epithelial cells also migrate along the suture tracks. They are either pulled out with the sutures or gradually disappear.

Once the cells stop moving on the wound surface, they start to reconstitute the basement membrane, which is essential in order for the epidermis to 'fix' to the dermis. Until the basement membrane is fully reconstituted, it is easy for epithelial cells to be sheared off the wound surface by mechanical forces (Cherry *et al.*, 2000).

Epithelialisation commences as early as the second day in closed wounds. However, in open wounds it is necessary for the wound cavity to be filled with granulation tissue before it can commence. There is a very variable time span for this stage.

1.4.4 Maturation

During maturation the wound becomes less vascularised as there is a reduction in the need to bring cells to the wound site. The collagen fibres are reorganised so that, instead of being laid down in a random fashion, they lie at right angles to the wound margins. During this process, collagen is constantly degraded and new collagen synthesised. The highest level of activity in this process occurs between days 14 and 21 (Cherry *et al.*, 2000). The scar tissue present is gradually remodelled and becomes comparable to normal tissue after a long period of time. The scar gradually flattens to a thin white line. This may take up to a year in closed wounds and very much longer in open wounds.

Tensile strength gradually increases. This is a way of describing the ability of the wound to resist rupture or dehiscence. Forester *et al.* (1969) found that at ten days an apparently well-healed surgical incision has little strength. During maturation it increases so that by three months the tensile strength is 50% that of normal tissue. Further work by Forester *et al.* (1970) compared surgical incisions where the skin edges were held together by tape with those where sutures were used. The findings showed that, when tape was used, the wounds regained 90% strength of normal tissue whereas sutured wounds only regained 70% strength.

1.5 IMPAIRED WOUND HEALING

Although the majority of wounds heal without problem, impaired healing may sometimes occur. Some of the different types of impaired healing are described here. Their management will be discussed elsewhere.

1.5.1 Hypertrophic scars

Hypertrophic scars occur when there is an excessive fibrous tissue response during the healing process resulting in excessive deposition of collagen and a thick wound scar (Munro, 1995). Cherry *et al.* (2000) suggest that the ratio of type I to type III collagen is lower than in normal skin. Hypertrophic scars are more common after traumatic injury, especially large burns. They occur shortly after the injury or surgery and remain limited to the area of the injury. They will generally flatten out with time, about one to two years.

1.5.2 Keloids

Keloids are similar to hypertrophic scars in that they are also the result of an excessive fibrous response but this time, the ratio of type I to type III collagen is much higher than in normal skin. Another difference is that keloids take some time to form and may occur years after the initial injury. They can range in size from small papules to large pendulous growths (Munro, 1995). Keloids more commonly occur in individuals aged between 10 and 30 (Cosman *et al.*, 1961) and in those with a darker skin (Placik & Lewis, 1992). Unfortunately, unlike hypertrophic scars, keloids do not gradually flatten out.

1.5.3 Contractures

Wound contraction is part of the normal healing process but occasionally contraction will continue after re-epithelialisation has occurred, resulting in scar contraction (Tredget *et al.*, 1997). Engrav *et al.* (1987) describe how this type of scar contracture can lead to joint contracture with subsequent loss of mobility, functional loss, delay in return to work and a poor cosmetic result, any of which may necessitate surgery.

1.5.4 Acute to chronic wounds

Wounds may be called 'chronic' because their underlying aetiology makes healing a very long process. A good example is the venous leg ulcer. However, some chronic wounds may have originally been acute wounds that have failed to heal over a long period of time, perhaps years. The original factor delaying healing may have been related to infection or local irritation, perhaps caused by a suture. Once these problems have been resolved, the wound still fails to heal, causing considerable misery to the patient.

The differences between acute and chronic wounds are still imperfectly understood. However, work by Phillips *et al.* (1998) did shed some light on the problem. They used cultured fibroblasts from human neonatal foreskin as a plated laboratory model and treated them with either chronic wound fluid (CWF) or bovine serum albumen (the control). They found that CWF inhibited the growth of the fibroblasts quite dramatically. The researchers concluded that this study gave some indication of how the microenvironment has a negative effect on the healing wound. As result of this work, other research groups have looked at wound exudate in more detail.

Trengrove *et al.* (1999) used wound fluid from venous leg ulcers at both non-healing and healing stages to measure MMP levels. They found elevated levels of MMPs at the non-healing stage, which decreased significantly as the ulcers started to heal ($p = 0.01$). The levels of MMPs in the healing ulcers were similar to those in acute wounds, thus suggesting that failure to heal may be linked to excessive matrix degradation. Ladwig *et al.* (2002) collected wound fluid from 56 pressure ulcers and found lower levels of MMP9 in those ulcers that went on to heal well compared with those that healed poorly.

Trengrove *et al.* (2000) undertook further studies of wound exudate from non-healing and healing leg ulcers. They found significantly higher concentrations of a number of proinflammatory cytokines or growth factors in the non-healing ulcers. They consider that wound healing is delayed in chronic wounds because of an impairment of inflammatory mediators rather than by any deficit of growth factors.

Premature ageing of fibroblasts may also be a problem. Mendez *et al.* (1998) investigated the characteristics of fibroblasts cultured from chronic venous ulcers and found signs of accelerated ageing or senescence in these cells. Senescent fibroblasts have reduced mobility, are less able to replicate, have abnormal protein production and do not respond well to growth factors. A small study of seven patients by Stanley and Osler (2001) compared the senescence rates in fibroblasts from chronic venous ulcers with fibroblasts from punch biopsies taken from the proximal thigh of the same patient. They found a significantly higher senescence rate in the fibroblasts from the leg ulcers ($p = 0.0001$).

1.6 CONCLUSION

This chapter has described 'normal' physiology. However, not all wounds heal without complication or delay and some of the differences between acute and chronic wound healing have been discussed. But many factors can affect the healing process and they will be considered in more detail in Chapter 2.

FURTHER READING

Cherry, G.W., Hughes, M.A., Ferguson, M.W.J., Leaper, D.J. (2000) Wound healing, in (eds) Morris, P.J., Wood, W.C., *Oxford Textbook of Surgery*, 2nd edn. Oxford University Press, Oxford.

Vander, A., Sherman, J., Luciano, D. (1998) *Human Physiology*, 7th edn. McGraw-Hill, Boston.

REFERENCES

Cherry, G.W., Hughes, M.A., Ferguson, M.W.J., Leaper, D.J. (2000) Wound healing, in (eds) Morris, P.J., Wood, W.C., *Oxford Textbook of Surgery*, 2nd edn. Oxford University Press, Oxford.

Cosman, B., Crikelair, G.F., Ju, M.C. *et al.* (1961) The surgical treatment of keloids. *Plastic and Reconstructive Surgery*, **27**, 335–358.

Engrav, L.H., Covey, M.H., Dutcher, K.D. *et al.* (1987) Impairment, time out of school and time out of work after burns. *Plastic and Reconstructive Surgery*, **79**, 927.

Forester, J.C., Zederfeldt, B.H., Hunt, T.K. (1969) A bioengineering approach to the healing wound. *Journal of Surgical Research*, **9**, 207.

Forester, J.C., Zederfeldt, B.H., Hunt, T.K. (1970) Tape-closed and sutured wounds: a comparison by tensiometry and scanning electron microscope. *British Journal of Surgery*, **57**, 729.

Gabbiani, G., Hajno, G., Ryan, G.B. (1973) The fibroblast as a contractile cell: the myofibroblast, in (eds) Kulonen, E., Pikkarainen, J., *The Biology of the Fibroblast.* Academic Press, London.

Greenhalgh, D. (1996) The role of growth factors in wound healing. *Journal of Trauma,* **41** (1), 159–167.

Harding, K.G., Morris, H.L., Patel, G.K. (2002) Healing chronic wounds. *British Medical Journal,* **324**, 160–163.

Irvin, T.T. (1987) The principles of wound healing. *Surgery,* **1**, 1112–1115.

Ladwig, G.P., Robson, M.C., Liu, R., Kuhn, M.A., Muir, D.F., Schultz, G.S. (2002) Ratios of activated matrix metalloproteinase-9 to tissue inhibitor of matrix matellopro-teinase-1 in wound fluids are inversely correlated with healing in pressure ulcers. *Wound Repair and Regeneration,* **10** (1), 26.

Martin, C.W., Muir, I.F.K. (1990) The role of lymphocytes in wound healing. *British Journal of Plastic Surgery,* **43**, 655–662.

Mendez, M.V., Stanley, A.C., Phillips, T.H., Murphy, M., Menzoian, J.O., Park, H.Y. (1998) Fibroblasts cultured from venous ulcers display cellular characteristics of senes-cence. *Journal of Vascular Surgery,* **28**, 1040–1050.

Munro, K.J.G. (1995) Hypertrophic and keloid scars. *Journal of Wound Care,* **4** (3), 143–148.

Orgill, D., Demling, R.H. (1988) Current concepts and approaches to wound healing. *Critical Care Medicine,* **16** (9), 899–908.

Phillips, T.J., Al-Amoudi, H.O., Leverkus, M., Park, H-Y. (1998) Effect of chronic wound fluid on fibroblasts. *Journal of Wound Care,* **7** (10), 527–532.

Placik, O., Lewis, V.L. (1992) Immunological associations of keloids. *Surgery, Gynaecol-ogy and Obstetrics,* **175**, 185–193.

Stanley, A., Osler, T. (2001) Senescence and the healing rates of venous ulcers. *Journal of Vascular Surgery,* **33**, 1206–1210.

Stopak, D., Harris, A.K. (1982) Connective tissue morphogenesis by fibroblast traction. 1. Tissue culture observations. *Developments in Biology,* **90** (2), 383–398.

Tomasek, J.J., Haaksma, C.J., Eddy, R.T. (1989) Rapid contraction of collagen lattices by myofibroblasts is dependent upon organised actin microfilaments. *Journal of Cell Biology,* **170**, 3410.

Tredget, E.E., Nedelec, B., Scott, P.G., Ghahary, A. (1997) Hypertrophic scars, keloids and contractures. *Surgical Clinics of North America,* **77** (3), 701–730.

Trengrove, M.K., Stacey, M.C., McCauley, S. *et al.* (1999) Analysis of the acute and chronic wound environments: the role of proteases and their inhibitors. *Wound Repair and Regeneration,* **7** (6), 442–452.

Trengrove, N.J., Bielefeldt-Ohmann, H., Stacey, M.C. (2000) Mitogenic activity and cytokine levels in non-healing and healing chronic leg ulcers. *Wound Repair and Regeneration,* **8** (1), 13–25.

Wagner, B.M. (1985) Wound healing revisited: fibronectin and company. *Human Pathol-ogy,* **16** (11), 1081.

Winter, G.D. (1962) Formation of the scab and the rate of epithelialisation of superficial wounds in the skin of the domestic pig. *Nature,* **193**, 293.

Chapter 2
The Management of Patients with Wounds

2.1 INTRODUCTION

This chapter looks at assessment of the patient with a wound and how appropriate care may be planned and evaluated. When caring for patients with wounds of all types, it is important to take a holistic approach, considering physical, psychological and spiritual care as they are inextricably linked. There are many factors that can affect the healing process. If they are taken into account when taking a history and assessing the patient, it may be possible to mitigate some of the effects. Nursing intervention is not able to resolve every problem (for example, age) but where nursing intervention can be effective, appropriate strategies are suggested.

2.2 PHYSICAL CARE

2.2.1 Nutrition

The precise relationship between wound healing and nutrition remains uncertain (Williams & Barbul, 2003). There is increasing evidence that nutritional deficit impairs healing, such as the study by Wissing *et al.* (2001) which followed up patients with leg ulceration identified in a previous study. Those patients whose ulcers were still open had significantly lower nutritional status compared with those whose ulcers had healed. A number of other studies have identified the impact of malnutrition on the healing of surgical wounds, burns and pressure ulcers (Andel *et al.*, 2003; Haydock & Hill, 1986; Mathus-Vliegen, 2004). The importance of nutrition in relation to pressure ulcer prevention and management is highlighted by the development of nutrition guidelines by the European Pressure Ulcer Advisory Panel (EPUAP, 2003).

Malnutrition is a pathological state that results from a relative or absolute deficiency or excess of one or more essential nutrients. As protein or carbohydrates are used in the largest quantities, they are usually the deficient nutrients. This is referred to as protein energy malnutrition or PEM. In her *Notes on Nursing, What it is and What it is Not*, Florence Nightingale (1974) said: 'Every careful observer of the sick will agree in this, that thousands of patients are annually starved in the midst of plenty, from want of attention to the ways which alone make it possible for them to take food'. More than a century later this statement is still true. McWhirter and Pennington (1994) assessed the nutritional status of 500 acutely ill patients and found 40% were undernourished on admission to hospital. Gallagher-Allred *et al.* (1996) reviewed studies involving 1327 patients which showed that 40–55% were malnourished and 12% were severely malnourished. Edington *et al.* (1996) surveyed community patients and found that 10% of cancer patients and 8% of those with chronic diseases were malnourished.

Overall, malnutrition is seldom recognised in hospital patients although it has a major impact on morbidity and mortality (Pablo *et al.*, 2003). Correia and Waitzberg (2003) undertook multivariate analysis of the impact of malnutrition on adult hospital patients and found mortality increased to 12.4%, compared with 4.7% in the well nourished. Hospital costs increased up to 308.9%. Older patients are at particular risk of malnutrition. Guigoz *et al.* (2002) identified malnutrition in 20% of hospitalised patients in a survey of more than 10 000 Swiss elderly people in the community, nursing homes and hospitals. Similar results were found in a Spanish study of hospital patients – 18.2% of patients had severe malnutrition (Cereceda *et al.*, 2003). Fortunately, politicians have been alerted to the importance of food and nutritional care in hospitals. The Council of Europe Committee of Ministers passed a resolution in 2003 that each member state should have national recommendations that encompass all aspects of nutritional care (Resolution RESAP(2003)3) (Committee of Ministers, 2003).

Nutritional status

The initial causes of malnutrition may be related to debilitating disease, especially of the gastrointestinal tract, old age, poverty or ignorance. Once admitted to hospital, other factors become relevant. An early study by Hamilton Smith (1972) found that patients were starved for up to 12 hours prior to surgery and for varying lengths of time afterwards. Chapman (1996) found little had changed in over 20 years. She found that patients fasted for periods ranging from 4 to 29 hours. A long period of preoperative starvation serves to compound the effects of trauma and surgery, both of which cause marked catabolism. This catabolic state usually lasts between 6 and 18 hours. Following this, the basal metabolic rate rises, leading to increased energy requirements. Unless adequate protein and carbohydrate are taken in to supply these needs, further tissue breakdown occurs, resulting in muscle wasting and a negative nitrogen balance. Lee (1979) suggests that the consequences of a negative nitrogen balance include poor wound healing, impaired immunocompetence and susceptibility to infection.

Whilst some patients will return to a normal diet fairly quickly and so redress the balance, others will receive only intravenous fluids. A litre of dextrose 5% contains approximately 150 calories. Normal saline does not contain any at all. These fluids obviously do not provide adequate calories to meet the body's requirements.

Burn patients are particularly at risk and may continue to be so for as long as four weeks (Sutherland, 1985). Trauma, burns and pain increase the metabolic rate, further diminishing the patient's nutritional status (Arturson, 1978).

Zinc, in particular, is burned up in large amounts during emotional or physical stress. Taylor (1999) studied 106 burn patients who received enhanced enteral nutrition (50% of energy and nitrogen requirements). There was a significantly greater incidence of infection and length of hospital stay when there was a delay of 24 hours in commencing the enhanced nutrition treatment. Zhou *et al.* (2003) randomly allocated severely burned patients to additional enteral glutamine (an amino acid) and found a 19% improvement in wound healing compared to controls, who had received standard feeds.

It is the responsibility of the nurse to see that patients have an adequate diet. Many patients have their mealtimes disrupted by medical ward rounds or being away from the ward undergoing investigations, although there is increased awareness of the need to have protected mealtimes. Older *et al.* (1980) saw food being placed beyond the reach of a patient and then removed later without the patient ever having the chance to actually eat any of it. Delmi *et al.* (1990), in their study of a group of elderly patients with fractured neck of femur, found that inadequate amounts of food were consumed. It should also be noted that 80% of patients in the study were malnourished on admission. Lewis *et al.* (1993) studied the diet of a small group of elderly patients with leg ulcers and found their intake was below the estimated average requirement for their age group and did not meet the requirements for healing their ulcers. A similar study by Sitton-Kent and Gilchrist (1993) of elderly hospitalised patients with chronic wounds found that they did not consume adequate levels of nutrients and in some instances had inadequate quantities on their plates. Many things can affect the appetite such as anxiety, altered mealtimes, cultural differences or malaise. It is obvious that a nutritional assessment of all patients should be made on admission and at regular intervals afterwards.

The Better Food Programme (DoH, 2001c) was introduced to try and address some of the problems described above. The Essence of Care document (DoH, 2001a) has provided best practice standards against which healthcare providers can benchmark their practice. It includes statements such as the following.

- Patients/clients receive the care and assistance they require with eating and drinking.
- Food that is provided by the service meets the needs of individual patients/clients.

Age

The cell metabolic rate slows with advancing years. There is also an increased risk of malnutrition. Exton Smith (1971) divided the causes of this into primary and secondary. Primary causes included ignorance, social isolation, physical disability, mental disturbance, iatrogenic disorder and poverty. Secondary causes were impaired appetite, masticatory inefficiency, malabsorption, alcoholism, drugs and increased requirements.

Disease

Many patients suffering from malignant disease have a reduced nutritional status. Stubbs (1989) found that one in four cancer patients experienced alterations in taste perception that affected their appetite and eating habits.

Drugs

Several drugs affect the nutritional status of patients. Methotrexate has an anti-vitamin effect which means that the enzyme that would normally bind a vitamin binds the drug instead. Methotrexate competes with folic acid and causes it to be excreted, thereby inhibiting DNA synthesis and cell replication (Holmes, 1986). Neomycin reduces the absorption of vitamins K and D. Para-aminosalicylic acid (PAS) and colchicine reduce the absorption of vitamin B12. A number of drugs can cause loss of appetite, which may lead to a diminished nutritional status. Examples are phenformin, metformin, indomethacin, morphine, digoxin and cancer drugs.

It should also be noted that patients not deemed to be at risk of undernutrition may fail to eat adequately. Brown (1991) studied the intake of patients who were considered to have no special dietary requirements. She found that 68% had intakes of less than 1000 kcal and large deficits of a range of vitamins and minerals. The deficit was caused by failure to eat the food provided. Adequate monitoring of patients' diets is essential as this group of patients are often missed.

It is important to identify those who are malnourished in order that appropriate steps can be taken to improve their nutritional status. A number of screening tools have been developed and some have been widely validated. One such is the Mini-Nutritional Assessment Tool (MNA), which has been used to assess elderly patients with leg ulceration (Wissing & Unosson, 1999). The first part of the MNA is a screening tool that identifies those who require more detailed assessment. The second part allows the assessor to identify those at risk of malnutrition and those who are actually malnourished, allowing the healthcare professional to develop an appropriate plan of care.

The British Association for Parenteral and Enteral Nutrition (BAPEN) launched the MUST screening tool in 2003 (Elia & Stratton, 2004). It is a five-step tool that has been validated for use with adults of all ages in both hospital and community settings. It allows the assessor to determine if a patient is at low, medium or high risk of malnutrition and provides appropriate management guidelines, depending on whether the patient is in hospital, a care home or the community. The guidance also provides information on how to calculate height for a patient who cannot be measured in the usual way. Further information can be obtained from www.bapen.org.uk.

Hunt (1997) and her colleagues have devised a nutritional assessment tool that considers various factors that can affect nutritional status. Patients are assessed according to their mental condition, weight, appetite, ability to eat, gut function, medical condition, including chronic wounds, and age. The tool provides a score that indicates whether the patient is nutritionally at risk. Use of a screening tool can be helpful in identifying those less obviously at risk of poor nutritional status than those discussed above.

● *Nursing assessment* ●

On admission:

● identify those at special risk using an appropriate screening tool.
● take a dietary history.
● observe for obvious signs of obesity, emaciation or muscle wasting.

● *Nursing intervention* ●

  Problem: Reduced nutritional status
  Goal: The patient will consume sufficient nutrients for his daily needs

The nutritional needs for each individual vary according to their age, sex, activity and the severity of any illness. If a patient has been assessed as having a reduced nutritional status or falls into a high-risk category, then his nutritional intake should be very carefully monitored. Each patient requires sufficient nutrients to support his basal metabolic rate, his level of activity and the metabolic response to trauma. Patients with heavily exuding wounds, such as fistulae or leg ulcers, may lose large amounts of protein without it being realised. Table 2.1 shows the nutrients required for wound healing and their sources.

The dietician will be able to help in assessing individual needs, so that very specific goals can be set. The goal set at the beginning of this section is of necessity broad but needs to be more clearly defined for each individual. If a patient is being cared for at home, the carer must also be involved. Many patients will eat better at home, where they can eat what they want, when they want to.

The elderly may have special problems or needs. Penfold and Crowther (1989) have provided helpful guidelines for assisting the elderly to maintain a good diet. One problem may be developing disability. The occupational therapist can give guidance on adapting cooking equipment. Another problem may be lack of education as to what constitutes a 'good' diet. An even simpler problem may be poorly fitting dentures. A new set of teeth may be all that is needed to allow an elderly person to maintain an adequate nutritional status.

For many people, the short period of starvation during surgery followed by a rapid return to an adequate diet will not be harmful and the body will quickly adapt. However, nurses need to be aware of the amount of food their patients actually eat. These days the plated meal system is widely used in hospitals and there has been little monitoring of the amount of food which patients actually eat. It is to be hoped that the benchmarking process discussed earlier will assist in resolving this problem. When assisting a patient to plan appropriate menus, it is helpful to bear in mind the sources of the nutrients particularly required for wound healing (see Table 2.1).

Some critically ill patients will not have an adequate intake without artificial feeding. This may take the form of a supplement or total nutrition, either by enteral or parenteral feeding. Enteral feeding is the more desirable way of providing nutrition but if the gastrointestinal tract is not functioning, then total

Table 2.1   The nutrients required for healing.

Nutrient	RDA*	Food source	Contribution
Carbohydrates	1600–3350 kcals	Wholemeal bread, wholegrain cereals, potatoes (refined carbohydrates are seen as 'empty' calories)	Energy for leucocyte, macrophage and fibroblast function
Protein	42–84 g	Meat, fish, eggs, cheese, pulses, wholegrain cereals	Immune response, phagocytosis, angiogenesis, fibroblast proliferation, collagen synthesis, wound remodelling
Fats	1–2% kcals	Dairy products, vegetable oil, oily fish, nuts	Provision of energy, formation of new cells
Vitamin A	750 µg	Carrots, spinach, broccoli, apricots, melon	Collagen synthesis and cross-linking, tensile strength of wound
B complex	3 mg	Meat (especially liver), dairy products, fish	Immune response, collagen cross-linking, tensile strength of wound
Vitamin C	30 mg	Fruit and vegetables (but easily lost in cooking)	Collagen synthesis, wound tensile strength, neutrophil function, macrophage migration, immune response
Vitamin E		Vegetable oils, cereals, eggs	Appears to reduce tissue damage from free radical formation
Copper		Shellfish, liver, meat, bread	Collagen synthesis, leucocyte formation
Iron	10–12 mg	Meat (especially offal), eggs, dried fruit	Collagen synthesis, oxygen delivery
Zinc	12–15 mg	Oysters, meat, whole cereals, cheese	Enhances cell proliferation, increases epithelialisation, improves collagen strength

* These recommended daily amounts are the requirements in health and may need to be increased (see text).

parenteral nutrition is necessary. Zainal (1995) discussed the issues around the feeding of critically ill patients and stressed the importance of starting feeds early. However, this must be done with caution as overfeeding the critically ill can cause major metabolic problems. Further problems may be caused by persisting with enteral feeding for a patient in septic shock with reduced splanchnic blood flow. The nutrition team should be involved in managing these patients.

Decision trees can also be used in planning care. They can be particularly helpful in providing guidance for less experienced staff and for setting a standard for care. The European Pressure Ulcer Advisory Panel has developed a decision tree to use alongside their nutrition guideline (Fig 2.1) which maps the essential elements of the guideline (Clark *et al.*, 2004).

● *Evaluation* ●

Evaluation may be achieved by regular weighing of the patient and reassessment using a nutritional screening tool. Gazzotti *et al.* (2003) used weighing and the MNA in a randomised trial to determine the effectiveness of nutritional supplements in preventing malnutrition.

2.2.2 Infection

Consideration of infection must include both systemic and localised wound infection. Systemic infection affects healing as the wound has to compete with more widespread infection for white cells and nutrients. Wound healing may not take place until after the body has dealt with the infection. Systemic infection is frequently associated with pyrexia which causes an increase in the metabolic rate, thus increasing catabolism or tissue breakdown.

All wounds are contaminated with bacteria, especially open wounds. This does not affect healing but clinical infection will certainly do so. Infection prolongs the inflammatory stage of healing as the cells combat the large numbers of bacteria. It also appears to inhibit the ability of fibroblasts to produce collagen (Senter & Pringle, 1985).

Infection in a burn wound increases the metabolic rate and thereby increases the period of negative nitrogen balance. Kinney (1977) has shown that there may be a loss of 20–30% of the initial body weight in the presence of major sepsis. Infection also causes pain, which raises the metabolic rate (Arturson, 1978).

A number of factors have been found to increase the risk of developing a wound infection. They are identified below.

Age

Moro *et al.* (1996) used logistical regression to identify factors associated with increased risk of surgical wound infection. They found that age greater than 85 years was a significant factor. A study using multivariate analysis (de Boer *et al.*, 1999) found age over 74 years to be the most important independent risk

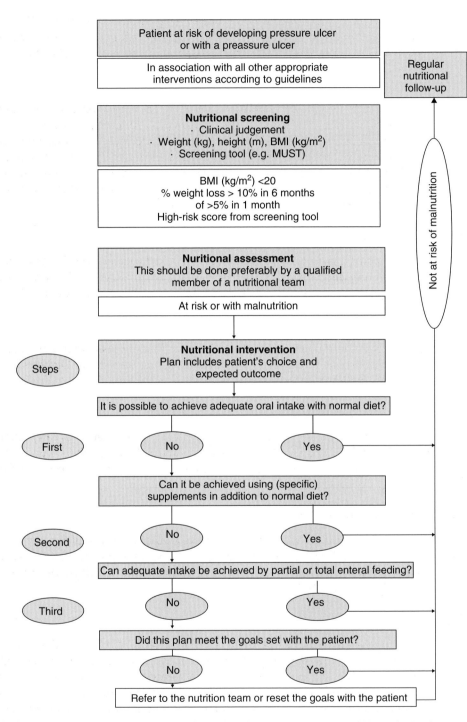

Fig. 2.1   Decision tree on nutrition in pressure ulcer prevention and treatment (reproduced by kind permission of the European Pressure Ulcer Advisory Panel).

factor for infection in over 10 000 orthopaedic patients. Pavlidis *et al.* (2001) compared local and systemic factors in 89 patients with abdominal wound dehiscence with a control group and found age over 65 years to be a significant factor.

Obesity

Martens *et al.* (1995) found obesity to be a significant factor in wound infection following caesarean section. These findings are supported by Moro *et al.* (1996), who found obesity to be a significant factor for infection in a wide range of surgical cases, and also by He *et al.* (1994) and Birkmeyer *et al.* (1998). Researchers in these latter two studies found a significantly higher incidence of sternal wound infection following bilateral internal mammary artery grafting and coronary artery bypass surgery respectively.

Nutritional status

Poor nutrition increases the infection risk. McPhee *et al.* (1998) found preoperative protein depletion to be a significant factor for wound infection in patients undergoing spinal surgery. (See also under Nutrition heading above.)

Diabetes

Borger *et al.* (1998) found diabetes to be a predictor of deep sternal wound infection for patients undergoing cardiac surgery. (See also under Diabetes Mellitus heading, p. 25.)

Special risks

Irradiation, steroids and immunosuppressive drugs cause greatly increased infection rates (Bibby *et al.*, 1986). Chmell and Schwartz (1996) found that preoperative chemotherapy was a significant factor in wound infection following musculoskeletal sarcoma resections.

Length of preoperative stay

The longer anyone is in hospital, the more chance there is that the patient's skin will become colonised by bacteria against which the patient has no resistance. A preoperative stay over four days was found to be an independent risk factor by de Boer *et al.* (1999).

Shave

It is impossible to carry out a shave without causing injury to the skin. Bacteria flourish and multiply rapidly in these minute cuts. Mishriki *et al.* (1990) and Moro *et al.* (1996) found shaving to be a significant factor in the development of infection. Mishriki *et al.* suggest that this is particularly so when contaminated and dirty procedures are undertaken and bacteria are shed on the skin. It is generally recommended that if a patient needs to be shaved preoperatively, it should be done just prior to surgery.

Type of surgery

Infection rates are much higher in some types of surgery than others. This is discussed in more detail in Chapter 6. The appearance of infected wounds will be discussed in Chapter 3.

- ● *Nursing assessment* ●

- ● Identify those at risk.
- ● Assess wound (see Chapter 3).
- ● Monitor temperature regularly.

Recently neural network analysis has been used to predict outcomes and identify those at higher risk of developing an infection. Lammers *et al.* (2003) undertook a study of a cohort of 1142 uncomplicated traumatic wounds. Clinicians undertaking the initial treatment of the wound were asked to estimate the likelihood of subsequent infection. Staff blinded to this prediction followed the wounds until the sutures were removed. Independent predictors were identified and used in the neural network analysis as input variables; infection was the output variable, in order to arrive at an equation for the analysis model. The researchers were able to use this as a diagnostic test for wound infection in this group of wounds. This type of data analysis has potential for the future as neural network analysis becomes more widely used.

- ● *Nursing intervention* ●

  Problem: Actual/potential risk of infection
  Goal: Prevention or early detection

The prevention of infection is the responsibility of all healthcare professionals. There are both general and specific measures that can be taken. Most health authorities have infection control policies that provide guidelines both to prevent infection and to reduce the risk of cross-infection. The infection control team, especially infection control nurses, can give advice and support.

Much has been written on the prevention of infection. The UK Department of Health developed guidelines entitled *Standard Principles for Preventing Infections in Hospitals* together with guidelines for preventing hospital-acquired infections (HAI) associated with the use of short-term indwelling urethral catheters in acute care and with central venous catheters in acute care (DoH, 2001b). It is intended that these guidelines are incorporated into local protocols. Within the first part of the guideline there are four standard principles.

- ● Hospital environmental hygiene.
- ● Hand hygiene.
- ● The use of personal protective equipment.
- ● The use and disposal of sharps.

The spread of infection is mostly by people from people. Thus, the simplest and most effective measure to prevent infection is good handwashing. A review by Larson and Kretzer of the period 1984–1994 found that researchers consistently reported that whilst the action of handwashing was carried out mostly at the appropriate times, the methods used were ineffective (Larson & Kretzer, 1995). Gould (1992) also supports this view but she suggests that there has been a failure to consider the reality of the situation in the clinical area. One example cited is that compliance is unlikely if the designated cleanser makes hands sore. Adequate facilities for handwashing are also necessary although alcohol handrub may be a useful alternative.

Tibballs (1996) observed doctors to obtain their handwashing rates and then asked a sample for their estimated frequency of handwashing prior to patient contact. There was a considerable difference between the estimated rate of 73% (range 50–90%) and the observed rate of 9%. It is also interesting to note that an editorial in the *British Medical Journal* by the Handwashing Liaison Group (1999) provoked 21 letters to the editor from seven different countries, not all of them in support of handwashing.

The DoH guideline recommendations for handwashing include either the use of soap and water or the use of alcohol-based handrub. Hands that are obviously soiled or could be grossly contaminated must be washed in soap and water. Handwashing is defined as having three stages: preparation, washing and rinsing, and drying. It is important to ensure that the soap or handrub touches all the surfaces of the hands. The guidelines also recommend regular use of an emollient hand cream in order to reduce skin dryness.

Identification of patients at risk of infection means that appropriate measures can be taken. Some particularly vulnerable patients may require extra measures. These may include the use of a single room with a positive pressure filtered air system, providing protective isolation, prophylactic drugs or special operating techniques such as a Charnley Howarth tent for orthopaedic procedures.

A more controversial prevention method is the use of supplemental oxygen. Greif *et al.* (2000) randomly allocated 500 patients undergoing colorectal surgery to one of two regimes of supplemental oxygen. They found that provision of supplemental oxygen during surgery and for two hours afterwards halved the infection rate. This approach seems promising but Gottrup (2000) suggested that the optimal treatment period has not been finally determined.

● *Evaluation* ●

Careful monitoring of vulnerable patients is essential. Monitoring a patient's temperature is a useful means of evaluation as a rise in temperature is often the first indication of infection. The use of clinical audit will identify areas where cross-infection may be a regular problem.

2.2.3 Smoking

Smoking causes vasoconstriction and is associated with Buerger's disease, a condition causing intermittent claudication and gangrene. Smoking may also act as an appetite depressant. Smokers have been found to be deficient in vitamins B1, B6, B12 and C. Smoking reduces subcutaneous oxygen tension significantly for up to 30–45 minutes after each cigarette. Synthesis of type I collagen has also been found to be reduced in smokers (Jorgensen *et al.*, 1998). A review of the effects of smoking on wound healing by Siana *et al.* (1992) found that nicotine affected macrophage activity and reduced epithelialisation and wound contraction. There is increasing evidence that smoking is associated with poor wound healing and increased complications. However, most studies undertaken in this area have looked at surgical wounds and there is little information regarding smoking and chronic wound healing (Sorensen, 2003).

Sorensen *et al.* (2002) studied the impact of smoking compared with non-smoking on 425 patients undergoing breast surgery. They found smoking was significantly associated with wound infection, skin flap necrosis and epidermolysis. The same group studied the impact of abstinence from smoking on healing of experimental incisional wounds in healthy individuals. They compared never-smokers with smokers randomised to either continue smoking or abstain from smoking for a four-week period. They found a significantly higher incidence of wound infection in the smokers compared with the never-smokers (12% versus 2%, $p < 0.05$). They also found there was a significant reduction in infection in the abstinent smokers compared with continuous smokers (Sorensen *et al.*, 2003). Manassa *et al.* (2003) undertook a retrospective study of 132 patients undergoing abdominoplasty and compared outcomes for smokers and non-smokers. They found a significant incidence of wound complications, including wound dehiscence (47.9% versus 14.8%, $p < 0.01$).

In reviewing the evidence on smoking and problems in wound healing, Sorensen (2003) suggests that there is a need for research into the impact of smoking on chronic wound healing. Further research is also required to determine the impact of abstinence on collagen production and delayed healing.

● *Nursing assessment* ●

Early identification of patients who smoke, especially prior to surgery.

● *Nursing intervention* ●

Problem: Patient who smokes about to undergo surgical intervention
Goal: Patient to abstain from smoking for a four-week period, two weeks before and two weeks after operation

Nurses can play a significant role in both educating patients about the harmful effects of smoking on a healing wound and encouraging them to abstain over the perioperative period. Prescription of nicotine patches may be helpful for some patients and additional support from helplines and other agencies may also be beneficial.

● *Evaluation* ●

Monitoring abstinence (or otherwise) may not be easy. It requires both honesty from the patient and respect from the nurse, whatever the outcome. Even if there are lapses, nurses should continue to encourage their patients to refrain from smoking.

2.2.4 Diabetes mellitus

Both Type I and Type II diabetes have been shown to be associated with delayed healing. King (2001) suggested that the most frequently quoted reason for delayed healing is infection as high glucose levels encourage proliferation of bacteria. McCampbell *et al.* (2002) found higher infection rates in 181 diabetic patients with burn injuries compared with 190 non-diabetic burn patients. There are, however, a number of other problems that may be encountered through each stage of the healing process in diabetics with deep wounds such as surgical incisions.

- Signs of inflammation may be limited because a thickened basement membrane causes a rigidity that prevents vasodilation (Renwick *et al.*, 1998).
- In addition, high glucose levels make erythrocytes, platelets and leucocytes more adhesive and they tend to stick together, filling the vascular lumen (Alberti & Press, 1992).
- There is decreased phagocytosis and poor chemotactic response in neutrophils although the precise reason is uncertain (King, 2001).
- Chbinou and Frenette (2004) found reduced levels of neutrophils, macrophages and angiogenesis in a diabetic animal model.
- Several studies have demonstrated that diabetics have abnormal fibroblasts with reduced capacity for proliferation and collagen synthesis. This results in abnormal cross-linking of collagen and reduced wound contraction, further prolonging the healing process (Hehenberger *et al.*, 1998; Leaper & Harding, 1998; Loots *et al.*, 1999).
- Also, diabetics deal with the stress of wounding (trauma or surgery) by producing increased levels of glucagons, cortisol and growth hormone, leading to raised levels of blood glucose and an increased need for insulin. If this situation is not corrected the patient can become catabolic. The body will start to break down proteins and fats, ultimately resulting in a state of negative nitrogen balance (Rosenberg, 1990).

- *Nursing assessment* •

Regular checks of blood glucose levels, the frequency depending on patient condition.

- *Nursing intervention* •

Actual/potential problem: Unstable glycaemic control increases potential for poor wound healing and infection in diabetic patients with surgical or traumatic wounds
Goal: Effective glycaemic control and uncomplicated wound healing

In planned procedures it is possible to ensure that the patient is adequately prepared and the diabetes well controlled. Obviously, this is not possible when a patient suffers traumatic injury. In either event, during any period of fasting the greatest risk is from hypoglycaemia and it may be necessary to commence a dextrose intravenous infusion. In the immediate postoperative or postinjury period the patient is at considerable risk of hyperglycaemia as a result of the stress of the event.

Perkins (2004) discussed this problem in relation to critically ill patients, in particular the danger of intensive insulin therapy resulting in hypoglycaemia. She proposed that effective interventions could only be achieved by multiprofessional teamwork and agreement of planned actions or protocols. Such an agreement would need to consider the frequency of monitoring for blood glucose and the level at which insulin therapy would be commenced. Perkins describes the regime that was set for the critically ill trauma patient: two-hourly monitoring with insulin therapy set to commence if blood glucose levels rose above 7 mmol/l. Insulin was to be administered according to a sliding scale in order to ensure titration. Obviously, this degree of intervention is not necessary or appropriate for every patient but the principle of team working and developing agreed, planned action can be applied to any situation where diabetic control is challenged because of stress.

● *Evaluation* ●

Regular monitoring of blood glucose levels will determine the effectiveness of care.

2.2.5 The physical effects of stress

Stress has a physiological effect. Stimulated by the release of adrenalin, a primary biochemical change in stress is an increased secretion of adrenocorticotrophic hormone (ACTH), which stimulates production of adrenal cortex hormones. In particular, ACTH regulates production of glucocorticoids, cortisol and hydrocortisone. Glucocorticoids cause the breakdown of body stores to glucose, raising the blood sugar, and reduce the mobility of granulocytes and macrophages, impeding their migration to the wound. In effect, this suppresses the immune system and reduces the inflammatory response. Glucocorticoids also increase protein breakdown and nitrogen excretion, which inhibits the regeneration of endothelial cells and delays collagen synthesis.

Kiecolt-Glaser and colleagues researched the effects of psychological stress on 13 women and found it significantly slowed the rate of healing when compared with a group matched for sex, age and income (Kiecolt-Glaser *et al.*, 1995). There would also seem to be an increased risk of wound infection in a stressed patient (Kiecolt-Glaser *et al.*, 2002). An animal model study found a significantly higher incidence of opportunistic infection compared with the control group as well as a 30% rate of delayed healing (Rojas *et al.*, 2002). Cole-King and Harding (2001) measured stress levels in 53 patients with leg ulcers that had been present for no more than three months. They found that of the 16 patients identified as having clinical anxiety, 15 had delayed healing and that all 13 patients with clinical depression also had delayed healing.

A great number of factors can cause stress and they will be discussed throughout the rest of this chapter.

2.2.6 Pain

Pain and stress are closely related because pain can increase stress and stress increases pain (Augustin & Maier, 2003). Hayward (1975) showed that preoperative information to reduce stress and anxiety resulted in less postoperative pain. Fear of pain can cause much anxiety to patients. Pracek *et al.* (1995) found that procedural pain experienced by burn patients in the early stages of their admission could be a causal factor in their ability to adjust after discharge. The greater the pain levels, the poorer the adjustment.

There has been increasing recognition of the effect of pain on patients with chronic wounds, especially leg ulceration (Ebbeskog & Ekman, 2001). Nemeth *et al.* (2003) surveyed leg ulcer patients for the prevalence of pain and found that approximately half of them suffered from pain to the extent that it impacted on their quality of life. Gibson and Kenrick (1998) graphically described the impact that the pain from a chronic condition (peripheral vascular disease) can have on the sufferer and the resulting sense of powerlessness.

There is a wealth of evidence that lack of adequate pain control is common. Carr (1997) described four barriers to effective pain control.

Lack of knowledge and inappropriate attitudes of healthcare professionals

A large study by the Royal College of Surgeons and College of Anaesthetists (1990) on pain after surgery found that nurses had insufficient commitment to providing adequate pain control and a lack of relevant knowledge; as a result up to 75% of patients experience moderate to severe postoperative pain. Field (1996) found that nurses consistently underestimated the pain suffered by their patients. Closs (1992) found that patients' sleep was disturbed by pain. In her study of 100 surgical patients, 49 said the pain was worse at night.

It is not only patients undergoing surgery who experience unrelieved pain. A study was undertaken by Chan *et al.* (1990) to determine the prevalence of chronic pain in diabetics. They found that chronic pain was more common in those suffering from diabetes than in those who did not. The pain was most commonly reported to be in the lower limbs. The researchers noted that there seemed to be little recognition of the problem or facilities to help resolve it. Hitchcock *et al.* (1994) surveyed over 200 individuals who suffered from chronic pain. They found that on average, the respondents suffered pain 80% of the time and 50% reported that their prescribed analgesia was inadequate.

Patients expect pain and patients may minimise their pain

Yates *et al.* (1995) studied older patients in long-term residential care. They found that these patients were resigned to having pain and expected that they would just have to tolerate it. They also reported being reluctant to discuss their pain for fear of being labelled a complainer. Carr and Thomas (1997) found similar results when they interviewed postoperative patients. Ward *et al.* (1996) discussed cancer patients' perceptions of pain and noted that many feared that they would become addicted to their analgesia. Others do not complain because they believe that 'good' patients should not complain. Also, pain to the cancer patient indicates further progression of the disease and the patient may be reluctant to report increased pain.

The organisation may inhibit the provision of good pain relief

Fagerhaugh and Strauss (1977) considered the organisational structure within which pain management takes place. They suggested that workload in the clinical area, lack of accountability and the complexity of the nurse–patient relationship were all factors that resulted in poor pain management. The acute pain team can play a major role in improving the standards of assessment and organisation of analgesia which result in improved pain control (Harmer & Davies, 1998). However, there can also be problems. Carr and Thomas (1997) suggest that ward nurses still fail to recognise their responsibilities for pain management and may abdicate their role to the pain management team. They also found that nurses tended to assume that 'high-tech' equipment, such as patient-controlled analgesia, automatically abolished pain and therefore pain assessment was not necessary.

Parsons (1992) gave an overview of studies of cultural aspects of pain and concluded that definitions of pain by both the sufferer and carer are shaped by cultural beliefs. In some cultures, free expression of feelings of pain is expected whereas in others it is unacceptable. There needs to be recognition of these cultural differences in order to manage pain successfully.

● Nursing assessment ●

Holzman and Turk (1986) describe pain as a unique experience for each individual. It therefore follows that only the patient can describe its presence and severity. Pedley (1996) reviewed some of the assessment tools that have been developed. She recommends the use of a visual analogue scale such as that in Figure 2.2. However, elderly people do not always find such a concept easy to use. Verbal analogue scales may be more suitable. This type of scale uses descriptions ranging from no pain through mild, moderate and severe to unbearable pain. Simons and Malaber (1995) considered the problem of patients who cannot communicate by speech and developed a method of assessing behaviour and body language.

● Nursing interventions ●

Problem: Inadequate pain control
Goal: The patient will be able to express feelings of comfort and relief from pain

Pain management is a big topic and can only be addressed briefly here. Pain at dressing change will be addressed in Chapter 3. Modern systems of drug delivery, such as slow-release drugs or intravenous pumps, provide constant pain relief that is more effective than the use of injections that have a bolus effect. Spinal infusion has been found to be effective for a small group of terminally ill patients for whom other methods failed (Hicks et al., 1994).

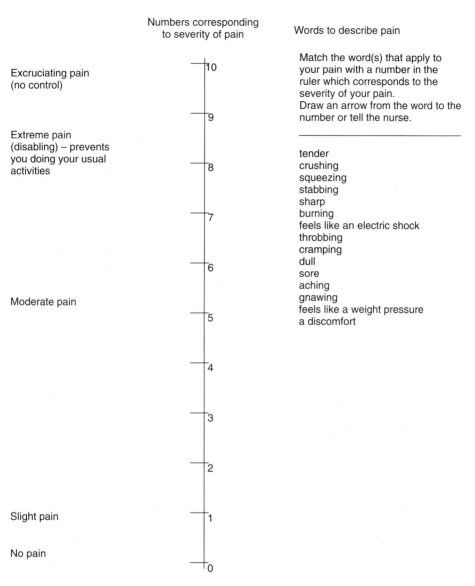

Numbers corresponding
to severity of pain

Words to describe pain

Match the word(s) that apply to
your pain with a number in the
ruler which corresponds to the
severity of your pain.
Draw an arrow from the word to the
number or tell the nurse.

Excruciating pain
(no control)

10

9

Extreme pain
(disabling) – prevents
you doing your usual
activities

8

tender
crushing
squeezing
stabbing
sharp
burning
feels like an electric shock
throbbing
cramping
dull
sore
aching
gnawing
feels like a weight pressure
a discomfort

7

6

Moderate pain

5

4

3

2

Slight pain

1

No pain

0

Fig. 2.2 A pain chart.

Music has been used as a distraction therapy to help reduce a patient's perception of pain in the immediate postoperative period (Taylor *et al.*, 1998). Relaxation has been successfully used as a technique to reduce pain in cancer patients (Sloman *et al.*, 1994) and in older men undergoing hip replacement (Parsons, 1994). Other strategies may be used to assist in pain relief. Measures such as turning, lifting or massage may be very comforting. Simple aids such as a bed cradle to reduce the weight of the bed clothes can be very effective.

● *Evaluation* ●

Regular use of a pain chart allows constant evaluation of the effectiveness of pain relief.

2.2.7 Sleeping

Most people consider sleep to be important as it provides a sense of refreshment and well-being. In recent years there has been considerable research on sleep and its effects. Sleep deprivation causes people to become increasingly irritable and irrational (Carter, 1985). They may complain of lassitude and loss of feelings of well-being. The sleep–activity cycle is part of the circadian rhythm. During wakefulness, the body is in a state of catabolism. Hormones such as catecholamine and cortisol are released. They encourage tissue degradation to provide energy for activity; in particular, protein degradation occurs in muscle.

Growth hormone is secreted from the anterior pituitary during sleep and stimulates protein synthesis and the proliferation of a variety of cells, including fibroblasts and endothelial cells (Lee & Stotts, 1990). Rose *et al.* (2001) reviewed the impact of burn injury on the sleep patterns of children and the need to aggressively treat growth hormone insufficiency. They speculate that improved sleep would improve growth hormone levels. However, Brandenberger *et al.* (2000) argue that the body is able to compensate during the day and the levels of growth hormone secreted over 24 hours remain much the same, regardless of any sleep deprivation.

There has been some reliance on animal studies to determine the impact of sleep deprivation and the surrogate measure, noise, on wound healing. Wysocki (1996) measured the impact of noise on wound healing and found that wounds healed more slowly compared with controls. Landis and Whitney (1997) studied the impact of 72 hours of sleep deprivation and found that there was no difference between experimental and control groups. It should be noted that these studies were undertaken on basically healthy animals and the findings may not be transferable to sick humans. Further studies, especially clinical studies, are needed to clarify the matter.

There is much evidence that sleep patterns are disturbed in hospital. Hill (1989) suggested that ward routines, such as early morning waking, prevent the patient getting adequate sleep. Also, many patients are disturbed during the night, especially in the intensive care unit. Woods (1972) observed cardiac surgery patients and noted that they were disturbed as many as 56 times during the first postoperative night. Morgan and White (1983) found that intensive care nurses were aware of the importance of sleep but failed to recognise when they were disturbing their patients unnecessarily.

Freedman *et al.* (1999) surveyed 203 patients immediately after discharge from different types of intensive care units and found that poor sleep quality was common to all units. They also found that sleep disruption was caused by human interventions, diagnostic testing and environmental noise. A further study from the same research centre investigated the impact of environmental noise on sleep. The sleep patterns of 22 medical patients in an intensive care unit were monitored for 24–48 hours continuously. Patients were found to sleep for short periods throughout a 24-hour timeframe with a mean number of sleep periods of 41+/–28 and the mean length of a sleep bout was 15+/–9 minutes. Overall, environmental noise was responsible for only 17% of sleep disturbances (Freedman *et al.*, 2001).

Other factors may also disturb sleep, as shown in a survey by Southwell and Wistow (1995) of 454 patients and 129 nurses across a variety of wards in three hospitals. Half the patients had difficulty in sleeping through the nights and did not get as much sleep as they wished. Many of the patients complained that the ward was too hot and the mattresses were uncomfortable and they disliked having plastic covers on both mattresses and pillows. Pain and worry were also likely to make sleeping more difficult. A variety of factors were found to disturb sleep including: other patients making a noise, nurses attending other patients, telephones ringing, lights in the ward, nurses talking to each other or to patients, having treatment including medication, toilets flushing or commodes being used, nurses' shoes making a noise. Patients on surgical wards reported more disturbances than other ward specialties. The authors of this study considered that nurses should be more aware of the need to ensure that patients get a good night's sleep.

● *Nursing assessment* ●

- Compare 'normal' with present patterns of sleep.
- Assess the ward environment – is it conducive to sleeping?
- Consider ward routines – do they allow the patient to follow any aspect of their usual routines or are they too rigid?

● *Nursing intervention* ●

Problem: Disruption of normal sleeping patterns
Goal: Patients are able to sleep a number of hours at night and state that they feel well rested

McMahon (1990) suggested four types of sleeplessness:

- difficulty getting to sleep.
- waking regularly during the night.
- waking early in the morning.
- sleeping for the normal length of time but not waking refreshed.

Various strategies can be employed to help patients resolve their specific problems. The provision of a milky drink can be beneficial, especially if the patient normally has one at bedtime. Some people may become hungry after having supper between 1700 and 1800 hours. They may ask their visitors to bring them in a snack. Whilst there is no evidence that food can induce sleep, it is difficult to sleep when hungry. Most people have specific routines that they follow each night. As much as possible, this same routine should be followed in hospital which can introduce a feeling of normality into a strange situation.

Some people find their sleep disrupted because of pain. This may be acute pain following trauma or surgery or a more chronic pain relating to a long-standing illness or condition. Adequate pain control is essential. Pain is a resolvable problem (see also section 2.2.6). The position of patients may affect their comfort so it is helpful to ensure that the patient is in a comfortable position, with a bell close to hand.

During the night, many fears that are suppressed during the day come to the surface. Sleep may be disturbed because of a particular anxiety. Nighttime is a quieter time on the ward so the nurse may have an opportunity to sit and listen and allow patients to express their fears and anxieties. Once this has happened, the patient may be able to return to normal sleep patterns.

Hospital routines can disrupt normal sleep patterns. The lights of a ward may go off late, around 2300 hours, and come on again at 0600 hours (Southwell & Wistow, 1995). Patients are woken for their drugs and a drink. It seems reasonable for more flexibility to be introduced, with a reduction of the 0600 drug round to the minimum and an arrangement not to wake those who would prefer to sleep later. Jarmon et al. (2002) experimented with flexible morning and evening medication times and found that patients were able to sleep for longer. Haddock (1994) found some patients benefited from using earplugs but they are not suitable for everyone. It should be possible, with careful planning, to provide an environment that is conducive to sleep, and a comfortable patient who is able to benefit from it.

● *Evaluation* ●

Patient questionnaires are a useful way of establishing the success or otherwise of the above plan.

2.2.8 Hypothermia

Anaesthesia for major surgery can lead to hypothermia as a result of decreased metabolic rate and impaired thermoregulation (Sellden, 2002). Recently, there has been increased understanding of the impact that even mild levels of intra-operative hypothermia can have on postoperative recovery. Schmied et al. (1996) randomised 60 patients undergoing total hip arthroplasties to either nor-mothermia (36.6°C) or mild hypothermia (35°C). They found that blood loss was significantly higher in the hypothermic group compared with the nor-mothermic patients.

Kurz et al. (1996) proposed that mild hypothermia increased the risk of wound infection because of vasoconstriction decreasing the level of tissue oxygen and impacting on neutrophil activity. To investigate this further, they undertook a double-blind randomised study of 200 patients undergoing col-orectal surgery. Patients were randomised to either the normothermic group (37°C) or the hypothermic group (34.4°C). They found that patients in the hypothermic group were three times more likely to develop a postoperative wound infection and had significantly longer hospital stay. Their sutures were also removed later than those in the normothermic group.

Mahoney and Odom (1999) reviewed the outcome costs for mildly hypothermic patients compared with normothermic patients undergoing a range of operations. They were able to pool the findings of the studies and undertake a meta-analysis. They found that mildly hypothermic patients were more likely to require blood transfusions and to develop wound infections and the cost of these adverse outcomes ranged between $2500 and $7000.

Plattner *et al.* (2000) tested an experimental warming bandage system and compared it with conventional gauze with elastic adhesive in 40 normothermic patients following elective abdominal surgery. The experimental bandage consisted of an adhesive shell and a foam frame surrounding a clear window. A heated card was inserted into the frame approximately 1 cm above the wound surface and left *in situ* for two hours at a time. Oxygen tension was measured via a probe inserted 2–3 cm laterally to the incision. Their results were unexpected. They found that the oxygen tension was considerably lower in those with a conventional dressing because of the pressure exerted by the elastic strapping. The warming device did not appear to benefit normothermic patients particularly, although it had potential for use for hypothermic patients.

Perioperative hypothermia is associated with a higher incidence of wound infection. This is of particular relevance in surgery where there is already a high risk of infection such as abdominal surgery. It is less likely to be important in surgery with a low risk of infection, such as neurosurgery. There are also procedures when cooling the patient is appropriate, such as during craniotomy.

2.2.9 Steroids

Glucocorticoids or corticosteroids are widely used in the treatment of inflammatory diseases. Although they produce effective anti-inflammatory outcomes, this can have a serious impact on wound healing. A review by Anstead (1998) highlighted the fact that glucocorticoids affect every stage of the healing process. This includes overall effects such as the increased risk of infection and dehiscence in surgical wounds, although this is probably dose dependent. Grunbine *et al.* (1998) studied 73 patients who had had a steroid injection following surgery to the foot or ankle and compared the outcome with those who did not. The use of a single dose of steroids made no difference to healing rates.

Anstead (1998) summarised the effects of glucocorticoids on wound healing as follows.

- Inflammation is suppressed because of a reduction in the numbers of neutrophils and macrophages and an impaired ability to digest phagocytosed material.
- Wound contracture is poor as a result of inhibition of fibroblast proliferation.
- Reduced wound strength, as collagen structure and cross-linking are affected.

- Epithelialisation is delayed and the cells are thin, producing a weak wound covering.

When there is planned wounding, such as surgery, it may be beneficial to reduce the level of glucocorticoids, especially preoperatively. Pollack (1982) suggests that doses of prednisolone greater than 40 mg/day have the greatest effect on wound healing. However, it may not be possible to change dosage levels and there has been considerable interest in the potential of vitamin A to counteract the unwanted side effects of glucosteroids. Vitamin A has been found to restore a normal inflammatory response (Ehrlich *et al.*, 1972) and also epithelial regeneration, fibroblast proliferation and collagen content (Talas *et al.*, 2003). However, although there have been a number of animal studies, there is a need to test the use of vitamin A clinically using controlled trials to determine what might be an appropriate dose and also to ensure that its use does not adversely affect the beneficial systemic outcomes of glucocorticoids (Anstead, 1998).

2.2.10 Radiotherapy

Radiation effectively destroys cancer cells as they are more radiosensitive than normal cells. A dosage high enough to kill cancer cells does not affect the surrounding cells. However, if the dosage has to be increased there is increased risk of normal tissue necrosing. Radiation has the potential to impact on wound healing and it would seem that the worst outcomes occur when radiotherapy is given before surgery.

Hillmann *et al.* (1997) found preoperative irradiation was an influencing factor in postoperative complications for patients with Ewing's sarcoma. Sassler *et al.* (1995) found major wound complications in patients undergoing head and neck surgery following an initial regime of chemotherapy and irradiation. They reported a 77% incidence of complications in patients undergoing surgery within one year of the regime compared with a 20% incidence after one year. Lin *et al.* (2001) found that a history of radiotherapy was a factor in wound-healing complications of breast reconstruction. Similar results were found by Wang *et al.* (2003) and O'Sullivan *et al.* (2002), when comparing pre- and postoperative radiotherapy. Both studies found a significantly higher rate of wound-healing complications when radiotherapy was given preoperatively.

Radiation may affect the healing of an existing wound or it may cause changes to the skin so that any later wound will heal slowly. The skin may show signs of damage from the radiation during treatment. This is known as a radiation reaction and will be discussed in Chapter 6.

Levenson *et al.* (1984) investigated the use of vitamin A supplements to counteract the effects of radiation on wound healing. In the animal model, they found that giving vitamin A supplements was effective. Good results were obtained if the supplementation was started prior to radiotherapy or up to two days after treatment.

2.3 PSYCHOLOGICAL CARE

Nurses have always excelled at the physical care of patients. It is only recently that the emotional needs of patients have been considered. Many situations may cause psychological distress, which may be described as stress. The physiological effects of stress and its effect on wound healing have already been described in section 2.2.5. Factors causing psychological distress may be defined as stressors. Those that may be particularly associated with wounded patients will be discussed in this section. It should be noted that other factors, not addressed here, can also act as stressors.

2.3.1 Anxiety

Lazarus and Averill (1972) stated that 'Anxiety results when a person is unable to fully comprehend the world around him'. This could be considered in relation to ill health. A further quotation from Frankenhaeuser (1967) adds to this: 'Information is necessary for comprehension, but the perception of this information can be modified by the expectations of the subject'. Many nurses will have seen patients who have not heard or have misunderstood what has been said to them because of their degree of anxiety.

Admission to hospital, whether planned or unplanned, can be a very stressful experience.

● *Nursing assessment* ●

Zigmond and Snaith (1983) designed a simple questionnaire, known as the Hospital Anxiety and Depression Score or HAD Score, that can identify the degree of stress being suffered and can be completed by patients. The questionnaire comprises a series of questions such as whether an individual is worried or able to relax and enjoy watching television. There is a choice of four answers to each question, such as 'most of the time' or 'seldom'. Most patients find it simple to use. Cole-King and Harding (2001) used the HAD Score to identify stress in 53 patients with leg ulcers and found it to be a useful research tool.

● *Nursing intervention* ●

Problem: Anxiety related to hospital admission
Goal: Patients will be able to express their specific anxieties

Many patients find their admission to hospital a very anxious time. Gammon (1998) compared the impact of hospital admission on patients with that of isolating a patient because of infection. All patients were assessed using the HAD Score and two other assessment tools to measure self-esteem (the Self-Esteem Scale) and a sense of control (the Health Illness (Powerlessness) Questionnaire) (Rosenburg, 1965; Roy, 1976). The isolated patients had significantly higher levels of anxiety and depression and lower levels of self-esteem and sense of control than the routine admission patients. However, results for all patients showed them to be outside normal levels, indicating that they were all suffering above normal levels of stress.

Communication is essential to address this problem. The initial assessment should provide both information and an opportunity for the patient to ask questions and express their feelings and concerns. Not everyone will always be able to discuss their anxieties immediately so there may be an ongoing process of building up a relationship over a period of time.

A study by McCabe (2004) investigated patients' experiences of nurse–patient communication. She noted that all the patients in the study frequently stated that nurses did not provide them with enough information and seemed to be more interested in tasks than in talking to patients. This was then excused by saying that the nurses were too 'busy'. McCabe analysed the findings from her study in terms of patient-centred communication and task-centred communication. Patient-centred communication involves attending behaviour and the patients in the study described this in terms of: giving time and being there, open/honest communication, genuineness, empathy and friendliness and humour. McCabe considered that nurses could have been using friendliness and humour as a means of maintaining a superficial level of communication to avoid the need to address emotional or difficult issues. She also considered that the culture of the organisation tended to discourage patient-centred communication.

Active listening is not a very safe occupation. The consequences may be emotionally painful to the nurse because of the difficult questions that may be asked. Many may feel inadequate or too inexperienced. Koshy (1989) describes active listening as 'the process of receiving and assimilating ideas and information from verbal and non-verbal messages and responding appropriately'. Tschudin (1991) emphasises the importance of not making assumptions. It is too easy for nurses to assume that they not only know the problem but also have the answers for dealing with it.

● *Evaluation* ●

Repetition of the assessment will enable the nurse to identify any reduction in stress levels.

Problem: Anxiety related to surgery
Goal: The patient's anxiety will be reduced by adequate preoperative preparation

There is now much greater awareness of the importance of providing good preoperative information. A Department of Health circular (1990) makes it clear that all patients have the right to understand their treatment and the risks involved. The role of the nurse is to ensure that each patient receives appropriate preoperative information about the surgery and what to expect in the postoperative period. Radcliffe (1993) has considered how a suitable strategy can be implemented. She suggests that oral information is reinforced with written leaflets, which can be a source of reference for both patients and relatives.

Doering *et al.* (2000) assessed the impact of providing a videotape of a patient undergoing a hip replacement from time of admission to discharge, purely from a patient's perspective. One hundred patients were randomly allocated to either the preparation group (shown the videotape) or a control group. They were assessed for levels of anxiety and pain for four days post surgery. The researchers found significantly lower levels of anxiety in the preparation group as well as a lower intake of analgesia, although there were no differences in the amount of pain. They considered that this was an effective method of providing information to patients.

● *Evaluation* ●

The patient should be able to describe the likely course of events in the perioperative and postoperative period.

Alternative therapies

Some alternative therapies have been successful in assisting patients to reduce anxiety. Marshall (1991) described the use of aromatherapy and relaxation techniques to reduce stress in dermatology patients. Dossey (1991) used case studies to discuss the benefits of guided imagery. This is a method of relaxation that encourages the patient to use their imagination to first identify the health problem and then to visualise how the treatment will work effectively. This may involve favourite scenes, music or other audiotapes. Ultimately patients have to visualise themselves in the final healed state. This technique should be used over a period of time, such as for two weeks prior to surgery, for it to be effective.

It is easy to dismiss such a concept as 'mumbo-jumbo' because it is alien to many healthcare professionals. However, Holden-Lund (1988) randomly allocated cholecystectomy patients to either guided imagery or period of quiet and those receiving guided imagery had significantly lower anxiety levels, cortisol levels and surgical wound erythema compared to the control group.

Therapeutic touch has been used in the USA for a number of years to reduce anxiety levels. Heidt (1981) used matched patient groups in a cardiovascular unit to receive therapeutic touch, casual touch or no touch. Those receiving therapeutic touch had significantly lower levels of anxiety compared with the other groups.

2.3.2 Motivation and education

Bentley (2001) discussed the importance of working in partnership with chronic wound patients in their own care. Such an approach can help to reduce the sense of powerlessness and loss of control felt by many patients. Bentley uses a case example of a patient with both pressure ulcers and a chronic leg ulcer to support her arguments. Rivera *et al.* (2000) used a similar approach to demonstrate how a model of behaviour modification was utilised to motivate and educate a patient with a diabetic foot ulcer. Such papers provide support for the importance of patient education. Unfortunately, there is limited research evidence of effective outcomes, mainly because of poor methodological quality, as demonstrated by the Cochrane review of the benefits of patient education in preventing diabetic foot ulceration (Valk *et al.*, 2003). The authors concluded that it appeared that patient education may reduce the incidence of ulceration and amputation but randomised controlled trials were needed to provide conclusive evidence.

Involving patients in their own care can reduce the risk of non-compliance and therefore it is useful to have a greater understanding of compliance and non-compliance. Nyatanga (1997) reviewed psychosocial theories of non-compliance and divided them into the following categories.

- *Perceptual theory* – people interpret the world based on what they already know. They may have pre-existing theories about their treatment.
- *Value clarification* – patients may consider the choices in relation to their treatment and choose whether to comply. An example would be a man choosing not to give up smoking despite knowing it increases his risk of leg amputation.
- *Attribution theory* – this relates to the locus of control. Patients who feel in control of their treatment or who see a link between their treatment and the healing of their wound are more likely to be compliant.
- *Cultural theories* – all individuals have a cultural understanding of their wound, its meaning and the treatment. This may lead them to decide not to follow all the treatment requirements, such as not wishing to take analgesia.
- *Health belief model* – patients may choose to engage in health-related behaviour if they believe that the benefits in terms of health gain outweigh the costs. For example, a leg ulcer patient may choose to wear a four-layer bandage that she finds hot and uncomfortable because she believes that it will heal her ulcer.

More recently, it has been recognised that the term 'compliance' does not reflect the move to increased patient autonomy and 'concordance' is now seen as a more accurate word to use. Moffatt (2004) has discussed concordance in relation to leg ulcer management and emphasised the importance of understanding the reasons why patients may not be concordant with their treatment plan. Physical reasons, such as bodily pain that reduces tolerance to treatment, or psychosocial issues, such as a patient's expectations of care, can have an impact on concordance. It is important to understand the patient's perspective when planning care so that they can truly become engaged in the healing process.

● *Nursing assessment* ●

Simple questioning can determine the level of relevant knowledge that a patient possesses.

● *Nursing intervention* ●

Problem: A lack of understanding of the care needed to promote wound healing
Goal: Patients demonstrate the ability to be self-caring and are able to explain their plan of care

In the climate of early discharge from hospital, many patients will return home with a wound that still requires dressing. If it is practicable, it is helpful to teach patients to undertake their own dressing. Monitoring and supervision by the district nurse or practice nurse would still be necessary. A planned education programme using short-term goals is the most effective. Information about allied care such as diet or exercise can also be incorporated into the programme. Patients with chronic wounds should be given information about their causes and possible prevention.

Some patients will have little motivation to carry on the plan of care once they have been discharged from hospital. Recognition of the reasons for the lack of motivation and good communication with the community staff may be of some help. A few patients will still fail to respond. It is necessary to accept that every patient has the right to choose not to comply with the care recommended by the healthcare team.

● *Evaluation* ●

The ability of the patient to undertake management of the wound will provide adequate evaluation of the effectiveness of the nursing care.

2.3.3 Body image

Body image is the mental picture that people have of themselves. Body image is also closely associated with self-esteem. Shipes (1987) suggests that self-esteem can be defined as the sum total of all we believe about ourselves. All patients with wounds have an altered body image which can have a profound effect on the person's self-esteem and motivation. Obvious types of wounds that can have these effects are those resulting in disfigurement, such as burns, head and neck surgery, mastectomy, amputation and ostomies. Many patients will also be suffering from anxiety about their prognosis. Chronic wounds can also affect body image, as shown in a study by Ebbeskog and Ekman (2001) who found that leg ulcer patients were embarrassed by their ulcer and bandages and hid them with clothing. The resultant stress can be so overwhelming that the patient may be unable to take in information, to share their feelings or to commence rehabilitation.

● *Nursing assessment* ●

Neil (2001) developed an assessment tool called the Stigma Scale to measure body image in relation to the skin. Users are asked to judge a series of 11 statements using a five-point Likert scale. This is a promising approach but a major limitation is that, as yet, the scale has been validated only by educated, mainly white, women and further work is required.

● *Nursing intervention* ●

Problem: Loss of self-esteem related to altered body image
Goal: Patients acknowledge change in body image and express their feelings about this change

In the early stages, following the circumstances that led to an altered body image, some patients appear to be quite euphoric. This is due to simple relief at having survived. After a while the patient's attitude is likely to change. Common problems that can occur include:

- a sense of loss, similar to bereavement.
- anxiety related to diagnosis, especially if it is cancer.
- loss of sexual function, which may be related to type of surgery or trauma or to either of the previous problems.
- withdrawal from social relationships with family or significant others, possibly due to a malodorous wound or any of the previous problems.

The role of the nurse is to assist the patient to develop a reintegrated body image (Burgess, 1994). This may be achieved in a variety of ways. Perhaps the most important is accepting patients as they are, at whatever stage they have reached. Allowing patients to express their feelings and providing them with matter-of-fact information, such as an honest appraisal of the progress of the wound, is beneficial. It is also essential to include family and/or significant others in the patient's care and in any education programme. Good management of the wound should prevent odour or leakage, which helps to boost confidence. Burgess also suggests that if patients are having difficulty coping, it may be necessary to emphasise the importance of the surgery for the health of the individual and the fact that it does not change them as a person.

As already discussed under Anxiety (section 2.3.1), preoperative information and counselling are most important. Kelly (1989) studied 67 patients who had undergone head and neck surgery. Generally, they said they were more anxious before surgery than after but 42% of men and 21% of women would have liked more information. Another study by Elspie et al. (1989) found that 41% of patients suffered psychological stress following major surgery for intraoral cancer.

In many areas, specialist nurses are employed to give help and support to patients, such as colorectal nurses or breast care nurses. They can build up a relationship with their patients which can give patients the confidence to express their feelings freely. In other circumstances, it may be a nurse who already has a good relationship with a patient who is able to provide this service.

● Evaluation ●

Regular evaluation of progress is important for patients with an altered body image. Learning to cope with the new image may take time and strategies may have to be changed along the way. This may be particularly true for those undergoing a series of plastic surgery operations who may have to cope with a constantly changing body image.

2.3.4 Other psychological problems

Fear

Fear is a common human experience that may be transitory or longer lasting. Illness may release many fears: fear of hospitalisation, fear of illness, fear of a life-threatening condition, fear of loss of affection of loved ones, fear of the mutilation of surgery. Such fear creates great stress within the sufferer. This may be made worse by the healthcare team failing to recognise when patients are experiencing fear and so not allowing them to express their feelings.

Grief

Grief is a normal process that allows adaptation to some major loss in a person's life. The wounded patient may have to come to terms with skin damage from burns, the loss of a limb or breast or other types of mutilating surgery (see also Body Image, section 2.3.3.). Kubler-Ross (1969) described various stages in the grief process. She related them to dying but they can be applied to all types of grief. The stages are: denial, isolation, anger, bargaining, depression and acceptance. Each person will progress through some or all of these stages at a different rate and not necessarily in the same sequence. By listening to the patient and accepting without judgement, the nurse can assist in this process and thus reduce the amount of stress suffered. This may be particularly difficult during the stage of anger as the aggression expressed by the patient is often directed at the main caregivers. Understanding of the cause of the aggression will help the nurse deal with this stage of grief.

Powerlessness

Taylor and Cress (1987) describe powerlessness as the 'perception of loss of control over what happens to oneself and one's environment'. This is a feeling experienced by many hospital patients as they are placed in the subservient 'patient role'. Even simple decisions such as when to eat or go to bed are taken away from the individual. There is pressure to conform and be a 'good' patient. Stockwell (1972) describes very graphically the fate of the unpopular patient who did not conform to the role the nurses desired from him. A 'good' patient will submit without question to treatment and will not ask too many questions. Although it is to be hoped that nursing has moved forward since 1972, many patients are still aware of their loss of status once they are in hospital. Some may feel depressed because of their feelings of learned helplessness. Others may feel quite euphoric to have survived, which may also be misinterpreted as a lack of compliance.

In a society where independence is prized, dependence on others may produce feelings of anger and frustration. Many patients remark that they feel a nuisance because they cannot care for themselves. It may also reduce feelings of self-worth. A common attitude of elderly people when asked to participate in a research project is that they will do so – because it will help others. Such a contribution is important to them as they feel that, despite their physical limitations, they can still make a contribution to the good of society.

● *Nursing assessment* ●

Although the precise problem may vary, the assessment is the same.

● Observe body language – does the patient look relaxed, tense, fidgety, withdrawn, hypoactive or hyperactive? Do they avoid eye contact?
● Conversation – does the patient talk excessively, not talk to anyone, ask questions?
● Do any of these terms describe the patient? Angry, confused, aggressive, confident, demanding, distrustful, anxious, fearful, critical, passive, depressed, euphoric, disorientated.

Katona and Katona (1997) proposed that a slightly different approach is required for assessing older people. They recommended the use of four simple questions.

● Are you basically satisfied with your life?
● Do you feel that your life is empty?
● Are you afraid that something bad is going to happen to you?
● Do you feel happy most of the time?

The patient would score a point for replying 'no' to the first and last questions and for replying 'yes' to the middle two. Anyone with a score of two or more is probably depressed.

● *Nursing interventions* ●

Although nurse training is providing improved knowledge of psychological care, it may be more appropriate for the patient to have further help from others such as a clinical psychologist, a psychiatric trained nurse, a chaplain or a trained counsellor.

Problem: Fear due to separation from loved ones or related to unfamiliarity
Goal: Patients identify the source(s) of their fear and are able to describe their feelings

Once the nurse recognises that the patient is very frightened, then strategies can be developed to allow the patient the opportunity of expressing their specific fears. Time may have to be set aside for 'casual' conversation, especially if the patient has few visitors. Assigning the same nurses to care for the patient can build up confidence. Involving the patient and, possibly, the family in all aspects of planning may be helpful. Patients with any sort of sensory loss will need orientation to the new surroundings.

Problem: Grieving related to loss of or disfigurement to a body part
Goal: Patients will allow themselves to experience the grieving process

A variety of strategies can be adopted to help the patient move through the grief process. Setting aside time to allow the patient to talk is very important.

However, it may be constructive to set time constraints as it can be exhausting for both the patient and the nurse. Patients may prefer to know that they have the undivided attention of the nurse for a set period of time each day, rather than an indeterminate amount of time occasionally. For some individuals, it may be appropriate for others to assist the patient in recognising and talking through their grief. In those situations, the nurse should be there to support and encourage.

> *Problem: Powerlessness related to feelings of loss of control of the environment*
> *Goal: The patent will express feelings of having a sense of control and will partici-*
> *pate in the planning of care*

Many healthcare workers fail to recognise the degree to which the 'system' takes charge of the individual once they pass through the doors of a hospital. Whilst in an emergency situation there may be some alteration of priorities, every patient is entitled to be treated with respect. Nurses can play an important role in assisting their patients to remain in control of as many areas of their lives as possible. Patient education not only promotes compliance but also allows the patient to participate in care, thus having a degree of control. Discussing with the patient when particular treatment should be given and involving them in planning care will reduce feelings of powerlessness.

A study by Efraimsson *et al.* (2003) demonstrates graphically how this can go wrong. They undertook a case study of discharge planning for an elderly patient. The patient and some of her family were invited to participate in the case conference. Observation showed that the clinical staff talked *about* rather than *with* the patient, using technical language, and they failed to answer questions posed by the patient or her children. In an interview with one of the researchers later, the patient revealed that she felt like on object during the discharge planning meeting and that she felt powerless. It is pointless to involve patients in the discharge planning process if we do not give them time and space to express their own feelings and desires.

● *Evaluation* ●

Evaluation of psychological care is not easy. Some indication can be obtained by repeating the assessment and by talking to the patient.

2.4 SPIRITUAL CARE

In recent years there has been increasing awareness of the importance of spiritual care within healthcare. Although much of it has centred around palliative care, as is evidenced in the NICE guideline *Improving Supportive and Palliative Care for Adults with Cancer* (NICE, 2004), it is seen to be wider than that, as discussed in the paper *NHS Chaplaincy: meeting the religious and spiritual needs of patients and staff* (DoH, 2003). A survey by King *et al.* (1999) of 250 patients admitted to a London teaching hospital found that 79% of patients professed some form of spiritual belief, although not all engaged in a religious activity. A survey undertaken of 1.75 million patients in American hospitals found that emotional and spiritual care was seen as largely ineffective and as an area that was in considerable need of improvement (Clark *et al.*, 2003).

NICE (2004) suggests that healthcare professionals frequently fail to recognise when patients need spiritual support. Spirituality is a concept that many nurses find difficult to define and they may feel unsure of what is required. Spirituality should not just be put into the framework of religion. Everyone, whether they believe in a God or not, has spiritual needs. Spirituality can be defined as that within us that responds to the infinite realities of life. Narayanasamy (1996) listed some indicators of spirituality which provide further clarity: a sense of purpose, hopefulness, creativity, joy, enthusiasm, courage, reverence, serenity, humour, providing meaning in struggle and suffering.

If the spiritual needs of individuals are not met or they experience a catastrophic event in their lives, the result is spiritual pain or distress. This acts as a stressor and thus can impact on wound healing. Kohler (1999) defined spiritual distress as the lack of meaning in one's life. In her study of French AIDS and cancer patients, Kohler found that nearly all of them expressed feelings of 'ill being' and raised questions about the meaning of life, death, pain or illness. Kawa *et al.* (2003) studied palliative care patients in Japan and described spiritual distress as consciousness of the gap between an individual's aspirations and their current situation. The patients in the study were distressed by the gap between their current situation and how they wanted to live or how they wanted to die or how they wanted to maintain relationships with others. Despite the cultural differences between the patient groups in these studies, there are obvious similarities in the factors causing their spiritual distress.

Cressey and Winbolt-Lewis (2000) worked with a group of chaplains and lay people to determine areas of potential distress where the patient can be left with feelings of isolation, fragmentation or despair. They are listed in Table 2.2. In the context of spiritual distress, acceptance also has significance. A patient may need reassurance that others, particularly family and friends, will accept them in the new role as a patient, especially if having to come to terms with a disfiguring wound. Finlay *et al.* (2000) suggest that patients perceive that healthcare professionals are too busy to discuss spiritual matters and so only disclose their distress when it becomes severe.

● *Nursing assessment* ●

Peterman *et al.* (2002) have developed a validated assessment tool to measure spiritual well-being, called the Functional Assessment of Chronic Illness Therapy – Spiritual Well-Being (FACIT-sp). This measures a sense of meaning and peace and also the role of faith in illness. However, it has only been validated with cancer patients. King *et al.* (2001) took a different approach and developed an assessment questionnaire that consistently differentiates between patients with high and low spiritual beliefs.

Villines and Harrington (1998) suggested a number of signs indicative of spiritual distress.

Table 2.2   Potential causes of spiritual distress (based on Cressey & Winbolt-Lewis, 2000).

Potential cause	Explanation
Being valued	Individuals need to feel loved and valued and have a sense of belonging. If this is not present, patients can feel isolated and fragmented
Finding meaning	Illness and suffering challenge preconceived ideas of the meaning of life and often provoke a search for further meaning. Until this is found the patient will suffer
Having hope	Hope is a major motivator and powerful life force. The loss of hope results in misery and melancholy
Emotions	Emotions are part of everyday life but the distressed patient may express feelings of fear, doubt or despair
Having dignity	Loss of privacy and dignity can be very distressing as can a failure to respect aspects of the many different cultures in today's society
Truth and honesty	Everyone is entitled to truth and honesty but this needs to be expressed with compassion and insight. Denying patients this right may result in tensions within their family and a 'conspiracy of silence'
Good communication	Failures of communication can cause distress and even offence
Death, dying, bereavement and loss	This often links to the need to find meaning and patients may ask 'why me?'
Religion	Patients can be very distressed by the lack of opportunity to follow their usual religious observances
Culture	For some, cultural observances are intertwined with their religious beliefs, yet we often fail to recognise them

- Crying.
- Expressions of guilt: 'I must have been very wicked to have to suffer all this'.
- Sleeping a great deal/not sleeping (afraid of not waking).
- Disrupted spiritual trust.
- Feeling remote from God or the higher power.
- Showing anger towards God/others.
- Loss of meaning and purpose in life: 'Why is this happening to me?'
- Challenged belief or value system.

The signs of spiritual despair include:

- loss of hope.
- refusal to communicate with loved ones.
- loss of spiritual belief.

- death wish.
- severe depression.

- *Nursing interventions* •

  Problem: Spiritual distress related to separation from religious or cultural ties or from a challenged belief or value system
  Goal: The patient will be able to identify the cause of spiritual distress and specify the assistance required to alleviate it

Cavendish *et al.* (2003) suggest that provision of spiritual care is part of nursing care, although nurses may not always be comfortable with the concept. Nurses are not always able to recognise the difference between spiritual needs and religious needs. Cressey and Winbolt-Lewis (2000) describe spiritual care as conveying to patients that they have value and are unconditionally regarded for who they are, regardless of illness, colour or creed.

The chaplaincy team is very much part of the multiprofessional network and can give much support to both the patients and staff by listening, comforting and counselling when necessary. However, nurses need to have some understanding of the range of spiritual care activities. There can be no standardised spiritual care as there is with postoperative physical care. In this situation, each patient must be cared for in the light of their unique needs. Fish and Shelly (1985) proposed the following activities: listening, empathy, vulnerability, humility and commitment.

- *Listening* – this is active listening, giving the patient full attention and noting all the non-verbal as well as verbal cues.
- *Empathy* – this allows the nurse to share the feelings of the patient without losing objectivity. This is essential to enable the patient to consider alternatives.
- *Vulnerability* – as nurses enter into and share patients' feelings, they become vulnerable. This may be painful but can also be rewarding.
- *Humility* – this is not easy. Few people want to admit that they do not have the answers in their particular field. A sense of humility will enable nurses to see that they can learn from their patients. Humility also allows nurses to accept themselves and their patients in all their human frailty.
- *Commitment* – being with a patient through all the difficult times, sharing the pain as well as the joys, involves considerable commitment.

Several studies have investigated spiritual coping mechanisms. Dein and Stygall (1997) undertook a review of religion and chronic illness and found that religion was a positive coping mechanism. A qualitative study using grounded theory found that 13 Christian patients undergoing open heart surgery sought comfort through prayer. They used two strategies: praying themselves and enlisting others to pray for them, especially for the times when they were unable to pray (Hawley, 1998). Narayanasamy (2002) interviewed 15 chronically sick people (nine Christians, two Hindus and four with no religious affiliation) and also found that prayer brought comfort as it gave both a sense of connectedness to God and also a sense of hope, strength and security. However, the author only found this sense of connectedness to God (or Hindu deities) amongst the Christians and Hindus in his sample.

● *Evaluation* ●

Just as spiritual assessment is very difficult, so too is evaluation of the outcomes of care. Narayanasamy (1996) suggests that spiritual integrity is one outcome that may be demonstrated as relief from spiritual pain or by restoration of the life principle. Resolution of the signs of spiritual distress or despair would indicate a positive outcome, as would an improved FACIT-sp score.

REFERENCES

Alberti, K., Press, C. (1992) The biochemistry of the complications of diabetes mellitus, in (eds) Keen, H., Jarrett, J., *Complications of Diabetes*. Edward Arnold, London.

Andel, H., Kamolz, L.P., Horauf, K., Zimpfer, M. (2003) Nutrition and anabolic agents in burned patients. *Burns*, **29** (6), 592–595.

Anstead, G.M. (1998) Steroids, retinoids and wound healing. *Advances in Wound Care*, **11**, 277–282.

Arturson, M.G.S. (1978) Metabolic changes following thermal injury. *World Journal of Surgery*, **2**, 203–213.

Augustin, M., Maier, K. (2003) Psychosomatic aspects of chronic wounds. *Dermatology and Psychosomatics*, **4** (1), 5–13.

Bentley, J. (2001) Promoting patient partnership in wound care. *British Journal of Community Nursing*, **6** (10), 493–500.

Bibby, B.A., Collins, B.J., Ayliffe, G.A.J. (1986) A mathematical model for assessing the risk of post-operative wound infection. *Journal of Hospital Infection*, **8**, 31–39.

Birkmeyer, N.J., Charlesworth, D.C., Hernandez, F. *et al.* (1998) Obesity and risk of adverse outcomes associated with coronary artery bypass surgery. Northern New England Cardiovascular Disease Study Group. *Circulation*, **97** (17), 1689–1694.

Borger, M.A., Rao, V., Weisel, R.D. *et al.* (1998) Deep sternal wound infection: risk factors and outcomes. *Annals of Thoracic Surgery*, **65** (4), 1050–1056.

Brandenberger, G., Gronfier, C., Chapotot, F., Simon, C., Piquard, F. (2000) Effect of sleep deprivation on overall 24 h growth hormone secretion. *Lancet*, **356** (9239), 1408.

Brown, K. (1991) Improving intakes. *Nursing Times*, **87** (20), 64–68.

Burgess, L. (1994) Facing the reality of head and neck cancer. *Nursing Standard*, **8** (32), 30–34.

Carr, E. (1997) Overcoming barriers to effective pain control. *Professional Nurse*, **12** (6), 412–416.

Carr, E., Thomas, V.J. (1997) Anticipating and experiencing post-operative pain: the patients' perspective. *Journal of Clinical Nursing*, **6**, 191–201.

Carter, D. (1985) In need of a good night's sleep. *Nursing Times*, **81** (46), 24–26.

Cavendish, R., Konecny, L., Mitzeliotis, C. *et al.* (2003) Spiritual care activities of nurses using Nursing Interventions Classification (NIC) labels. *International Journal of Nursing Terminologies and Classifications*, **14** (4), 113–124.

Cereceda, F.C., Gonzalez, G.I., Antolin, J.F.M. *et al.* (2003) Detection of malnutrition on admission to hospital. *Nutricion Hospitalaria*, **18** (2), 95–100.

Chan, A.W., Macfarlane, I.A., Bowsher, D. (1990) Chronic pain in patients with diabetes mellitus: comparison with a non-diabetic population. *Pain Clinic*, **3** (3), 147–159.

Chapman, A. (1996) Current theory and practice: a study of pre-operative fasting. *Nursing Standard*, **10** (18), 33–36.

Chbinou, N., Frenette, J. (2004) Insulin-dependent diabetes impairs the inflammatory response and delays angiogenesis following Achilles tendon injury. *American Journal of Physiology – Regulatory Integrative and Comparative Physiology*, **286** (5), R952–957.

Chmell, M.J., Schwartz, H.S. (1996) Analysis of variables affecting wound healing after musculoskeletal sarcoma resections. *Journal of Surgical Oncology*, **61**, 185–189.

Clark, M., Schols, J.M.G.A., Benati, G. *et al.* (2004) Pressure ulcers and nutrition: a new European guideline. *Journal of Wound Care*, **13** (7), 267–272.

Clark, P.A., Drain, M., Malone, M.P. (2003) Addressing patients' emotional and spiritual needs. *Joint Commission Journal on Quality and Safety*, **29** (12), 659–670.

Closs, S.J. (1992) Patients' night time pain, analgesic provision and sleep after surgery. *International Journal of Nursing Studies*, **29** (4), 381–392.

Cole-King, A., Harding, K.G. (2001) Psychological factors and delayed healing in chronic wounds. *Psychosomatic Medicine*, **63**, 216–220.

Committee of Ministers (2003) *Resolution ResAP(2003)3 on Food and Nutritional Care in Hospitals*. Council of Europe, Brussels.

Correia, M.L., Waitzberg, D.L. (2003) The impact of malnutrition on morbidity, mortality, length of hospital stay and costs evaluated through a multivariate model analysis. *Clinical Nutrition*, **22** (3), 235–239.

Cressey, R.W., Winbolt-Lewis, M. (2000) The forgotten heart of care: a model of spiritual care in the National Health Service. *Accident and Emergency Nursing*, **8**, 170–177.

De Boer, A.S., Mintjes-de Groot, A.J., Severijnen, A.J., van den Berg, J.M.J., van Pelt, W. (1999) Risk assessment for surgical-site infections in orthopaedic patients. *Infection Control and Hospital Epidemiology*, **20** (6), 402–407.

Dein, S., Stygall, J. (1997) Does being religious help or hinder coping with chronic illness? A critical review. *Palliative Medicine*, **11**, 291–299.

Delmi, M., Rapin, C.H., Bengoa, J.M. (1990) Dietary supplementation in elderly patients with fractured neck of femur. *Lancet*, **235**, 1013–1016.

Department of Health (1990*) Health Service Management – Patient Consent to Examination and Treatment*. NHS Management Executive, London.

Department of Health (2001a) *The Essence of Care*. Department of Health, London.

Department of Health (2001b) *Standard Principles for Preventing Infections in Hospitals*. Department of Health, London.

Department of Health (2001c) Better hospital food panel launched. Department of Health, London.

Department of Health (2003) *NHS Chaplaincy: meeting the religious and spiritual needs of patients and staff*. Department of Health, London.

Doering, S., Katzlberger, F., Rumpold, G. *et al.* (2000) Videotape preparation of patients before hip replacement surgery reduces stress. *Psychosomatic Medicine*, **62** (3), 365–373.

Dossey, B. (1991) Awakening the inner healer. *American Journal of Nursing*, **Aug**, 31–34.

Ebbeskog, B., Ekman, S.L. (2001) Elderly persons' experiences of living with a venous leg ulcer: living in a dialectal relationship between freedom and imprisonment. *Scandinavian Journal of Caring Sciences*, **15**, 235–243.

Edington, J., Kon, P., Martyn, C.N. (1996) Prevalence of malnutrition in patients in general practice. *Clinical Nutrition*, **15**, 60.

Efraimsson, E., Rasmussen, B.H., Gilje, F., Sandman, P.O. (2003) Expressions of power and powerlessness in discharge planning: *Journal of Clinical Nursing*, **12**, 707–716.

Ehrlich, H.P., Tarver, H., Hunt, T.K. (1972) Effects of Vitamin A and glucocorticoids upon inflammation and collagen synthesis. *Annals of Surgery*, **177**, 222–227.

Elia, M., Stratton, R. (2004) On the ESPEN guidelines for nutritional screening 2002. *Clinical Nutrition*, **23** (1), 131–132.

Elspie, C.A., Freedlander, E., Campsie, L.M. *et al.* (1989) Psychological distress at follow-up after major surgery for intraoral cancer. *Journal of Psychosomatic Research*, **33** (4), 441–448.

Exton-Smith, A.N. (1971) Nutrition of the elderly. *British Journal of Hospital Medicine*, **5**, 639–645.

European Pressure Ulcer Advisory Panel (EPUAP) (2003) *Nutritional Guidelines for Pressure Ulcer Prevention and Treatment*. EPUAP, Oxford.

Fagerhaugh, S.Y., Strauss, A. (1977) *Politics of Pain Management: staff–patient interaction*. Addison-Wesley, London.

Field, L. (1996) Are nurses still underestimating patients' pain post-operatively? *British Journal of Nursing*, **5** (13), 778–784.

Finlay, I.G., Ballard, P.H., Jones, N., Searle, C., Roberts, S. (2000) A person to have around. What value do patients want from a hospice chaplain? *Journal of Health Care Chaplaincy*, **3** (2), 41–52.

Fish, S., Shelley, J.A. (1985) *Spiritual Care: the nurse's role*. InterVarsity Press, Downers Grove, IL.

Frankenhaeuser, M. (1967) Some aspects of research in physiological psychology, in (ed.) Levi, L., *Emotional Stress, Physiological and Psychological Reactions – medical, industrial and military implications*. Karger, Basel.

Freedman, N.S., Kotzer, N., Schwab, R.J. (1999) Patient perception of sleep quality and etiology of sleep disruption in the intensive care unit. *American Journal of Respiratory and Critical Care Medicine*, **159** (4 Pt 1), 1155–1162.

Freedman, N.S., Gazendam, J., Levan, L., Pack, A.I., Schwab, R.J. (2001) Abnormal sleep/wake cycles and the effect of environmental noise on sleep disruption in the intensive care unit. *American Journal of Respiratory and Critical Care Medicine*, **163**, 451–457.

Gallagher-Allred, C.R., Voss, A.C., Finn, S.C., McCamish, M.A. (1996) Malnutrition and clinical outcomes: a case for medical nutrition therapy. *Journal of the American Dietetic Association*, **96** (4), 361–366.

Gammon, J. (1998) Analysis of the stressful effects of hospitalisation and source isolation on coping and psychological constructs. *International Journal of Nursing Practice*, **4** (2), 84–96.

Gazzotti, C., Arnaud-Battandier, F., Parello, M. *et al.* (2003) Prevention of malnutrition in older people during and after hospitalisation. *Age and Ageing*, **32** (3), 321–325.

Gibson, J.M.E., Kenrick, M. (1998) Pain and powerlessness: the experience of living with peripheral vascular disease. *Journal of Advanced Nursing*, **27**, 737–745.

Gottrup, F. (2000) Prevention of surgical wound infections. *New England Journal of Medicine*, **342** (3), 202–204.

Gould, D. (1992) Hygienic hand decontamination. *Nursing Standard*, **6** (32), 33–36.

Greif, R., Akca, O., Horn, E.P., Kurz, A., Sessler, D.I. (2000) Supplemental peri-operative oxygen to reduce the incidence of surgical wound infection. *New England Journal of Medicine*, **342** (3), 161–167.

Grunbine, N., Dobrowolski, C., Bernstein, A. (1998) Retrospective evaluation of post-operative steroid injections on wound healing. *Journal of Foot and Ankle Surgery*, **37** (2), 135–144.

Guigoz, Y., Lauque, S., Vellas, B.J. (2002) Identifying the elderly at risk for malnutrition. The Mini Nutritional Assessment. *Clinics of Geriatric Medicine*, **18** (4), 737–757.

Haddock, J. (1994) Reducing the effects of noise in hospital. *Nursing Standard*, **8** (43), 25–28.

Hamilton Smith, A. (1972) *Nil by Mouth*. RCN Publications, London.

Handwashing Liaison Group (1999) Hand washing; a modest measure with big effects. *British Medical Journal*, **318**, 686.

Harmer, M., Davies, K.A. (1998) The effect of education, assessment and a standardised prescription for post-operative pain management. The value of clinical audit in the establishment of acute pain services. *Anaesthesia*, **53** (5), 424–430.

Hawley, G. (1998) Facing uncertainty and possible death: the Christian patients' experience. *Journal of Clinical Nursing*, **7** (5), 467–478.

Haydock, D.A., Hill, G.L. (1986) Impaired wound healing in surgical patients with varying degrees of malnutrition. *Journal of Enteral and Parenteral Nutrition*, **10** (6), 550–554.

Hayward, J. (1975) *Information – a prescription against pain*. RCN Publications, London.

He, G.W., Ryan, W.H., Acuff, T.E. *et al.* (1994) Risk factors for operative mortality and sternal wound infection in bilateral internal mammary artery grafting. *Journal of Thoracic and Cardiovascular Surgery*, **107** (1), 196–202.

Hehenberger, K., Heilborn, J.D., Brismar, K., Hansson, A. (1998) Inhibited proliferation of fibroblasts derived from chronic diabetic wounds and normal dermal fibroblasts treated with high glucose is associated with increased formation of l-lactate. *Wound Repair and Regeneration*, **6** (2), 135–141.

Heidt, P. (1981) Effect of therapeutic touch on anxiety level of hospitalised patients. *Nursing Research*, **30** (1), 32–37.

Hicks, F., Simpson, K.H., Tosh, G.C. (1994) Management of spinal infusions in palliative care. *Palliative Medicine*, **8** (4), 325–332.

Hill, J. (1989) A good night's sleep. *Senior Nurse*, **9** (5), 17–19.

Hillmann, A., Ozaki, T., Rube, C. *et al.* (1997) Surgical complications after pre-operative irradiation of Ewing's sarcoma. *Journal of Cancer Research and Clinical Oncology*, **123** (1), 57–62.

Hitchcock, L.S., Ferrell, B.R., McCaffery, M. (1994) The experience of chronic nonmalignant pain. *Journal of Pain and Symptom Management*, **9** (5), 312–318.

Holden-Lund, C. (1988) Effects of relaxation with guided imagery on surgical stress and wound healing. *Research Nursing Health*, **11** (4), 235–244.

Holmes, S. (1986) Nutritional needs of medical patients. *Nursing Times*, **82** (16), 34–36.

Holzman, A.D., Turk, D.C. (1986) *Pain Management*. Pergamon Press, Oxford.

Hunt, A. (1997) Assessment and planning for older people. *Nursing Times*, **93** (21), 74–78.

Jarmon, H., Jacobs, E., Walter, R., Witney, C., Zielinski, V. (2002) Allowing the patients to sleep: flexible medication times in an acute hospital. *International Journal of Nursing Practice*, **8** (2), 75–80.

Jorgensen, L.N., Kallehave, F., Christensen, E., Siana, J.E., Gottrup, F. (1998) Less collagen production in smokers. *Surgery*, **123** (4), 450–455.

Katona, C.L., Katona, P.M. (1997) Geriatric depression scale can be used in older people in primary care. *British Medical Journal*, **315** (7117), 1236.

Kawa, M., Kayama, M., Maeyama, E. *et al.* (2003) Distress of inpatients with terminal cancer in Japanese palliative care units: from the point of view of spirituality. *Supportive Care in Cancer*, **11** (7), 481–490.

Kelly, R. (1989) *A study of patients who have had surgery in the head and neck region*, Paper given at the RCN Research Scotland Symposium, November.

Kiecolt-Glaser, J.K., Marucha, P.T., Malarkey, W.B., Mercado, A.M., Glaser, R. (1995) Slowing of wound healing by psychological stress. *Lancet*, **346** (8984), 1194–1196.

Kiecolt-Glaser, J.K., McGuire, L., Robles, T.F., Glaser, R. (2002) Emotions, morbidity and mortality: new perspectives from psychoneuroimmunology. *Annual Review of Psychology*, **53**, 83–107.

King, L. (2001) Impaired wound healing in patients with diabetes. *Nursing Standard*, **15** (38), 39–45.

King, M., Speck, P., Thomas, A. (1999) The effect of spiritual beliefs on outcome from illness. *Social Science and Medicine*, **48** (9), 1291–1299.

King, M., Speck, P., Thomas, A. (2001) The Royal Free interview for spiritual and religious beliefs: development and validation of a self-report version. *Psychological Medicine*, **31** (6), 1015–1023.

Kinney, J.M. (1977) The metabolic response to injury, in (eds) Richards, J.R., Kinney, J.M., *Nutritional Aspects of the Critically Ill*. Churchill Livingstone, Edinburgh.

Kohler, C. (1999) The nursing diagnosis of spiritual distress, a necessary re-evaluation. *Recherche en Soins Infirmiers*, **56**, 12–72.

Koshy, K.T. (1989) I only have ears for you. *Nursing Times*, **85** (30), 26–29.

Kubler-Ross, E. (1969) *On Death and Dying*. Macmillan, London.

Kurz, A., Sessler, D.I., Lenhardt, R. (1996) Perioperative normothermia to reduce the incidence of surgical-wound infection and shortened hospitalisation. *New England Journal of Medicine*, **334** (19), 1211–1215.

Lammers, R.L., Hudson, D.L., Seaman, M.E. (2003) Prediction of traumatic wound infection with a neural network derived decision model. *American Journal of Emergency Medicine*, **21** (1), 1–7.

Landis, C.A., Whitney, J.D. (1997) Effects of 72 hours sleep deprivation on wound healing in the rat. *Research in Nursing and Health*, **20**, 259–267.

Larson, E., Kretzer, E.K. (1995) Compliance with handwashing and barrier precautions. *Journal of Hospital Infection*, **30** (Suppl), 88–106.

Lazarus, R.S., Averill, J.R. (1972) Emotion and cognition with special reference to anxiety, in (ed.) Spielberger, C.D., *Anxiety: current trends in theory and research*. Academic Press, New York.

Leaper, D.J., Harding, K.G. (1998) *Wounds: biology and management*. Oxford University Press, Oxford.

Lee, H.A. (1979) Why enteral nutrition? *Research and Clinical Forums*, **1**, 15–24.

Lee, K.A., Stotts, N.A. (1990) Support of the growth hormone-somatomedin system to facilitate wound healing. *Heart Lung*, **19** (2), 157–163.

Levenson, S.M., Gruber, C.A., Rettura, G., Gruber, D.K., Demetriou, A.A., Seifter, E. (1984) Supplemental Vitamin A prevents acute radiation-induced deficit in wound healing. *Annals of Surgery*, **200**, 494–512.

Lewis, B.K., Hitchings, H., Bale, S., Harding, K.G. (1993) Nutritional status of elderly patients with venous ulceration of the leg – report of a pilot study. *Journal of Human Nutrition and Dietetics*, **6**, 509–515.

Lin, K.Y., Johns, F.R., Gibson, J., Long, M., Drake, D.B., Moore, M.M. (2001) An outcome study of breast reconstruction: presurgical identification of risk factors for complications. *Annals of Surgical Oncology*, **8** (7), 596–591.

Loots, M.A., Lamme, E.N., Mekkes, J.R., Bos, J.D., Middelkoop, E. (1999) Cultured fibroblasts from chronic diabetic wounds on the lower extremity (non-insulin-dependent diabetes mellitus) show disturbed proliferation. *Archives of Dermatological Research*, **291** (2–3), 93–99.

Mahoney, C.B., Odom, J. (1999) Maintaining intraoperative normothermia: a meta-analysis of outcomes with costs. *American Association of Nurse Anaesthetists Journal*, **67** (2), 307–308.

Manassa, E.H., Hertl, C.H., Olbrisch, R.R. (2003) Wound healing problems in smokers and non-smokers after 132 abdominoplasties. *Plastic and Reconstructive Surgery*, **111** (6), 2082–2087.

Marshall, M. (1991) Stress management in dermatology patients. *Nursing Standard*, **5** (24), 29–31.

Martens, M.G., Kolrud, B.L., Faro, S., Maccato, M., Hammill, H. (1995) Development of wound infection or separation after caesarian delivery. Prospective evaluation of 2431 cases. *Journal of Reproductive Medicine*, **40** (3), 171–175.

Mathus-Vliegen, E.M. (2004) Old age, malnutrition and pressure sores: an ill-fated alliance. *Journals of Gerontology Series A-Biological Sciences and Medical Sciences*, **59** (4), 355–360.

McCabe, C. (2004) Nurse–patient communication: an exploration of patients' experiences. *Journal of Clinical Nursing*, **13**, 41–49.

McCampbell, B., Wasif, N., Rabbitts, A., Staiano-Coico, L., Yurt, R.W., Schwartz, S. (2002) Diabetes and burns: a retrospective study. *Journal of Burn Care and Rehabilitation*, **23** (3), 157–166.

McMahon, R. (1990) Sleep therapies. *Surgical Nursing*, **3** (5), 17–20.

McPhee, I.B., Williams, R.P., Swanson, C.E. (1998) Factors influencing wound healing after surgery for metastatic disease of the spine. *Spine*, **23** (6), 726–732.

McWhirter, J.P., Pennington, C.R. (1994) Incidence and recognition of malnutrition in hospital. *British Medical Journal*, **308** (6934), 945–948.

Mishriki, S.F., Law, D.J.W., Jeffery, P.J. (1990) Factors affecting the incidence of postoperative wound infection. *Journal of Hospital Infection*, **16**, 223–230.

Moffatt, C.J. (2004) Perspectives on concordance in leg ulcer management. *Journal of Wound Care*, **13** (6), 243–248.

Morgan, H., White, B. (1983) Sleep deprivation. *Nursing Mirror*, **157** (14) (Suppl), 8–11.

Moro, M.L., Carrieri, M.P., Tozzi, A.E., Lana, S., Greco, D. (1996) Risk factors for surgical wound infections in clean surgery: a multicentre study. Italian PRINOS Study Group. *Annals of Italian Chirugia*, **67** (1), 13–19.

Narayanasamy, A. (1996) Spiritual care of chronically ill patients. *British Journal of Nursing*, **5** (7), 411–416.

Narayanasamy, A. (2002) Spiritual coping mechanisms in chronically ill patients. *British Journal of Nursing*, **11**, 1461–1470.

National Institute for Clinical Excellence (NICE) (2004) *Improving Supportive and Palliative Care of Adults with Cancer.* NICE, London.

Neil, J.A. (2001) The Stigma Scale: measuring body image and the skin. *Plastic Surgical Nursing*, **21** (2), 79–81, 87.

Nemeth, K.A., Harrison, M.B., Graham, I.D., Burks, S. (2003) Pain in pure and mixed aetiology venous leg ulcer: a three-phase point prevalence survey. *Journal of Wound Care*, **12** (9), 336–340.

Nightingale, F. (1974) *Notes on Nursing. What it is and What it is not.* Blackie and Son, Glasgow and London (first published 1859).

Nyatanga, B. (1997) Psychosocial theories of patient non-compliance. *Professional Nurse*, **12** (5), 331–334.

Older, M.W.J., Edwards, D., Dickerson, J.W.T. (1980) A nutrient survey in elderly women with femoral neck fracture. *British Journal of Surgery*, **67**, 884.

O'Sullivan, B., Davis, A.M., Turcotte, R. *et al.* (2002) Peroperative versus postoperative radiotherapy in soft-tissue sarcoma of the limbs: a randomised trial. *Lancet*, **359** (9325), 2235–2241.

Pablo, A.M., Izaga, M.A., Alday, L.A. (2003) Assessment of nutritional status on hospital admission: nutritional scores. *European Journal of Clinical Nutrition*, **57** (7), 824–831.

Parsons, E.P. (1992) Cultural aspects of pain. *Surgical Nurse*, **5** (2), 14–16.

Parsons, G. (1994) The benefits of relaxation in the control of pain. *Nursing Times*, **90** (19), 11–12.

Pavlidis, T.E., Galatianos, I.N., Papaziogas, B.T. *et al.* (2001) Complete dehiscence of the abdominal wound and incriminating factors. *European Journal of Surgery*, **167** (5), 351–354.

Pedley, H. (1996) The nurse's role in pain assessment and management in a coronary care unit. *Intensive and Critical Care Nursing*, **12**, 254–260.

Penfold, P., Crowther, S. (1989) Causes and management of neglected diet in the elderly. *Care of the Elderly*, **1** (1), 20–22.

Perkins, C. (2004) Improving glycaemic control in a metabolically stressed patient in ICU. *British Journal of Nursing*, **13** (11), 652–657.

Peterman, A.H., Fitchett, G., Brady, M.J., Hernandez, L., Cella, D. (2002) Measuring spiritual well-being in people with cancer: the functional assessment of chronic illness therapy-Spiritual Well-Being Scale (FACIT-sp). *Annals of Behavioral Medicine*, **24** (1), 49–58.

Plattner, O., Akca, O., Herbst, F. *et al.* (2000) The influence of 2 surgical bandage systems on wound tissue oxygen tension. *Archives of Surgery*, **135** (7), 818–822.

Pollack, S.V. (1982) Wound healing IV. Systemic medications affecting wound healing. *Journal of Dermatology and Surgical Oncology*, **8**, 667–671.

Pracek, J.T., Patterson, D.R., Montgomery, B.K., Heimbach, D.M. (1995) Pain, coping and adjustments in patients with burns: preliminary findings from a prospective study. *Journal of Pain and Symptom Management*, **10** (6), 446–455.

Radcliffe, S. (1993) Pre-operative information: the role of the ward nurse. *British Journal of Nursing*, **2** (6), 305–309.

Renwick, P., Vowden, K., Wilkinson, D., Vowden, P. (1998) The pathophysiology and treatment of diabetic foot disease. *Journal of Wound Care*, **7** (2), 107–110.

Rivera, E., Walsh, A., Bradley, M. (2000) Using behaviour modification to promote wound healing. *Home Healthcare Nurse*, **18** (9), 579–587.

Rojas, I.G., Padgett, D.A., Sheridan, J.F., Marucha, P.T. (2002) Stress-induced susceptibility to bacterial infection during cutaneous wound healing. *Brain, Behaviour and Immunity*, **16** (1), 74–84.

Rose, M., Sanford, A., Thomas, C., Opp, M.R. (2001) Factors altering the sleep of burned children. *Sleep*, **24** (1), 45–51.

Rosenberg, C.S. (1990) Wound healing in the patient with diabetes mellitus. *Nursing Clinics of North America*, **25** (1), 247–261.

Rosenburg, M. (1965) *Society and the Adolescent Self Image*. University Press, Princeton, NJ.

Roy, C. (1976) Decision making by the physically ill and adaptation to illness. Health-Illness (Powerlessness) Questionnaire, in US Department of Health, Education and

Welfare, *Instruments for Measuring Nursing Practice and Other Health Care Variables*, Vol 1 and 11. US Department of Commerce, National Technical Information Services, Washington.

Royal College of Surgeons and College of Anaesthetists (1990) *Commission on the Provision of Surgical Services: Report of the Working Party on Pain after Surgery*. Royal College of Surgeons and College of Anaesthetists, London.

Sassler, A.M., Esclamado, R.M., Wolf, G.T. (1995) Surgery after organ preservation therapy. *Archives of Otolaryngology-Head and Neck Surgery*, **121** (2), 162–165.

Schmied, H., Kurz, A., Sessler, D.I., Kozek, S., Reiter, A. (1996) Mild hypothermia increases blood loss and transfusion requirements during total hip arthroplasty. *Lancet*, **347** (8997), 289–292.

Sellden, E. (2002) Peri-operative amino acid administration and the metabolic response to surgery. *Proceedings of the Nutrition Society*, **61** (3), 337–343.

Senter, H., Pringle, A. (1985) *How Wounds Heal*. Calmic Medical Division of the Wellcome Foundation, London.

Shipes, E. (1987) Psycho-social issues, the person with an ostomy. *Nursing Clinics of North America*, **22** (2), 291–302.

Siana, J.E., Frankild, S., Gottrup, F. (1992) The effect of smoking on tissue function. *Journal of Wound Care*, **1** (2), 37–41.

Simons, W., Malaber, R. (1995) Assessing pain in elderly patients who cannot respond verbally. *Journal of Advanced Nursing*, **22** (4), 663–669.

Sitton-Kent, L., Gilchrist, B. (1993) The intake of nutrients by hospitalised pensioners with chronic wounds. *Journal of Advanced Nursing*, **18**, 1962–1967.

Sloman, R., Brown, P., Aldana, E. *et al.* (1994) The use of relaxation for the promotion of comfort and pain relief in persons with advanced cancer. *Contemporary Nurse*, **3** (1), 6–12.

Sorensen, L.T. (2003) Smoking and wound healing. *EWMA Journal*, **3** (1), 13–15.

Sorensen, L.T., Horby, J., Friis, E., Pilsgaard, B., Jorgensen, T. (2002) Smoking as a risk factor for wound healing and infection in breast cancer surgery. *European Journal of Surgical Oncology*, **28** (8), 815–820.

Sorensen, L.T., Karlsmark, T., Gottrup, F. (2003) Abstinence from smoking reduces incisional wound infection: a randomised, controlled trial. *Annals of Surgery*, **238** (1), 1–5.

Southwell, M.T., Wistow, G. (1995) Sleep in hospitals at night: are patients' needs being met? *Journal of Advanced Nursing*, **21**, 1101–1109.

Stockwell, F. (1972) *The Unpopular Patient*. Royal College of Nursing, London.

Stubbs, L. (1989) Taste changes in cancer patients. *Nursing Times*, **85** (3), 49–50.

Sutherland, A.B. (1985) Nutrition and general factors influencing infection in burns. *Journal of Hospital Infection*, **6** (suppl. B), 31–42.

Talas, D.U., Nayci, A., Atis, S. *et al.* (2003) The effects of corticosteroids and vitamin A on the healing of tracheal anastomoses. *International Journal of Pediatric Otorhinolaryngology*, **67** (2), 109–116.

Taylor, C.M., Cress, S.S. (1987) *Nursing Diagnosis Cards*. Springhouse Corporation, Pennsylvania.

Taylor, L.K., Kuttler, K.L., Parks, T.A., Milton, D. (1998) The effect of music in the postanaesthesia care unit on pain levels in women who have had abdominal hysterectomies. *Journal of Perianesthesia Nursing*, **13** (2), 88–94.

Taylor, S.J. (1999) Early enhanced enteral nutrition in burned patients is associated with fewer infective complications and shorter hospital stay. *Journal of Human Nutrition and Dietetics*, **12** (2), 85–91.

Tibballs, J. (1996) Teaching hospital medical staff to hand wash. *Medical Journal of Australia*, **164**, 395–398.

Tschudin, V. (1991) Just four questions. *Nursing Times*, **87** (39), 46–47.

Valk, G.D., Kriegsman, D.M.W., Assendelft, W.J.J. (2003) Patient education for preventing diabetic foot ulceration (Cochrane Methodology review). *The Cochrane Library*, Issue 4. John Wiley & Sons Ltd, Chichester.

Villines, B., Harrington, J. (1998) A spiritual needs protocol. *American Journal of Nursing*, **98** (1), 28.

Wang, Z., Qiu, W., Mendenhall, W.M. (2003) Influence of radiation therapy on reconstructive flaps after radical resection of head and neck cancer. *International Journal of Oral and Maxillofacial Surgery*, **32** (1), 35–38.

Ward, S.E., Berry, P.E., Misiewicz, H. (1996) Concerns about analgesics among patients and family caregivers in a hospice setting. *Research in Nursing and Health*, **19** (3), 205–211.

Williams, J.Z., Barbul, A. (2003) Nutrition and wound healing. *Surgical Clinics of North America*, **83** (3), 571–596.

Wissing, U., Unosson, M. (1999) The relationship between nutritional status and physical activity, ulcer history and ulcer-related problems in patients with leg and foot ulcers. *Scandinavian Journal of Caring Science*, **13** (2), 123–128.

Wissing, U., Ek, A.C., Unosson, M. (2001) A follow-up study of ulcer healing, nutrition and life situation in elderly patients with leg ulcers. *Journal of Nutrition, Health and Ageing*, **5** (1), 37–42.

Woods, N. (1972) Patterns of sleep in post-cardiotomy patients. *Nursing Research*, **21**, 347–352.

Wysocki, A.B. (1996) The effect of intermittent noise exposure on wound healing. *Advances in Wound Care*, **9** (1), 35–39.

Yates, P., Dewar, A., Fentiman, B. (1995) Pain: the views of elderly people living in long-term residential care settings. *Journal of Advanced Nursing*, **21** (4), 667–674.

Zainal, G. (1995) Nutritional demands. *Nursing Times*, **91** (38), 57–59.

Zhou, Y.P., Jiang, Z.M., Sun, Y.H., Wang, X.R., Ma, E.L., Wilmore, D. (2003) The effect of supplemental enteral glutamine on plasma levels, gut function and outcome in severe burns: a randomised, double-blind, controlled clinical trial. *Journal of Enteral and Parenteral Nutrition*, **27** (4), 241–245.

Zigmond, A.S., Snaith, R.P. (1983) The Hospital Anxiety and Depression Scale. *Acta Psychiatrica Scandinavica*, **67**, 361–370.

Chapter 3
General Principles of Wound Management

3.1 INTRODUCTION

This chapter will discuss, in broad detail, the general principles of wound management. Specific care of chronic and acute wounds will be considered in later chapters. The products mentioned in this chapter will be described in more detail in Chapter 4.

The ability to make an accurate assessment of a wound is an important nursing skill. It should be carried out in conjunction with an assessment of the patient as discussed in Chapter 2. The aim of the assessment is twofold. It will provide baseline information of the state of the wound, so that progress can be monitored, and will also ensure that an appropriate selection of wound management products is made. Keast *et al.* (2004) consider that accurate and comprehensive wound assessment requires meticulous and consistent clinical observation. To that end, they have proposed a mnemonic, 'MEASURE', to provide a framework for assessment (see Table 3.1). In addition, wound classification, the position of the wound and the environment of care also need to be determined. These factors provide the framework for wound assessment and will be discussed next, followed by the MEASURE framework.

3.2 WOUND ASSESSMENT

3.2.1 Wound classification

Wounds can be classified as chronic, acute and postoperative wounds.

Chronic wounds have been described as being of long duration or frequent recurrence (Fowler, 1990). Typical examples are pressure ulcers and leg ulcers. Patients may have multifactorial problems that affect their ability to heal their wounds.

Acute wounds are usually traumatic wounds. They may be cuts, abrasions, lacerations, burns or other traumatic wounds. They usually respond rapidly to treatment and heal without complication.

Postoperative wounds are intentional acute wounds. They may heal by first intention, where the skin edges are held in approximation. Sutures, clips or tape may be used. Some surgical wounds are left open to heal by second intention, usually to allow drainage of infected material. Donor sites are also open wounds.

Table 3.1   MEASURE: a framework for wound assessment (from Keast *et al.*, 2004).

	Parameter	Parameter content
M	Measure	Length, width, depth and area
E	Exudate	Quantity and quality
A	Appearance	Wound bed, tissue type and amount
S	Suffering	Pain type and level
U	Undermining	Presence or absence
R	Re-evaluate	Monitoring all parameters regularly
E	Edge	Condition of wound edge and surrounding skin

There may be related factors to be considered when managing each of these types of wounds, such as the relief of pressure for pressure ulcers. The care of chronic wounds will be considered in Chapter 5 and of acute wounds in Chapter 6.

Traditionally, some wounds have been classified according to depth. This type of classification is widely used in the USA but is generally only used to describe burns or, occasionally, pressure ulcers in the UK. Wounds are described in relation to the tissues that are damaged or destroyed. Figure 3.1 illustrates the different depths of tissue damage.

Erosion is the term used to describe the loss of one or two layers of epithelial cells. There is no depth to this type of wound.

Superficial wounds are wounds where the epidermis has been damaged.

Partial-thickness wounds occur when the epithelium and part of the dermis are destroyed. Hair follicles and sweat glands are only partially damaged. This type of wound is sometimes subdivided into partial-thickness and deep partial-thickness wounds. When these wounds have a large surface area, hair follicles and sweat glands produce epithelial cells during the epithelialisation stage which form islets of cells on the wound surface, thus speeding the healing process.

Full-thickness wounds have all of the epidermis and dermis destroyed. Deeper tissues such as muscle or bone may also be involved. Healing may take longer to establish in these wounds.

3.2.2   The position of the wound

The position of a wound should be noted as part of the assessment. It may be an indicator of potential problems, such as risk of contamination in wounds in the sacral region or problems of mobility caused by wounds on the foot. Another aspect to consider is the fact that a dressing may stay in place very well on one part of the body but not on another.

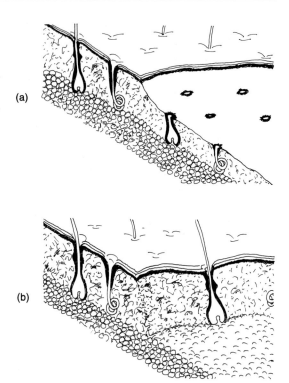

Fig. 3.1   The degree of tissue damage in wounds of differing depth. (a) A partial-thickness wound: islets of living epithelium remain around hair shafts and sweat ducts. (b) A full-thickness wound: no living epithelia remain in the injured area.

3.2.3 The environment of care

Consideration must be given to the environment in which care is to be given. Harding (1992) proposed a wound-healing matrix which includes consideration of the environment and carer. The management of a wound can be affected by the circumstances of the patient. For example, the timing of a dressing change may not be particularly important for a patient in hospital but for a patient at home, perhaps a young mother with children to get to school, timing may be critical. Flexibility may be important for a patient with a long-standing wound who has to return to work. It may be helpful to arrange for the occupational health nurse in the patient's place of employment to carry out the dressing change, thus reducing the frequency of clinic attendance.

Not all wound management products are available in the community. Hospital nurses need to ensure that the product selected can be continued after discharge home. If a non-skilled person is to provide some of the wound care for a patient, adequate time must be allowed for teaching the individual appropriate routines. Adequate monitoring of care must also be established.

3.2.4 M = Measure

The size and shape of a wound may alter during the healing process. In the early stages as necrotic tissue and/or slough are removed, the wound appears to increase in size because the actual extent of the wound was originally masked by the necrotic tissue. Monitoring of wound shape is important to guide dressing selection. A cavity wound requires a different dressing to a shallow wound. Some dressings are not appropriate for use if there is a sinus present. Accurate nursing records are essential for monitoring progress.

This section considers the various ways in which measurement of a wound may be undertaken. Some of them are not really appropriate for use in busy areas but may have value in a research study. Others are very expensive and beyond the budget of most nurses. Whatever type of measurement is used, it should be undertaken on a regular basis, the frequency depending on the type of wound. Chronic wounds should be measured every 2–4 weeks as little change is likely to be seen by more frequent measurement. However, acute wounds progress much more rapidly so measurement should be done at each dressing change.

Simple linear measurement

The very simplest method of measuring a wound is to measure it at its greatest length and breadth and to measure the depth if appropriate. If a wound is a relatively regular shape, such as the example shown in Figure 3.2, then this can be a fairly successful method. It is also likely to be more accurate if the wound edges are marked to indicate the measurement points. A probe can be used if the wound is a very irregular shape or has sinus formation.

There are several drawbacks to using this type of measurement. Goldman and Salcido (2002) suggest that the method has limited sensitivity to changes in wound size and it also provides limited information about the shape of a wound. The more people involved, the greater the risk of the measurement not being on the same spot each time. Even if the same person does the measurement each time, it still may not be replicated accurately; this is known as sampling error. If necrotic tissue or slough is present, the true wound size will become apparent as debridement occurs. Wound measurement will show that the wound has increased in size and can give a misleading picture of wound progress. Measurement gives no indication of wound appearance. Despite these drawbacks, Kantor and Margolis (1998) found a significant correlation between simple wound measurements and measurement using planimetry, except for

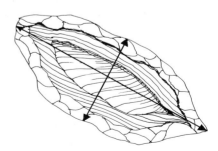

Fig. 3.2   Measurement of a regular-shaped wound.

wounds larger than 40^2 cm, and suggested that simple measurements could be used to monitor wound progress.

Simple measurement is best used on small, surgically induced cavities that are regular in shape and should heal rapidly. More comprehensive data would be obtained if used in conjunction with a nursing chart.

Measurement of surface area

Flanagan (2003a) reviewed the varying methods of wound measurement and found that measuring true surface area and monitoring the percentage reduction of wound surface area over time are the most useful methods. The most frequently used system for surface area measurement is that of tracing a wound. A variety of materials may be used, the commonest being acetate paper. One presentation of acetate paper is the lesion measure, samples of which are supplied by several dressing manufacturers. They are usually fairly small sheets with a series of circles on them. The centre circle is 1 cm in diameter and is surrounded by concentric circles that increase in size by 2 cm increments. This gives some estimate of measurement in the tracing.

The surface area of a wound can be calculated quite accurately by placing the tracing over squared paper and counting the number of whole squares or by using computerised planimetry. Successive tracings can be compared to show any difference in wound size. If necrotic tissue or slough is present then an initial increase in size will occur as debridement progresses.

More recently, sophisticated computerised methods have been developed that can measure surface area. Lagan *et al.* (2000) compared planimetry and digitising and found that digitising based on wound tracings gave a significantly higher level of repeatability than planimetry. Keast *et al.* (2004) described a portable digital tablet (Visitrak™) that can be used in conjunction with wound tracings. A tracing can be placed on the digital tablet and a special stylus used to trace over the wound outline. The system calculates the surface area and percentage reduction in wound size from previous measurements. Clinical evaluation of the digital tablet is in progress.

Another system is a specialised computer software package for use with a digital camera (Verge Videometer™ [VeV]). A photograph is taken and downloaded onto a computer where the program calculates the wound surface area. Thawer *et al.* (2002) compared tracings and planimetry with VeV and found excellent intrarater and interrater reliability in 45 chronic wounds. However, it must be noted that there is potential for inaccuracy when using a system involving a digital camera if the wound is over a curved part of the body such as the leg.

Flanagan (2003a) noted that errors can occur when undertaking wound tracings, particularly in identifying the wound margin. She suggested that establishing a simple protocol could help to improve accuracy. As with wound measurement, the tracing will show the increase or decrease in size without any explanation, as it does not provide information on wound appearance or depth.

If the acetate sheet is placed in direct contact with the wound, it will need cleansing with alcohol spray or similar. Some centres use plastic bags so the underside can be discarded and the side with the tracing retained. Some acetates are provided with disposable backing paper.

Tracing is best used on fairly straightforward shallow wounds. Ideally it should be used in combination with an assessment chart. Lucas *et al.* (2002) recommend using both tracings and photography to monitor wound healing.

Measuring volume

When wounds are deep, it may be useful to measure wound volume. Theoretically, it is possible to calculate the volume by measuring the wound depth (using a sterile swab) and multiplying by the surface area. However, there are inherent errors in this method (Goldman & Salcido, 2002). Deep wounds are rarely cuboid in shape, may not have a uniform depth, and sinus formation or undermining may be present. If the base of the wound is filled with necrotic debris, it must first be cleansed from the wound before undertaking any measurements (Keast *et al.*, 2004). Various methods have been used to measure wound volume but they are not simple, valid or reliable (Keast *et al.*, 2004).

The most practical method of monitoring changes in wound volume is to measure and record the depth at the deepest part of the wound and to note the amount of dressing required to fill the cavity.

3.2.5 E = Exudate

The amount of wound exudate varies during the healing process. In a normally healing wound, there is considerable exudate at the inflammatory stage and very little at epithelialisation. A copious exudate may indicate a prolonged inflammatory stage or infection. In their review of the role of exudate in the healing process, Vowden and Vowden (2003) consider the differences between acute and chronic wound exudate and conclude that chronic wound exudate has the potential to become a barrier to healing. Unfortunately, it is not possible to assess a wound and immediately determine if wound exudate is an actual barrier to healing.

Keast *et al.* (2004) suggest that exudate can be measured in terms of quantity, quality and odour. Falanga (2000) proposed a scoring system for wound exudate quantity that provides some qualification with the aim of achieving standardisation. Thus:

- 1 = minimal (dressings last up to one week).
- 2 = moderate (dressings changed every 2–3 days).
- 3 = heavy (dressings changed at least daily).

An alternative method to quantify exudate was used by Browne *et al.* (2004a) in a multicentre study assessing dressing performance in the presence of heavy exudate (called the WRAP Study). The research team used the TELER® system of clinical indicators (Le Roux, 1993) to measure exudate leakage. A clinical indi-

Table 3.2 Exudate leakage using TELER indicator (from Browne *et al.* (2004a). Reproduced by kind permission of TELER Ltd).

Code	Exudate leakage
5	No leakage between routine/planned dressing change
4	Exudate leakage within 2 hours of next dressing change
3	Exudate leakage within 8 hours of next dressing change
2	Exudate leakage within 24 hours of dressing change
1	Exudate leakage within 8 hours of dressing change
0	Exudate leakage within 2 hours of dressing change

cator is an ordinal measuring scale with six reference points that measure change. Each reference point is clinically significant, with 0 being the worst possible outcome and 5 the best. Table 3.2 shows the clinical indicator for exudate leakage when the planned frequency of dressing change is every two days. Exudate is considered to leak if it strikes through the outer bandage or strapping. Although this system measures exudate leakage rather than exudate amount, it still has clear clinical relevance.

Falanga (2000) considered that there is little benefit in scoring the quality of wound exudate. However, there may be some benefit in using clearly defined terminology to describe exudate quality. It may be of particular importance in postsurgical wounds where there is a potential risk of postoperative bleeding. Therefore the terms 'serous', 'serosanguinous', 'sanguinous', 'seropurulent' and 'purulent' may be useful.

Odour is much more difficult to measure in any objective way. Odour may be indicative of infection but wound odour also increases as necrotic tissue debrides by autolysis. Some dressings such as hydrocolloids may produce a foul-smelling odour when they are removed. It must also be remembered that many patients are distressed by wound odour and may feel embarrassment, disgust or shame (Hack, 2003). In a further paper on the WRAP project, Browne *et al.* (2004b) describe a clinical indicator to quantify odour (see Table 3.3). Browne *et al.* (2004b) used it in conjunction with a patient-focused indicator to determine the impact of odour on the patient, thus making it an even more powerful tool.

3.2.6 A = Appearance

The appearance of the wound gives an indication of the stage of healing that it has reached or of any complication that may be present. Open wounds or wounds healing by second intention can be categorised as:

Table 3.3   TELER indicator to quantify odour (from Browne *et al.* (2004b). Reproduced by kind permission of TELER Ltd).

Code	Odour
5	No odour
4	Odour is detected on removal of the dressing
3	Odour is evident on exposure of the dressing
2	Odour is evident at arm's length from the patient
1	Odour is evident on entering room
0	Odour is evident on entering house/ward/clinic

- necrotic.
- infected.
- sloughy.
- granulating.
- epithelialising.

Some wounds may fit into more than one category and so present as 'mixed' wounds. Before assessing a wound, the nurse should ensure that all the old dressing has been removed. Many modern dressings form a gel, which may give a misleading impression of the wound unless it is first cleaned away.

Necrotic wounds (see Fig. 3.3)

When an area of tissue becomes ischaemic for any length of time, it will die. The area may form a necrotic eschar or scab which can be black or brown in colour. Some necrotic tissue may present as a thick slough that can be brown, grey or off-white. When assessing these wounds it is important to remember that the wound may be more extensive than is apparent. The eschar or slough masks the true size of the wound. Intervention is needed for these wounds to heal.

Infected wounds (see Fig. 3.4)

All wounds are colonised with bacteria. This does not delay healing or mean that wounds will automatically become infected. If infection occurs, the clinical signs of infection will usually be present which are pain, heat, swelling, erythema and pus. The signs may vary slightly according to the bacteria causing the infection. Usually there is localised erythema or redness which may be restricted to just one part of the wound, such as at one end of a suture line, or may spread to a large area around the wound. Associated with the erythema is heat in the adjacent tissue that will also feel hotter than the skin at a distance from the wound. Oedema or swelling around the wound is also present. The

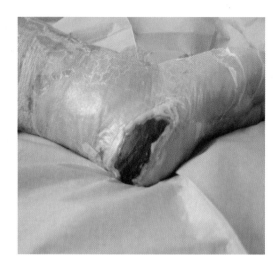

Fig. 3.3 A necrotic wound.

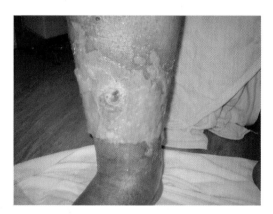

Fig. 3.4 An infected wound.

colour of the exudate and the slough on the wound surface depend on the bacteria causing the infection. There is usually a heavy exudate as the body rushes extra neutrophils and macrophages to the affected area and also tries to 'wash' the bacteria away. The exudate may have an offensive odour and can be the first indication of infection. Patients may also complain of increased pain.

However, chronic wounds do not always have such clear clinical signs. Cutting and Harding (1994) proposed additional criteria to those discussed above.

- Delayed healing (compared with expected rate, may be for other reasons).
- Discolouration: relates to wound bed.
- Friable granulation tissue that bleeds easily.
- Unexpected pain or tenderness.
- Pocketing or bridging at the base of the wound.
- Abnormal odour.
- Wound breakdown.

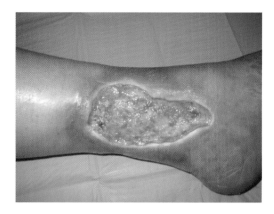

Fig. 3.5 A sloughy wound.

Cutting (1998) studied the use of these criteria and compared his clinical opinion with microbiological cultures on the wounds of 40 patients attending a wound clinic. He found that eight times out of nine, his decisions about infection were corroborated by the microbiological culture and also on the 31 occasions when he deemed infection was not present. This study demonstrates the potential value of using these criteria in clinical practice, although it must also be acknowledged that the researcher is both knowledgeable and experienced and this undoubtedly had an impact on the outcome.

Gardener *et al.* (2001a) further developed these signs and symptoms into a checklist with definitions for each sign and symptom. The checklist was submitted to a panel of six experts in chronic wounds for content validation and then tested for reliability using two nurses to assess 36 chronic wounds in three healthcare sites, using different nurses on each site. Perfect agreement using kappa statistics was achieved for increased pain, oedema, wound breakdown, delayed healing and friable granulation tissue; substantial agreement was achieved for erythema, purulent exudate, serous exudate, discolouration; only moderate agreement was achieved for foul odour and heat; pocketing was not observed. In a further aspect to the study, they also undertook microbiological cultures from the wounds (Gardener *et al.*, 2001b). They found the signs proposed by Cutting and Harding to be better indicators of chronic wound infection than the classic signs. However, increasing pain and wound breakdown were both sufficient indicators for infection without the other symptoms and have good interrater reliability.

Sloughy wounds (see Fig. 3.5)

Slough is typically a white/yellow colour. It is most often found as patches on the wound surface, although it may cover large areas of the wound. It is made up of dead cells that have accumulated in the exudate. It can be related to the end of the inflammatory stage in the healing process. Neutrophils have only a short lifespan and may die faster than they can be removed. Given the right

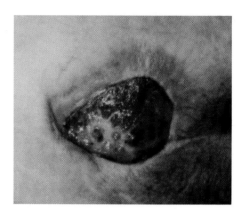

Fig. 3.6   A granulating wound.

environment for healing, the macrophages are usually capable of removing the slough and it disappears as healing progresses. Harding (1990) refers to a yellow fibrinous membrane that develops on the surface of some wounds. It is not stuck fast but can be easily removed. The membrane has no effect on healing and recurs if removed. He describes it as a variant on the normal.

Granulating wounds (see Fig. 3.6)

Granulation tissue was first described by John Hunter in 1786. It relates quite well to the stage of reconstruction in the healing process. The wound colour is red. The tops of the capillary loops cause the surface to look granular, hence the name. It should be remembered that the walls of the capillary loops are very thin and easily damaged, which explains why these wounds bleed easily. Regular, careful measurement will show a reduction in wound volume as the cavity fills with new tissue and contracts inwards.

Epithelialising wounds (see Fig. 3.7)

As the epithelia at the wound margins start to divide rapidly, the margin becomes slightly raised and has a bluey-pink colour. As the epithelia spread across the wound surface, the margin flattens. The new epithelial tissue is a pinky-white colour. In shallow wounds with a large surface area, islets of epithelialisation may be seen. The progress of epithelialisation may be easily identified as the new cells are a different colour from those of the surrounding tissue.

Recording wound appearance

Wound appearance can be recorded in a number of ways. The simplest is the written word but this is also likely to be the most subjective and open to misuse and misinterpretation. Common examples are 'wound healing well' or 'wound a bit sloughy'. Neither of these assessments has much value when trying to monitor wound progress accurately. In an attempt to overcome this problem,

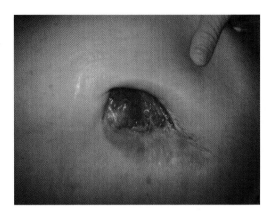

Fig. 3.7   An epithelialising wound.

some investigators use percentages to determine the quantity of each tissue type on the wound surface. This method has not been thoroughly tested but although still subjective, it is more precise than the previously described method.

Romanelli (1997) described the use of a colour reflectance analyser to determine the levels of granulation tissue in a wound. In a study evaluating methods of debridement in 32 patients with sloughy venous leg ulcers, he found chromatic measurement of the wound bed to be a reliable measurement tool. It was able to accurately measure the percentages of slough and granulation tissue in the wound. However, this type of equipment is not readily available in most clinical areas and it takes time to set up and use.

The old adage 'A picture is worth a thousand words' may not be strictly true in relation to photographs of wounds but photography does address some of the criticisms of the previous methods. A photograph provides clear evidence of the appearance of a wound and some suggestion of its size, especially if a rule is incorporated to provide a scale. Houghton *et al.* (2000) investigated the validity and reliability of using photography to assess wound status in comparison to a pressure ulcer assessment tool. They concluded that it was a valid and reliable tool for assessing wounds on the trunk and lower extremities. When managing chronic wounds, regular photographs can provide real encouragement to both patients and carers. It should be remembered that the depth of a wound is not demonstrated in a photograph, as it does not accurately record wounds on curved surfaces.

There are three types of camera in use for medical purposes: 35 mm camera, Polaroid camera and digital camera. Generally, it is hospital photographers who use 35 mm cameras rather than individual clinicians. Nechala *et al.* (1999) compared 35 mm cameras with Polaroid and digital cameras and found that the 35 mm camera produced the highest quality hard copies. Kokoska *et al.* (1999) found similar results in their comparison of 35 mm and digital cameras. Nechala *et al.* (1999) also found the 35 mm camera was the most economical per hard copy. The main disadvantage of the 35 mm camera is that it takes much longer to generate a photograph than the other camera types. Another disadvantage is that it is not possible to be certain of the quality or accuracy of an individual photograph until the film is developed. It is also important to determine how individual patients will be identified if using a film with large numbers of exposures. One issue many nurses have to consider if planning to purchase a camera is the need for an ongoing budget to pay for films and development.

Polaroid cameras have been very popular with nurses, especially in the community. The major advantage of this camera is that the hard copy is produced immediately and can be shown to the patient and immediately placed in the notes (Nechala *et al.*, 1999). Whilst the quality may not be as good as more powerful cameras, it is adequate for most needs, especially if a light lock lens is used to enable close-ups. There is still an ongoing cost for the purchase of films.

Increasingly, digital cameras are being used in clinical practice. They are gradually improving in quality and becoming cheaper. After initial training has been given, they have been found to be easy to use and focus and to transfer to computer to provide digital images. There are no ongoing costs as the film-card can be reused many times. However, access to a computer with a large memory on the hard drive is necessary, as the images require a large storage capacity. Once downloaded, the images can be utilised to produce hard copies, which can be displayed on the screen for teaching purchases or incorporated into a PowerPoint presentation. Galdino *et al.* (2000) monitored the costs of converting a large plastic surgery to digital photography rather than using the hospital photographic department. All the medical staff, including junior doctors, were supplied with their own camera and film-card. Over a five-year period, the authors estimated they would save $63950. The main disadvantages of digital cameras are the initial training to use them successfully and that it is possible to manipulate the image and to falsely enhance the results (Nechala *et al.*, 1999).

Hayes and Dodds (2003) successfully incorporated use of a digital camera into clinical practice in a hospital vascular clinic. They utilise a shared electronic patient record to communicate with primary care teams via the NHSnet, so that all involved can see the digital images. They recommend using standardised lighting and background and using the same patient position and that patient identification codes, the date and a calibration scale should be included within the digital image.

Not all nurses have access to a camera. It may be possible to obtain one on a short-term loan if a dressing trial is being undertaken.

Several factors need to be considered if the purchase of a camera is planned. Nechala *et al.* (1999) considered that it was important to determine the reason for requiring a camera before making a choice of camera type. If high-quality hard copies are required, a 35 mm camera is the best option. If speed is important then a Polaroid camera should be chosen and if digital images are required, then a digital camera is best. Other questions to answer are as follows.

- Who will pay for films and developing?
- Is the proposed camera capable of taking close-up pictures?

- Who will be using the camera?
- How can pictures be taken from the same angle and distance each time?
- How will patient consent be recorded? Some hospitals have a consent form for photography, others accept that implied consent is sufficient for routine photography.
- How will the images be stored to protect patient confidentiality?

Photographs provide good visual evidence of wound appearance. If a camera is not readily available, photography is best only considered for complicated or unusual wounds.

3.2.7 S = Suffering

Moffatt (2002) suggested that within chronic wound management, there is a need to focus on the patient, particularly their pain control. Unfortunately, pain assessment is rarely part of routine wound assessment despite the fact that many wounds are associated with pain (Krasner, 1995). Increased pain may be an indicator of infection and this must always be excluded in the first instance. Pain has been discussed in Chapter 2 and pain assessment should part of the overall patient assessment. This section will focus on local wound factors in relation to pain.

Dressing change and wound management activities such as debridement may cause pain. An international survey of practitioners was undertaken across 11 countries to investigate their views on wound pain (Moffatt et al., 2002). Dressing removal was identified as the time of greatest pain, with adherent dressings being seen as a major contributing factor. Szor and Bourguignon (1999) surveyed 32 patients with pressure ulcers for pain using the McGill Pain Questionnaire. They found that 28 (87.5%) had pain at dressing change and 12 (42%) had continuous pain both at rest and during dressing changes. Sadly, only two patients were receiving analgesia.

It is well recognised that burn patients suffer considerable pain at dressing change (Latarjet, 2002). Nagy (1999) investigated the impact on nurses of having to inflict pain on burn patients during dressing changes. She found that the commonest strategy was distancing by the nurse, which had the side effect of the nurses becoming less concerned about controlling pain. But if nurses developed a strategy of engaging with the pain, they saw it as a challenge to ensure good pain control. Taal et al. (1999) undertook a validation study of a pain anxiety scale specifically for burn patients. The scale included items such as 'I find it impossible to relax when my burns are being treated' and 'I am frightened of the pain during and/or after the treatment'. They found high levels of reliability and internal consistency and suggest that the scale could be used as a method of assessing therapeutic interventions.

Senecal (1999) stresses the importance of assessment and that it should include the type of pain and pain intensity. Krasner (1995) put forward a model of chronic wound experience that divides wound pain into three types: non-cyclical acute wound pain, such as sharp debridement; cyclical acute wound pain, such as dressing changes; chronic wound pain, which is persistent and constant. Pain intensity can be measured by means of a variety of visual analogue scales as discussed in Chapter 2. It may also be useful to identify any factors related to dressing change, such as dressing type, that may impact on pain levels. The frequency of reassessment should also be identified.

3.2.8 U = Undermining

In this part of their assessment framework, Keast *et al.* (2004) discuss assessment of the internal wound area. This is relevant in cavity wounds and it is important to identify any undermining, tunnelling or sinus tracts. A sterile swab can be used to probe under the wound edges to measure the extent of undermining. If it is extensive it may be helpful to mark the area on the surface of the skin using a pen. This will facilitate future assessments and assist in evaluating any change.

3.2.9 R = Re-evaluate

The purpose of re-evaluating a wound is to check for any signs of complications and to monitor progress towards achieving short-term goals, such as debridement and the overall goal of healing. This may be achieved by checking the wound for complications such as infection at each dressing change and regularly assessing selected wound parameters such as reduction in wound size. The frequency of assessment will vary according to wound type but for most chronic wounds, it should be every 1–2 weeks. Acute wounds may need to be assessed more frequently.

Flanagan (2003b) reviewed the methods for measuring wound healing and concluded that percentage reduction in size was the most useful indicator of wound progress as this can differentiate between healing and non-healing wounds in the first few weeks of treatment. Kantor and Margolis (2000) measured percentage reduction in wound size for 104 patients with venous leg ulcers and found that percentage change in the first four weeks of treatment predicted the healing outcome at 24 weeks. In a small study of nine patients with grade 4 pressure ulcers, Brown (2000) found that healing did not progress in a linear fashion and suggested that plotting wound-healing curves could be useful; that is, multiple measurements of percentage reduction in wound area from baseline, measured over time.

This type of accurate measurement may not be necessary for everyday clinical practice but it has considerable value in research. Specialist centres may be able to invest in some of the digitised systems that can provide this type of information very easily, as discussed in section 3.2.4, but they are not available to all. In general clinical practice, wounds should be regularly assessed every 1–4 weeks and progress towards treatment goals evaluated.

3.2.10 E = Edge

This final stage of the MEASURE assessment process refers to the need to assess the wound margins and the surrounding skin. The wound margin provides useful information indicative of both aetiology and healing status. For example, a punched-out appearance and a sharp margin is indicative of an arterial ulcer. A raised edge of epithelial cells on a wound with residual slough, such as can be seen in Figure 3.7, is indicative of a wound that is starting to heal, whereas Figure 3.4 shows no indication of any activity on the wound margin.

Nurses often neglect to assess the skin surrounding a wound and yet much useful information can be obtained. Erythema and heat may be indicative of infection. Erythema alone may be caused by allergy to the dressing (contact dermatitis), as shown in Figure 3.8. Induration may indicate further pressure damage around an existing pressure ulcer. Maceration can occur in the presence of heavy uncontrolled exudates; if this situation persists over time, irritant dermatitis may develop (Fig. 3.9). Fragile skin must be treated with caution and is at risk of damage if dressings and tapes are selected unwisely. Dry scaly skin should also be identified as scales can build up around the wound and cause problems.

Comment

Wound assessment is highly complex and is an important clinical skill. The use of uniform concepts and terms can assist in ensuring a consistent approach to the subject.

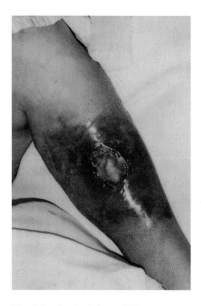

Fig. 3.8 Contact dermatitis.

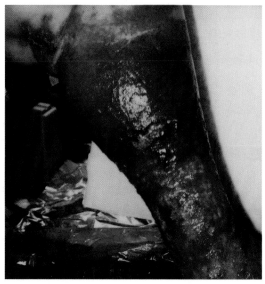

Fig. 3.9 Irritant dermatitis.

3.3 MANAGING WOUNDS

A great deal has been written about wound management but in order to make sense of what is proposed, it is helpful to understand the competing theories of wound management. They are moist wound healing and wound bed preparation.

3.3.1 Moist wound healing

The concept of moist wound healing was first introduced by George Winter in 1962. He compared the effect of leaving superficial wounds exposed to form a scab with the effect of applying a vapour-permeable film dressing, using an animal model (Winter, 1962). Epithelialisation was twice as fast in those wounds covered with a film dressing; this was because the dressing maintains humidity on the wound surface and the epithelial cells are able to slide across the surface of the wound. In contrast, epithelial cells in the exposed wounds had to burrow beneath the scab, dried exudate and layers of dessicated cells to find a moist layer to allow movement across the wound.

Little notice was taken of Winter's work until the 1980s when a number of clinical studies confirmed his findings and identified other benefits as well. Local wound pain was found to be considerably reduced in a moist environment (Eaglstein, 1985; May, 1984). The moist environment was also shown to enhance natural autolytic processes, thus aiding the breakdown of necrotic tissue (Freidman & Su, 1983; Kaufman & Hirshowitz, 1983).

Following these studies, there was a dramatic change in the methods of wound management and many new occlusive wound management products have been developed such as alginates, foams, hydrocolloids and hydrogels.

Schultz *et al.* (2003) summarised the benefits of a moist wound environment as follows:

- assists epidermal migration.
- promotes alterations in pH and oxygen levels.
- maintains an electrical gradient.
- retains wound fluid on the wound surface.

However, although these outcomes are of undoubted benefit to acute wounds, questions were being raised as to their usefulness in chronic wound management. Much of the research into the moist wound environment has been undertaken on acute, superficial wounds and does not address all the issues presented by chronic wounds, which tend to be deeper, with larger amounts of exudate and a greater bacterial burden. Thus a further wound management theory was required.

3.3.2 Wound bed preparation

The theory of wound bed preparation (WBP) has developed in part because of increasing understanding of the differences between acute and chronic wound exudate and the potentially harmful constituents of chronic wound fluid (see Chapter 1) and in part following clinical experience of using bio-engineered skin products. Falanga (2000) proposed that it was inappropriate to utilise expensive, sophisticated products on a poorly prepared wound. As a minimum, a wound should have a well-vascularised wound bed, minimal bacterial burden and little or no exudate before an effective outcome can be achieved. Further debate has led to a consensus paper (Schultz *et al.*, 2003), which has provided the following definition:

> 'Wound bed preparation is the management of the wound to accelerate endogenous healing or to facilitate the effectiveness of other therapeutic measures.'

WBP has four aspects: debridement, management of exudate, resolution of bacterial imbalance and undermined epidermal margin (Schultz *et al.*, 2003). Falanga (2004) has utilised the work of Schultz *et al.* (2003) to develop a framework called TIME to provide a comprehensive approach to chronic wound care. The terms in the framework have been modified by the European Wound Management Association WBP Advisory Board to maximise their use in different languages (Box 3.1). Figure 3.10 shows how the TIME framework can be used within a holistic approach to care.

Tissue management

This aspect of the TIME framework refers to the need to debride necrotic and sloughy tissue. Debridement may be achieved in a number of ways.

- Autolytic debridement utilises the ability of macrophages to phagocytose debris and necrotic tissue. Hydrocolloids and hydrogels are widely used to promote autolytc debridement as they provide a moist environment that enhances macrophage activity. Alginates are also used in the presence of moisture.
- Biosurgery or larval therapy has recently regained popularity and is widely used in the UK. Sterile maggots of the fly *Lucilia sericata* secrete enzymes that break down necrotic tissue to a semi-liquid form that the maggots can ingest, leaving only the healthy tissue (Thomas, 2001).
- Enzymatic debridement also ensures autolysis through the use of enzymes such as elastase, collagenase and fibrinolysin. These enzymes cleave through the collagen holding necrotic tissue to the wound bed, thus debriding the

---

Box 3.1   The TIME framework (based on Falanga, 2004).

T = Tissue management
I = Inflammation and infection control
M = Moisture balance
E = Epithelial (edge) advancement

Reproduced by kind permission of Radical Education Partnership.

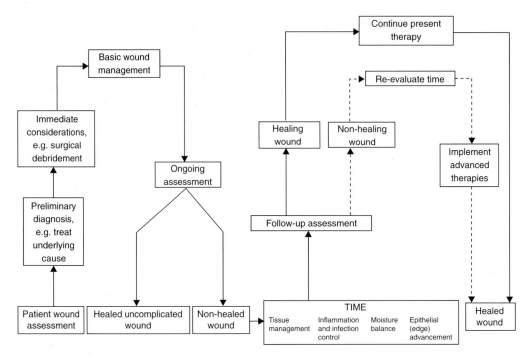

Fig. 3.10   Pathway showing how wound bed preparation is applied to practice (from Falanga 2004, reproduced by kind permission of Medical Education Partnership Ltd).

wound (Douglass, 2003). Although widely used in North America and mainland Europe, enzymes are rarely used in the UK.

- Mechanical debridement has been more popular in North America than elsewhere. Methods include wet-to-dry dressing, high-pressure wound irrigation and whirlpool baths. There is little evidence to support their use and they have the potential to cause harm. Wet-to-dry dressings are saline-soaked gauze swabs that are allowed to dry out and stick to the wound. They lift off slough and eschar when removed but also cause pain to the patient and may damage newly formed tissue. High-pressure irrigation can actually drive bacteria deeper into a wound rather than washing it off. Whirlpool footbaths can potentially spread infection elsewhere on the foot and may be difficult to decontaminate between patients (Schultz *et al.*, 2003).
- Sharp or surgical debridement is the fastest method. It is of particular benefit when managing diabetic foot ulcers in preventing the build-up of callus. However, it is not suitable for all situations. As there is potential for harm, such as excessive bleeding, it should be undertaken by a competent, trained professional (Fairbairn *et al.*, 2002).

Inflammation and infection control

Chronic wounds are always colonised with bacteria but if the numbers increase this may ultimately result in infection. Sibbald (2001) described the importance of maintaining a bacterial balance where the wound may be contaminated or colonised but this does not impact on healing. He also discussed the issue of deep and superficial infections. If healing does not result from topical therapy, systemic antibiotics may be necessary, especially if a deep infection is present. Schultz *et al.* (2003) emphasise the importance of debridement as it can reduce the bacterial burden by removing devitalised tissue, which is a focus for bacteria, and creating a more active wound. Using maggots for debridement is particularly useful, as they have been found to ingest and destroy bacteria, including MRSA (Thomas, 2001). Topical antiseptics such as slow-release silver and iodine have been shown to be beneficial but should only be used for two weeks (Edmonds *et al.*, 2004; Moffatt *et al.*, 2004). Topical antibiotics are not recommended because of the risk of bacterial resistance.

Moisture balance

A major criticism of the moist wound-healing theory is that there is no information about what constitutes the correct level of moisture on the wound surface. Wounds can produce widely varying quantities of exudate. Heavily exuding wounds may cause maceration of the surrounding skin as well as soggy dressings and a very distressed patient. On the other hand, wounds with little or no exudate may become dessicated. A balance between the two is required. Moisture balance in the presence of heavy exudate can be achieved in a variety of ways.

- Use of highly absorbent dressings. There are a number of highly absorbent dressings available and selection depends on the type, position and size of the wound and the wound bed status. Alginates, foams and hydrofibre dressings are widely used; they absorb exudate and may also have moisture vapour transmission capability. Capillary action dressings are multilayered and able to conduct exudate away from the wound surface.
- The use of appliances such as 'bag systems'. This may be by means of a stoma bag or a specialist wound appliance. These systems are useful in wounds that constantly seep but they only contain the problem, rather than solving it. However, they may be more effective and comfortable for the patient than bulky dressings that frequently leak (Vowden & Vowden, 2003).
- Compression is an effective method of controlling wound exudate in leg ulceration as compression reduces chronic venous hypertension. It can be achieved by the use of compression bandages or by intermittent compression therapy. This treatment is limited to leg ulcers where there is a venous component and will be discussed further in Chapter 5.
- Topical negative pressure therapy (TNP) is increasingly being applied to heavily exuding wounds of all types. It has also been suggested that use of TNP can reduce the bacterial burden of a wound (Morykwas *et al.*, 1997).

Whatever method of moisture balance is used, it is important to care for the skin surrounding the wound. Excessive moisture can cause maceration or irritant dermatitis (Cutting & White, 2002). Various strategies may be used, depending on the method used to manage the exudate. Creams containing zinc provide an effective barrier and are frequently used with heavily exuding leg ulcers. They are soothing to macerated skin but would be inappropriate where adhesive strapping is used close to the wound margin, such as with TNP. Skin sealants are particularly useful under adhesive dressings as they protect the skin from the adhesives as well as the exudate. Another strategy is to use a hydrocolloid dressing, first cutting a hole the shape of the wound in the dressing wafer and then applying it as a border around the wound, as is used in biosurgery.

Epithelial (edge) advancement

A healing wound not only has a wound bed filled with healthy granulating tissue but also evidence of epithelialisation at the wound margins. For many wounds, achieving debridement of necrosis and slough and bacterial and moisture balance will stimulate the wound to heal. However, Falanga (2004) suggests that the problems of impaired MMP metabolism or cell senescence (discussed in Chapter 1) may prevent this last phase of healing, although there is need for more research in this area. As shown in Figure 3.10, this may be the time to re-evaluate the wound and to consider the implementation of advanced therapies such as growth factors or tissue-engineered products (Schultz *et al.*, 2003).

Comment

Both these theories of wound management have moved our understanding forward. It is too simplistic to suggest that moist wound-healing theory should be used for the management of acute wounds and WBP for chronic wounds. Nurses should have an understanding of the underlying principles of both concepts and utilise them appropriately following a comprehensive patient and wound assessment.

3.3.3 Pain management

As discussed in section 3.2.7, pain management is often neglected in wound care. Accurate assessment will determine the type and intensity of pain, allowing appropriate strategies to be developed. Senecal (1999) proposed incremental steps to determine suitable analgesia and stressed the importance of regular administration. However, many patients are reluctant to take regular analgesia and may need to be encouraged to do so. Latarjet (2002) discussed the difference between background pain and procedural pain in burn patients. He considered that it is possible to achieve zero background pain but this is difficult during dressing changes. If additional medication is given before dressing changes, sufficient time must be allowed for the analgesia to take effect. If pain is not controlled, it may be useful to involve the pain team.

Briggs and Torra i Bou (2002) discussed additional strategies to reduce pain. They emphasise the importance of reducing anxiety and spending time explaining to the patient what will happen and the level of pain to expect. It is also important to select appropriate dressings that will maintain moisture balance and minimise pain and trauma on removal. If dressings have adhered to the wound, then it may be necessary to soak them off. If dressings persistently adhere to the wound, an alternative dressing should be considered.

3.4 DOCUMENTATION

In order to judge the progress of a wound, it is essential to keep accurate records. Good documentation will help to ensure continuity of care. Poor documentation has been implicated in frequent alterations of dressing type, according to the whim of individual nurses, as shown in a study by Rundgren *et al.* (1990). They followed the progress of 101 patients with a variety of wounds over a five-month period. They found that from week to week about 30% of the patients were receiving a different treatment; 65% of the wounds did not heal and were having treatment for the whole of the study period. They concluded that this lack of continuity was related to poor documentation, impatience and a lack of understanding of the healing process.

The European Tissue Repair Society (ETRS) has produced several statements in relation to wound management, including one on documentation (ETRS, 2003). This statement is given in full below.

- Adequate and accurate documentation of all patients with wounds should take place. This should include core information with additional information recorded depending on wound type.
- Core information should be recorded at least monthly and include:
  a) Wound size by:
     i)   Tracing.
     ii) Measurement.
     iii) Photography.
  b) Wound bed colour (black, green, yellow, pink, red)
     i) Percentage of wound bed.
     ii) Photography.
  c) Wound depth, using grading scale of initial assessment and detailing tissue at wound base
  d) Surrounding skin:
     i) Healthy.
     ii) Unhealthy.
  e) Exudate – composition and volume:
     i)   Nil.
     ii) Normal.
     iii) Excessive.
  f) Pain – continuous/dressing change/occasional

g) An evaluation of treatment effect with the outcome graded as wound:
   i)   Healing.
   ii) Static.
   iii) Deteriorating.
h) The reason for non-healing indicated, e.g. infection, and the reason for treatment changes documented

3.5 EVALUATING THE DRESSING

Nurses should be prepared to objectively evaluate the dressings they use, particularly if they are using new dressings, although traditional dressings should not be exempt from evaluation. When evaluating a dressing, various aspects need to be considered.

- Patient comfort.
- Ease of application.
- Effectiveness.
- Cost.

Patient comfort is of primary importance for any wound management product. It can be very distressing for a patient when the application of a dressing is painful. Eusol is a well-known example of a lotion which causes pain on application (see Chapter 4).

Other products may adhere to the wound and cause discomfort to patients when they move and pain when the dressing is removed. A dressing that fails to provide sufficient absorbency and allows leakage of exudate can cause considerable inconvenience, as well as promoting feelings of insecurity in the patient. Although different nurses may carry out the dressing, the patient is always present. Any evaluation should involve the patient. Many like to take an interest and can provide valuable information on new products.

Ease of application means that a dressing can be applied easily and so will stay in place. When using any new product, it may take a little practice to develop the most effective method of application. The nurse should be prepared to try a dressing over a period of time on a variety of wounds (unless contraindicated) and on different parts of the body. This will allow a more comprehensive evaluation.

Effectiveness is most important. If a product does not promote healing, then it does not matter if it is comfortable or easy to apply. Before a product becomes available for general use, it should have undergone stringent laboratory tests to check for safety. The ETRS (2003) has developed standards for clinical trials in wound healing that can guide the development of study protocols. Nurses may find particular difficulties in undertaking a clinical trial. Hunt (1983) suggested that these included a lack of control over the admission and discharge of patients, staffing patterns, the large numbers of nurses involved in patient care and the variations in patterns of care across healthcare providers. If nurses are to evaluate the effectiveness of any dressing they use, they need to be aware of any research that has been published and any relevant systematic reviews. This will be discussed further in Chapter 7.

Cost is an important factor in all aspects of care and should be considered when evaluating any dressing. However, not only the unit cost is relevant. The overall costs should be considered. One example is a study by Thomas and Tucker (1989) who compared the use of paraffin tulle and an alginate (Sorbsan™) and found a reduced overall cost using Sorbsan™, despite the fact that the unit cost is greater than that of tulle.

REFERENCES

Briggs, M., Torra i Bou, J.E. (2002) Pain at wound dressing changes: a guide to management, in European Wound Management Association (EWMA) Position Document, *Pain at Wound Dressing Changes*. MEP Ltd, London.

Brown, G.S. (2000) Reporting outcomes for stage IV pressure ulcer healing: a proposal. *Advances in Skin and Wound Management*, **13** (6), 277–283.

Browne, N., Grocott, P., Cowley, S. *et al.* (2004a) The TELER system in wound care research and post market surveillance. *EWMA Journal*, **4** (1), 26–32.

Browne, N., Grocott, P., Cowley, S. *et al.* (2004b) Woundcare research for appropriate products (WRAP) validation of the TELER method involving users. *International Journal of Nursing Studies*, **41**, 559–571.

Cutting, K. (1998) Identification of infection in granulating wounds by registered nurses. *Journal of Clinical Nursing*, **7**, 539–546.

Cutting, K., Harding, K.G. (1994) Criteria for identifying wound infection. *Journal of Wound Care*, **3** (4), 198–201.

Cutting, K., White, T. (2002) Maceration of the skin and wound bed. 1 Its nature and causes. *Journal of Wound Care*, **11** (7), 275–278.

Douglass, J. (2003) Wound bed preparation: a systematic approach to chronic wounds. *British Journal of Community Nursing*, **8** (6) (suppl), S26–S34.

Eaglstein, W.H. (1985) Experiences with biosynthetic dressings. *Journal of the American Academy of Dermatology*, **12**, 434–440.

Edmonds, M., Foster, A.V.M., Vowden, P. (2004) Wound bed preparation for diabetic foot ulcers, in European Wound Management Association (EWMA) Position Document, *Wound Bed Preparation in Practice*. MEP Ltd, London.

European Tissue Repair Society (ETRS) (2003) ETRS Working Group Statements. *ETRS Bulletin*, **10** (2&3), 10–13.

Fairbairn, K., Grier, J., Hunter, C., Preece, J. (2002) A sharp debridement procedure devised by specialist nurses. *Journal of Wound Care*, **11** (10), 371–375.

Falanga, V. (2000) Classification for wound bed preparation and stimulation of chronic wounds. *Wound Repair and Regeneration*, **8** (5), 347–352.

Falanga, V. (2004) Wound bed preparation: science applied to practice, in European Wound Management Association (EWMA) Position Document, *Wound Bed Preparation in Practice*. MEP Ltd, London.

Flanagan, M. (2003a) Improving accuracy of wound measurement in clinical practice. *Ostomy and Wound Management*, **49** (10), 28–40.

Flanagan, M. (2003b) Wound measurement: can it help us monitor progression to healing? *Journal of Wound Care*, **12** (5), 189–194.

Fowler, E. (1990) Chronic wounds: an overview, in (ed.) Krasner, D., *Chronic Wound Care: a clinical sourcebook for healthcare professionals*. Health Management Publications Inc., King of Prussia, PA.

Freidman, S., Su, D.W.P. (1983) Hydrocolloid occlusive dressing management of leg ulcers. *Archives of Dermatology*, **120**, 1329–1331.

Galdino, G.M., Swier, P., Manson, P.N., Vander Kolk, C.A. (2000) Converting to digital photography: a model for a large group or academic practice. *Plastic and Reconstructive Surgery*, **106** (1), 119–124.

Gardener, S.E., Frantz, R.A., Troia, C. *et al.* (2001a) A tool to assess clinical signs and symptoms of localised infection in chronic wounds: development and reliability. *Ostomy and Wound Management*, **47** (1), 40–47.

Gardener, S.E., Frantz, R.A., Doebbeling, B.N. (2001b) The validity of the clinical signs and symptoms used to identify localised chronic wound infection. *Wound Repair and Regeneration*, **9** (3), 178–186.

Goldman, R.J., Salcido, R. (2002) More than one way to measure a wound: an overview of tools and techniques. *Advances in Skin and Wound Care*, **15** (5), 236–243.

Hack, A. (2003) Malodorous wounds – taking the patient's perspective into account. *Journal of Wound Care*, **12** (8), 319–321.

Harding, K.G. (1990) Wound care: putting theory into practice, in (ed.) Krasner, D., *Chronic Wound Care: a clinical sourcebook for healthcare professionals*. Health Management Publications Inc., King of Prussia, PA.

Harding, K.G. (1992) The wound-healing matrix. *Journal of Wound Care*, **1** (3), 40–44.

Hayes, S., Dodds, S. (2003) Digital photography in wound care. *Nursing Times*, **99** (42) (Wound Care Suppl), 2–3.

Houghton, P.E., Kincaid, C.B., Campbell, K.E., Woodbury, M.G., Keast, D.H. (2000) Photographic assessment of the appearance of chronic pressure and leg ulcers. *Ostomy and Wound Management*, **46** (4), 20–30.

Hunt, J. (1983) Product evaluation. *Nursing*, **2** (12) (suppl), 6–7.

Kantor, J., Margolis, D.J. (1998) Efficacy and prognostic value of simple wound measurements. *Archives of Dermatology*, **134** (12), 1571–1574.

Kantor, J., Margolis, D.J. (2000) A multicentre study of percentage change in venous leg ulcer area as a prognostic index of healing at 24 weeks. *British Journal of Dermatology*, **142** (5), 960–964.

Kaufman, C., Hirshowitz, B. (1983) Treatment of chronic leg ulcers with Opsite. *Chirurgica Plastica*, **7**, 211–215.

Keast, D.H., Bowering, C.K., Evans, A.W., Mackean, G.L., Burrows, C., D'Souza, L. (2004) MEASURE: a proposed framework for developing best practice recommendations for wound assessment. *Wound Repair and Regeneration*, **12** (3) (suppl), S1–S17.

Kokoska, M.S., Currens, J.W., Hollenbeak, C.S., Thomas, J.R., Stack, B.C. (1999) Digital vs 35-mm Photography: to convert or not to convert? *Archives of Facial Plastic Surgery*, **1** (4), 276–281.

Krasner, D. (1995) The chronic wound pain experience: a conceptual model. *Ostomy and Wound Management*, **41**, 20–25.

Lagan, K.M., Dusoir, A.E., McDonough, S.M., Baxter, G.D. (2000) Wound measurement: the comparative reliability of direct versus photographic tracings analysed by planimetry versus digitising techniques. *Archives of Physical Medicine and Rehabilitation*, **81** (8), 1110–1116.

Latarjet, J. (2002) The management of pain associated with dressing changes in patients with burns. *EWMA Journal*, **2** (2), 5–9.

Le Roux, A.A. (1993) TELER: the concept. *Physiotherapy*, **79** (11), 755–758.

Lucas, C., Classen, J., Harrison, D., De, H. (2002) Pressure ulcer surface area measurement using instant full-scale photography and transparency tracings. *Advances in Skin and Wound Care*, **15** (1), 17–23.

May, S.R. (1984) Physiology, immunology and clinical efficacy of an adherent polyurethane wound dressing Opsite, in (ed.) Wise, D.L., *Burn Wound Coverings*, Vol.II. CRC Press, Boca Raton, FL.

Moffatt, C.J. (2002) Pain at wound dressing changes, in European Wound Management Association (EWMA) Position Document, *Pain at Wound Dressing Changes*. MEP Ltd, London.

Moffatt, C.J., Franks, P.J., Hollinworth, H. (2002) Understanding wound pain and trauma: an international perspective, in European Wound Management Association (EWMA) Position Document, *Pain at Wound Dressing Changes*. MEP Ltd, London.

Moffatt, C., Morison, M.J., Pina, E. (2004) Wound bed preparation for venous leg ulcers, in European Wound Management Association (EWMA) Position Document, *Wound Bed Preparation in Practice*. MEP Ltd, London.

Morykwas, M.J., Argenta, L.C., Shelton-Brown, E.I., McGuirt, W. (1997) Vacuum-assisted closure: a new method for wound control and treatment: animal studies and basic foundation. *Annals of Plastic Surgery*, **38** (6), 553–562.

Nagy, S. (1999) Strategies used by burn nurses to cope with the infliction of pain on patients. *Journal of Advanced Nursing*, **29** (6), 1427–1433.

Nechala, P., Mahoney, J., Farkas, L.G. (1999) Digital two-dimensional photogrammetry: a comparison of three techniques of obtaining digital photographs. *Plastic and Reconstructive Surgery*, **103** (7), 1819–1825.

Romanelli, M. (1997) Objective measurement of venous ulcer debridement and granulation with a skin colour reflectance analyser. *Wounds*, **9** (4), 122–126.

Rundgren, A., Nordehammar, A., Bjornestol, A., Magnusson, H., Nelson, C. (1990) Pressure sores in hospitalised geriatric patients. Background factors, treatment, long-term follow-up. *Care – Science and Practice*, **8** (3), 100–103.

Schultz, G.S., Sibbald, R.G., Falanga, V. *et al.* (2003) Wound bed preparation: a systematic approach to wound management. *Wound Repair and Regeneration*, **11** (2) (suppl), S1–S28.

Senecal, S. (1999) Pain management of wound care. *Nursing Clinics of North America*, **34** (4), 847–860.

Sibbald, R.G. (2001) What is the bacterial burden of the wound bed and does it matter? in (eds) Cherry, G.W., Harding, K.G., Ryan, T.J., *Wound Bed Preparation*. Royal Society of Medicine Press, London.

Szor, J.K., Bourguignon, C. (1999) Description of pressure ulcer pain at rest and at dressing change. *Journal of Wound, Ostomy and Continence Nursing*, **26** (3), 115–120.

Taal, L.A., Faber, A.W., van Loey, N.E.E., Reynders, C.L.L., Hofland, H.W.C. (1999) The abbreviated burn specific pain anxiety scale: a multicentre study. *Burns*, **25**, 493–497.

Thawer, H.A., Houghton, P.E., Woodbury, G., Keast, D., Campbell, K. (2002) A comparison of computer-assisted and manual wound size measurement. *Ostomy and Wound Management*, **48**, 46–53.

Thomas, S. (2001) Sterile maggots and the preparation of the wound bed, in (eds) Cherry G.W., Harding K.G., Ryan T.J., *Wound Bed Preparation*. Royal Society of Medicine Press, London.

Thomas, S., Tucker, C.A. (1989) Sorbsan in the management of leg ulcers. *Pharmaceutical Journal*, **243**, 706–709.

Vowden, K., Vowden, P. (2003) Understanding exudate management and the role of exudate in the healing process. *British Journal of Nursing*, **12** (20) (suppl), 4–13.

Winter, G.D. (1962) Formation of the scab and the rate of epithelialisation of superficial wounds in the skin of the domestic pig. *Nature*, **193**, 293.

Chapter 4
Wound Management Products

4.1 INTRODUCTION

There are many wound management products available and much conflicting advice on how they should be used. Many nurses have a great interest in this subject and take a justifiable pride in the acquired skills that facilitate dressing change. Recent developments have demonstrated a need to change or adapt traditional practices.

Wound management products include topical agents as well as dressings and also what have been described as 'advanced dressings'. A topical agent is one which is applied to a wound. A dressing is a covering on a wound that is intended to promote healing and protect from further injury. Advanced products are much more sophisticated dressings compared to those in everyday practice. The Department of Health divides dressings into primary and secondary. A primary dressing is that which is used in direct contact with the wound. A secondary dressing is superimposed over the primary dressing. The use of all these products will be discussed in this chapter.

4.2 THE DEVELOPMENT OF DRESSINGS THROUGH THE AGES

In *L'Ingenue* (1767) Voltaire described history as a 'tableau of crimes and misfortunes'. A study of the dressings used through the ages suggests that there may be some truth in this. Some of the treatments used on the wounded were bizarre, if not horrific, whilst others are still familiar today.

4.2.1 Early days

The earliest record of any dressing can be found on the Edwin Smith Papyrus. Edwin Smith was an American Egyptologist who bought the papyrus from a trader in Luxor in 1862. He was unable to translate it and its contents were unknown until a complete translation was published in 1930 (Zimmerman & Veith, 1961). The papyrus is dated at around 1700 BC but it is a copy of original manuscripts that date back to around 3000–2500 BC. A variety of dressings are mentioned including grease, honey, lint and fresh meat, which was valued for its haemostatic properties. Adhesive strapping was made by applying gum to strips of linen (Forrest, 1982).

As the power of Ancient Egypt waned, the Greek civilisation gradually developed. Amongst the men who made their mark at this time was Hippocrates. He lived from about 460 to 377 BC. Hippocrates laid the basis for scientific medicine with his emphasis on careful observation. For the most part, Hippocrates considered that wounds should be kept clean and dry. He recommended tepid water, wine and vinegar for cleansing wounds. If a wound showed signs of inflammation, he suggested applying a cataplasm or poultice to the area around the wound to soften the tissues and to allow free drainage of pus (Zimmerman & Veith, 1961). Hippocrates also used propolis, a hard resinous material produced by bees, to help in the healing of sores and ulcers (Trevelyn, 1997). Hippocrates gave the first definition of healing by first intention, where the skin edges are held in approximation to each other, and secondary intention where there is tissue loss and the skin edges are far apart.

Some of these concepts can also be found in the writings of Sushruta, an Indian surgeon who lived some time between the sixth century BC and the sixth century AD. His surgical textbook, the 'Sushruta Samhita', was used as a basis by later writers. Sushruta described 14 different types of dressings made from silk, linen, wool and cotton (Zimmerman & Veith, 1961). He also placed great emphasis on the importance of cleanliness. Meade (1968) describes Sushruta's recommendations for the management of wounds involving the intestines. First black ants were applied and then the intestines were washed in milk and lubricated with clarified butter before they were returned to their normal position. He differed from Hippocrates on the matter of the most appropriate diet for patients. Sushruta considered meat, normally forbidden to Hindus, an important factor whereas Hippocrates recommended the restriction of food and gave his patients only water to drink (Zimmerman & Veith, 1961).

The influence of Greek physicians continued on into the time of the Roman Empire. Oil and wine were commonly applied to wounds. Reference to this was made by the Gospel writer Luke, when he was recording the parable of the Good Samaritan (Luke, Ch.10, v.34, New Testament). Luke describes the Good Samaritan pouring oil and wine onto the wounds and then applying bandages.

Celsus compiled a history of the development of medicine from the time of Hippocrates to the first century AD, with great detail of the practices of his time. Although it is believed that Celsus was not a physician, he was the first to give a definition of inflammation. He listed the cardinal signs as redness, heat, pain and swelling. He advocated the cleansing of wounds to remove foreign bodies before suturing. He also expected wounds to suppurate; that is, to form pus (Meade, 1968). A Roman scholar, Pliny, described the use of propolis to soften induration and reduce swelling. He also wrote that it healed sores when healing seemed impossible (Trevelyn, 1997).

It is, however, Galen who stands out as the person whose work had lasting impact. Galen (129–199 AD) was surgeon to the gladiators in Pergamun and later physician to the Emperor Marcus Aurelius. He wrote many books, some of which survived him and were seen as the ultimate in medical knowledge for many centuries. He is particularly known for his theory of 'laudable pus' (*pus bonum et laudabile*), which holds that the development of pus is necessary for healing and should, therefore, actively be promoted. Galen found the application of writing ink, cobwebs and Lemnian clay to wounds to be efficacious (Forrest, 1982). When reviewing his achievements, Duin and Sutcliffe (1992) considered that although in some ways Galen considerably expanded medical knowledge, he also held it back for a thousand years.

4.2.2 The Dark Ages and early Middle Ages

After the fall of the Roman Empire, cultural influence moved eastwards and the Arab doctors of Islam further developed medical knowledge. However, their wound care was based on Galenic teaching. A number of doctors, such as Rhazes and Albucassis, translated Galen's writings into Arabic but the most famous was Ali Ibn Al-Husain-al-Sina (980–1037), also known as Avicenna to the Western world. Avicenna wrote the *Canon Medicina*, translating Galen's work and adding his own commentary (Dealey, 2002). Ultimately it was translated into both Hebrew and Latin and became the foremost medical textbook in the Middle East, North Africa and Europe up until the seventeenth century (Guthrie, 1945). Avicenna proposed treating pressure ulcers with white lead ointment, covering the bed with salix leaves and preventing the patient from sleeping on his back (Kanal, 1975). He also advised the use of astringents such as cooked honey and myrrh to reduce the amount of exudate in wounds with tissue loss.

Medical knowledge swept across the Middle East, through North Africa and into Spain and southern Italy with the spread of Islam and the Islamic Empire. Thus the teaching of the Arab doctors influenced many of the developments in Europe, including reinforcing the pre-eminence of Galen. It must also be recognised that during this time the Church supplied most of the healthcare provision outside the home, resulting in the Church having control over many aspects of medicine, such as giving support to Galenic teaching.

Salerno in southern Italy was the first European university to have a medical school, which was founded in the ninth century (Forrest, 1982). Unlike most other universities of the time, Salerno was not under ecclesiastical control and so was able to incorporate surgery into the curriculum at a time when the clergy were prohibited from practising it (Zimmerman & Veith, 1961). Salerno was the leading centre for surgical training in the eleventh century and during this time the *Surgery of Roger* was written. It was translated into 15 other languages and was used up to the sixteenth century (Paterson, 1988). Roger advocated the use of lard in head wounds, either applied directly or soaking cloth in molten lard for deep wounds. He did not recommend cleaning wounds but used dressings made from eggs and water, tow and salt and bandages of fine linen cloth (Paterson, 1988).

One of the expert surgeons who graduated from Salerno was Hugo of Lucca (1160–1257). He went on to found the School of Surgery at Bologna University (Dealey, 2003). Although none of his writings have survived, he was considered to be a very innovative surgeon. His famous pupil, Theodoric (also known at Teodrico Borgognoni) (1205–1296?), completed his *Chirurgia* or surgical textbook in 1267, which he stated was based in Hugo's teaching. Theodoric disagreed with the concept of 'laudable pus' as he considered that it prolonged healing. He advocated cleaning a wound with wine, debriding it and removing all foreign matter, approximating the wound edges and holding them in place using compresses of lint soaked in warm wine and then binding them in place. The dressing was then to be left *in situ* for 5–6 days, unless there was excessive heat or pain (Borgognoni, 1955). He proposed that chronic wounds should be cleansed with honey mixed with wine and water of holm-oak or vine ashes; alternatively, sea water could be used to cleanse and dry a wound. Unfortunately, his ideas were discredited and gradually disappeared until the twentieth century when they were again discovered in Italy (Popp, 1995).

One of the people influenced by Theodoric's teaching was Henri de Mondeville (1260–1320). He was a French doctor who trained in Paris and Montpellier as a physician, before going to Bologna to learn surgery from Theodoric (Gerster, 1910). He was highly respected as a man of profound erudition and moral character and became surgeon to King Phillippe le Bel of France in 1301. De Mondeville also wrote a *Chirurgie*, which drew on the work of Avicenna for anatomy and Theodoric for wounds. Unfortunately, de Mondeville was not a tactful person and he commenced his treatise on wounds by first describing and then condemning the common practices of the day that promoted 'laudable pus'. Unsurprisingly, he failed to influence his contemporaries who tried to put pressure on him to abandon his treatment (Dealey, 2004).

A close successor to de Mondeville was Guy de Chauliac (1300–1368). He followed a similar pattern to de Mondeville, training in Toulouse, Montpellier and Paris before travelling to Bologna to study anatomy (Johnson, 1989). It was when de Chauliac was in Bologna that he became strongly influenced by Galen's writing. This is reflected in his *Grande Chirurgie* in which he quoted Galen 890 times (Johnson, 1989). When writing about wound care, he rejected the ideas of Theodoric and de Mondeville and proposed treatments such as the use of tents (drains) and meshes (packing) to hold wounds open and oily salves to promote pus formation. De Chauliac's book was highly successful, having numerous editions and translations, and it became the primary surgical textbook for 200 years. He had so great an influence that his critics consider that he set back progress in wound management for up to six centuries, although not every commentator takes such a harsh view (Johnson, 1989).

4.2.3 Late Middle Ages and Renaissance

Kirkpatrick and Naylor (1997) have described the contents of a surgical treatise dated 1446 and believed to be the work of Thomas Morstede (1380–1450) who was a London surgeon. The work provides detailed information about the classification of ulcers and their treatment. The step-by-step approach describes how to enlarge the mouth of the ulcer, then the processes of mortification (debridement), mundification (cleansing) and fleshing (encouragement of granulation tissue). Recipes for the various topical applications are provided for the reader. They include items such as sage leaves, wormwood, white

Gascony wine, alum and honey for mundification. The recipe for a treatment for fleshing involved stirring the mixture for the length of time it took to say two Creeds (articles of belief for Christian faith).

Ambroise Paré (1510–1590) was the most famous surgeon of the Renaissance period (Zimmerman & Veith, 1961). He rose from a poor background with little education to become surgeon to four successive French kings, ultimately gaining the titles Premier Chirurgien and Conseiller du Roi. However, it is as a military surgeon that Paré is best known. With the discovery of gunpowder, warfare changed. Gunshot wounds were believed to be poisonous. In order to treat them, surgeons began to undertake more amputation of limbs. The standard practice was to use boiling oil to cauterise the stump. Paré is famous for using a mixture of egg yolks, oil of roses and turpentine instead. He is also well known for his saying 'Je le pensait, Dieu le guarist', which is generally translated as 'I dressed him, God healed him' (Zimmerman & Veith, 1961). Paré proposed using a dressing composed of rock alum, verdigris, Roman vitriol, rose honey and vinegar, boiled together to form a paste, on traumatic wounds (Linker & Womack, 1969). He treated a severe pressure ulcer by encouraging the patient, feeding him, providing pain relief and sleep-inducing medication and pressure relief by means of a small pillow (Levine, 1992). Paré wrote numerous books, all in the vernacular rather than Latin. Some of his later writings are considered to be classics.

4.2.4 The seventeenth, eighteenth and early nineteenth centuries

Another doctor worthy of mention is the German surgeon Lorenz Heister (1683–1758). Heister was exceedingly well educated in languages and the humanities as well as medicine and surgery at a time when most of his colleagues had little education or training and charlatans abounded (Zimmerman & Veith, 1961). He developed his skills working as a military surgeon and became a professor of anatomy and surgery at the University of Helmstadt in 1719. He wrote a *General System of Surgery* in three parts on the doctrine and management of: I) Wounds of all kinds, II) Several operations, and III) Bandages (Heister, 1768). Heister used lint dressings dipped in alcohol or oil of turpentine to treat haemorrhage or spread with a sound digestive ointment or balsam to heal wounds. He suggested that wound edges should not be closed, in order to allow pus to drain. He believed that all bandages should be made from clean linen that had been softened by repeated use (Bishop, 1959). His book was translated into numerous languages, including English, and ran to ten editions.

Many of the developments in wound management seem to be associated with wounds from battles. One development was that of debridement, possibly originated by Henri Francois LeDran (1685–1770) in order to relieve the constriction of soft tissues, believed to be caused by inflammation following gunshot wounds (Helling & Daon, 1998). However, other surgeons across Europe suggested caution in its use. John Hunter (1728–1793), the famous English surgeon, disagreed with the practice as he did not believe that wounds should be made larger in order to remove extraneous matter. He thought that suppuration would bring it to the surface (Zimmerman & Veith, 1961). During the Napoleonic wars, several French surgeons advocated the use of debridement, particularly in the care of gunshot wounds (Helling & Daon, 1998). However, its use was sporadic and most wounds were not explored and after the fall of Napoleon and his empire, the concept was almost entirely forgotten.

4.2.5 Mid-nineteenth and early twentieth century developments

The Crimean War led to a huge demand for dressings. Various types of dressings were produced in the workhouses, which were a source of cheap labour. Charpie was made from unravelled cloth. Oakum was old rope which had been unpicked and teased into fluff; it became popular with doctors during the American Civil War as they considered it to be very absorbent (Bishop, 1959). Tow was made from broken, ravelled flax fibres. Lint is linen that has been scraped on one side. The production of this dressing was mechanised. All of these dressings were washed and reused many times so they gradually became quite soft but they were not very absorbent.

Sheets of cotton wool retained by cotton bandages were used during the Franco-Prussian wars, but Joseph Sampson Gamgee (1828–1886) was the person who further developed its use. He noted that cotton wool could be made absorbent by removing the oily matter within it. He then conceived the idea of covering the cotton wool with unbleached gauze to make dressing pads or Gamgee tissue (Lawrence, 1987). Gamgee tissue is still available today.

In 1867, Lister introduced the use of carbolic acid and revolutionised surgery and surgical wound management. When he realised that carbolic caused skin irritation, he developed a method of impregnated carbolic gauze that became the first antiseptic dressing (Bishop, 1959). The use of antiseptics and concept of asepsis spread rapidly across Europe.

During the course of the First World War, severely wounded soldiers had to wait several days before receiving more than a simple field dressing. As a result, many wounds became infected and gangrenous. Antiseptics were developed to help resolve this problem. In particular, two similar antiseptic solutions came into use: Eusol (Edinburgh University Solution of Lime) and Dakin's solution. Other antiseptics such as iodine, carbolic acid and mercury and aluminium chloride were also available.

Sinclair and Ryan (1993) have reviewed some of the medical literature of 1915 to identify thinking at that time on the use of antiseptics. Bond (1915) considered that it was important to apply a 'germicide' as early as possible to wounds that were almost certain to be infected. British soldiers were advised to carry tincture of iodine so that they could apply it immediately to any gunshot wounds (Mayo-Robson, 1915). However, Herzog (1915), writing of the German experience in the battlefield, reported that he had seen a number of soldiers suffering from dermatitis of the skin around the wound as a result of the indiscriminate use of iodine.

Deparge, a Belgian surgeon of note, recognised that merely introducing antiseptics into war wounds was insufficient and he revived the concept of wound debridement (Helling & Daon, 1998). He believed that such devastating wounds, often covered in mud and dirt and receiving only minimal surgery, encouraged the development of soft tissue infections. He formulated a set of principles for managing them that involved exploring the wound and excision of all contaminated and contused tissue, followed by leaving the wound open and irrigating it with Dakin's solution. He also favoured the use of delayed primary closure or secondary closure if bacteria were present. Deparge's use of debridement has had a major impact on trauma surgery (Helling & Daon, 1998).

At this time, Lumiere devised a dressing called tulle gras, a gauze impregnated with paraffin. Sphagnum moss was also used as it was found to be twice as absorbent as cotton wool. It could also be impregnated with antiseptics and sterilised. Eupad was a dressing designed for use on leg ulcers. It was a Eusol preparation, made up with a mixture of boracic and bleach. Another popular type of dressing was Emplastrums which were made of white leather spread with a plaster mass, to which some type of medication was often added (Turner, 1986).

During the Second World War an American neurosurgeon called Eldridge Campbell was with a field hospital in Italy. In 1943 there was a great deal of heavy fighting and many casualties. Some of the Italian doctors caring for these patients proposed a method of wound care that involved cleansing and debriding the wound and then suturing it. This was contrary to the current practice of the day, which recommended packing with Vaseline gauze and immobilisation. Campbell was impressed by this method of healing and eventually traced its origins back to the thirteenth century and Theodoric. In describing this fascinating piece of medical history, Popp (1995) concludes that it demonstrates the problems of entrenched views that are not questioned, such as the teachings of Galen, and the dangers of summarily dismissing new ideas.

4.2.6 The British Pharmaceutical Codices

The first British Pharmaceutical Codex was published in 1907. It provided information on all the drugs and medicinal preparations in common use throughout the British Empire. Turner (1986) has reviewed the dressings listed in the earliest British Pharmaceutical Codices and compared them with more recent lists of dressings in the British Pharmacopoeia. He found that the list from 1923 contains much that is familiar today. Table 4.1 compares the 1923 list with the 1980 list, showing that little had changed in the intervening years. Gauzes, cotton wool pads and bandages can be seen as very popular methods of wound care. Turner suggests that it is only in the last 30 years that any attempt has been made to design materials that are actually functional. Prior to that, dressings were made from materials that happened to come to hand.

Table 4.1   Comparison of surgical dressings 1923 and 1980.

1923		1980	
Gauzes, medicated and unmedicated	(23)	Gauze products	(11)
Cotton wools, medicated and unmedicated	(15)	Cotton wool pads (eye)	(1)
Tows, medicated and unmedicated	(14)	Dressing pads	(2)
Lints, medicated and unmedicated	(8)	Impregnated gauze	(3)
Gauze and cotton tissues	(2)	Gauze and cotton tissues	(2)
Jaconet, oiled silk, etc.	(4)	Ribbon gauze	(3)
Bandages	(9)	Bandages	(15)
Emplastrums	(32)	Adhesive pads	(2)
		Foams	(3)
		Contact layers	(2)
		Absorbent cotton	(2)
		Medicated bandages	(4)

Numbers in parentheses indicate number of different types available within each category.

4.3 TRADITIONAL TECHNIQUES

Today nurses expect to perform the vast majority of dressings, other than simple first aid treatments applied in the home or workplace. But this was not always the case. Originally, dressing changes were undertaken by doctors. Eventually, medical students, particularly on surgical wards, were trained to change dressings. By the 1930s, the task was given to experienced sisters and ultimately, it became a recognised nursing task.

During the 1930s and 1940s, as the care of wounds gradually came into the nursing domain, much mystique became attached to the subject. This was exaggerated with the development of an aseptic, usually non-touch, technique. Merchant (1988) has reviewed the literature on this subject and concluded that the procedure developed in the 1940s was still being used at the time she was writing, despite the change to a central sterile supply system. Most hospitals had changed to this system by the early 1970s.

In the early days, large water sterilisers were used for preparing the equipment for an aseptic procedure. One was usually found on every ward. It was the task of the night nurses to boil all the metal bowls, receivers and gallipots, ready for the morning dressing round. The dressings were packed in drums and sent to a central point for sterilising. It was left to the ward sister to choose what went into the drum. Commonly, gauze squares, cotton wool balls and wadding were used. In many hospitals nurses wore masks and gowns, a practice that gradually disappeared. Usually two nurses carried out the dressing, a clean nurse and a dirty nurse. Much attention was paid to the position of the equipment on top of the trolley and to the frequency and timing of handwashing.

All wounds were redressed once or twice daily. The wound was thoroughly cleaned using cotton wool balls and forceps. The method of wiping across the wound surface varied from hospital to hospital. The Hippocratic principle of keeping wounds clean and dry became adapted to 'allowing wounds to dry up'. Mostly gauze preparations were used but gradually all sorts of dubious practices crept in. There have been reports of Marmite, eggs and even toast used on wounds (Dobrzanski *et al.*, 1988; Johnson, 1987).

A wide variety of pharmaceutical preparations have also been applied without any recognition of the need for evidence-based care. Murray (1988) found that within her health authority, an amazing selection of pharmaceutical products were in use: 18 different cleansing agents, 53 substances left in contact with open wounds and 24 products used for packing wounds. Millward (1989) found 19 different substances being used on pressure ulcers within one hospital. Walsh and Ford (1989) have discussed the rituals in nursing, much of which can be applied to wound care. The common reasons for choosing a dressing could be listed as:

- We always do it that way here.
- Sister said so.
- I have used this dressing for the last 30 years, why should I change?

Many older nurses will have been trained to use these ritualistic methods. It is only recently that there has been a critical evaluation of these methods and changes made to a more evidence-based approach.

4.4 THE USE OF LOTIONS

A variety of lotions are used in wound care, primarily for wound cleansing. The aims of wound cleansing are to remove any foreign matter such as gravel or soil, to remove any loose surface debris such as necrotic tissue and to remove any remnants of the previous dressing. A study by Thomlinson (1987) considered the various ways in which swabs could be wiped across the wound surface. The results showed that the action of cleansing did not reduce the number of bacteria on the wound surface but simply redistributed them.

4.4.1 Antiseptics

After saline, the commonest type of lotion in use is an antiseptic. An antiseptic can be defined as a non-toxic disinfectant, which can be applied to skin or living tissues and has the ability to destroy vegetative compounds, such as bacteria, by preventing their growth. If antiseptics are simply used to wipe across the wound surface, they will have little effect. They need to be in contact with bacteria for about 20 minutes before they actually destroy them (Russell *et al.*, 1982). In some instances they can be applied in the form of soaks or incorporated into dressings, ointments or creams.

Research using experimental wounds in the animal model has demonstrated that antiseptics have toxic effects that need to be weighed against any advantages obtained from their use. In the late 1980s and early 1990s there was considerable debate about antiseptics and their widespread use dramatically reduced. Since the introduction of the concept of wound bed preparation (discussed in Chapter 3), antiseptics have made something of a comeback as they are seen to have a place in achieving bacterial balance (Schultz *et al.*, 2003).

Each of the common antiseptics will be listed in turn and their advantages and disadvantages discussed.

Cetrimide

Cetrimide is useful for its detergent properties, particularly for the initial cleansing of traumatic wounds or the removal of scabs and crusts in skin disease. It should not be used in contact with the eye. It is rapidly inactivated by organic material. Two dangers should be noted: it can cause skin irritation and sensitivity, and, it is very easy for it to become contaminated by bacteria, especially *Pseudomonas aeruginosa*. It is mostly only used in accident and emergency departments for initial cleansing of wounds rather than as a routine cleanser. It is available as a cream or as a lotion in combination with chlorhexidine. Morgan (1993) suggests that cetrimide should be used with caution in restricted circumstances rather than as a general cleanser.

Chlorhexidine

Chlorhexidine is used in a variety of aqueous formulations. It is effective against Gram-positive and Gram-negative organisms. Brennan *et al.* (1986) found that it has a low toxicity to living cells. Tatnall *et al.* (1990) undertook a similar study to identify the toxicity of several antiseptics when used on cultured keratinocytes (used for grafts). They found chlorhexidine to be the least toxic but considered that antiseptics should not be used over these graft sites. Kearney *et al.* (1988) found that chlorhexidine could maintain its antimicrobial levels for a period of time when impregnated into a dressing. However, its efficacy is rapidly diminished in the presence of organic material such as pus or blood (Reynolds, 1982). Mengistu *et al.* (1999) tested chlorhexidine in different strengths against a range of Gram-negative bacteria and found that a significant number were only inhibited by high concentrations of chlorhexidine. They concluded that it was more suitable for disinfection and hospital hygiene rather than wound care.

Hydrogen peroxide

Hydrogen peroxide 3% (10 vols) has an oxidising effect that destroys anaerobic bacteria. However, it loses its effect when it comes in contact with organic material such as pus or cotton gauze. Lineaweaver *et al.* (1985) showed that hydrogen peroxide was cytotoxic to fibroblasts unless diluted to a strength of 0.003%. This dilution is not effective against bacteria. O'Toole *et al.* (1996) found that even in concentrations 1000-fold less than 3% dilution, it inhibits keratinocyte migration and proliferation. Bennett *et al.* (2001) found that 3% hydrogen peroxide significantly reduced neodermal regeneration and fibroblast proliferation compared to controls (untreated wounds) in an animal model study. There is also a report of an incident where an air embolism occurred after irrigation with hydrogen peroxide (Sleigh & Linter, 1985). Rees (2003) reviewed the evidence on hydrogen peroxide and concluded that it was unsuitable for use in cleaning wounds in A&E. Hydrogen peroxide is no longer widely used as there is no evidence to demonstrate its efficacy and there are a number of other more suitable alternatives.

Iodine

Iodine is a broad-spectrum antiseptic and is available as an alcohol and an aqueous solution. The aqueous solution is used in wound care, usually as povidone iodine 10%, which contains 1% available iodine. It is used as a skin disinfectant and to clean grossly infected wounds. McLure and Gordon (1992) and Michel and Zach (1997) found it to be effective against methicillin-resistant *staphylococcus aureus*.

Several studies have questioned the value of using povidone iodine. It is cytotoxic to fibroblasts unless diluted to 0.001%, retards epithelialisation and lowers the tensile strength of the wound (Lineaweaver *et al.*, 1985). Brennan and Leaper (1985) found that povidone iodine 5% damaged the microcirculation of the healing wound but a 1% solution was innocuous. In contrast, Bennett *et al.* (2001) found that povidone iodine significantly increased fibroblast proliferation and slightly increased neodermal regeneration and epithelialisation. Becker (1986) reported that when operating on contaminated head and neck cases, he irrigated 18 with povidone iodine and 17 with isotonic saline; 28% of wounds became infected, all of which had been irrigated with povidone iodine.

Povidone iodine has been used within the wound bed preparation model of wound management. Consequently, Selvaggi *et al.* (2003) reviewed and reappraised the role of iodine and concluded that most of the evidence is confusing, especially as a mixture of *in vitro* and animal models have been used as well as different preparations. They conclude that povidone iodine has been shown to be an effective antibacterial that is superior to other products and seems to have no problem with resistance. Zhou *et al.* (2002) proposed that a slow-release form of iodine might overcome the toxicity problems. They tested cadexomer iodine using both *in vitro* methods and a variety of chronic wounds. They found no evidence of toxicity in the *in vitro* study. After 2–3 weeks of treatment, all 16 chronic wounds showed increased debridement, decreased exudate, increased granulation tissue and reduced wound size.

Povidone iodine is available in ointment, spray and powder form and impregnated into dressings. Iodine should not be used for patients with thyroid disease or those who are sensitive to the product.

Potassium permanganate

Potassium permanganate 0.01% is mostly used on heavily exuding eczematous skin conditions, generally associated with leg ulceration. It is most easily used in the form of tablets. One tablet dissolved in four litres of water provides a 0.01% solution. The affected limb is generally placed in a container holding the fluid for approximately 15 minutes. It is mildly deodorising and has slight disinfectant properties. It has been found to cause staining of the skin. There is little evidence to demonstrate its efficacy (Anderson, 2003).

Proflavine

Proflavine has a mild bacteriostatic effect on Gram-positive organisms but not on Gram-negative bacteria. There has been little research to demonstrate its value. Although it is available as a lotion it is mostly used as an aqueous cream. However, proflavine is not released from the cream into the wound so has no effect on the bacteria. Foster and Moore (1997) compared the use of proflavine-soaked gauze packs with cellulose-based fibre dressing in surgical cavity wounds. They found that the proflavine packs were significantly more painful to remove and patients required analgesia prior to removal.

Silver

Silver has been used as an antiseptic in wound care for many years in the form of silver nitrate. It is still used in this format in some burns units in North America. However, it is extremely caustic, stains the skin black and prolonged use causes hyponatraemia, hypokalaemia and hypocalcaemia. To overcome these problems, a cream, silver sulphadiazine, was developed and has been very successful in controlling burn wound infections (Lansdown, 2004). However, the combination of cream and exudate makes dressing removal messy so it is usually undertaken in a hydrotherapy unit, which can be a source of cross-infection (Tredget et al., 1998). As a result, there is increasing interest in the use of silver-coated dressings of varying types.

Wright et al. (1998a) tested the bactericidal effect of silver in three modalities: liquid (silver nitrate), cream (silver sulphadiazine) and a silver-coated dressing. All products were effective at killing bacteria. The silver-coated dressing was the most efficacious against a wider range of bacteria and silver nitrate the least efficacious. Tredget et al. (1998) compared a silver-coated dressing, changed daily, with the standard procedure of covering a burn with gauze and moistening it with 0.5% silver nitrate every two hours. They found that the silver-coated dressing caused significantly less pain on removal and had substantially less infection. Also, the wound only required attention every 24 hours and could have been left for 48 hours, reducing dressing and nursing time costs. Silver dressings will be discussed in more detail in section 4.6.

Sodium hypochlorite

Sodium hypochlorite comes in several forms, the commonest being Eusol, Dakin's solution and Milton. It was originally used on heavily infected wounds during the First World War. Dakin suggested that to be effective, it should be used in large volumes (Thomas, 1990).

Several research studies have been undertaken which suggest that the hypochlorites may have few beneficial effects and do much harm. Bloomfield and Sizer (1985) found they cause irritation to both the wound and the surrounding skin. They were found to have a cumulative effect, causing redness, pain and oedema, and to prolong the inflammatory stage of healing. They are cytotoxic to fibroblasts, unless diluted to a strength of 0.0005%, and retard epithelialisation (Lineaweaver *et al.*, 1985). Brennan and Leaper (1985) found that they caused considerable damage to the microcirculation of the wound. The antiseptic effect is lost when the solution comes in contact with organic material such as pus or gauze. A study describing the use of Eusol and liquid paraffin on leg ulcers was undertaken by Daltrey and Cunliffe (1981) who found no significant evidence of antibacterial activity. Bennett *et al.* (2001) found that half-strength sodium hypochlorate had a mixed effect on wound repair, with no impairment of fibroblast proliferation but decreased vascular density. However, at that strength it was ineffective as an antimicrobial.

Carneiro and Nyawawa (2003) randomly allocated Eusol or phenytoin powder to treat 102 leg ulcers. They found that there was a significant reduction in pain, exudate levels and wound size in the phenytoin group compared with the Eusol group. This study was undertaken in Tanzania and many of the ulcers were due to animal bites. These ulcers were found to heal fastest. The authors concluded that phenytoin was more suitable than Eusol, especially as it is cheap and easily applied.

Humzah *et al.* (1996) surveyed 124 plastic surgeons in the UK regarding their views on the use of Eusol. They had responses from 95 (77%) of the surgeons. Analysis of the responses found that 82% still used Eusol when it was available and the majority (88%) used it for sloughy wounds. Since this survey was undertaken, the use of Eusol has reduced even further. It is interesting to consider that where alternatives have replaced Eusol, its use has not been missed at all. Overall, Eusol is an outmoded product whose disadvantages far outweigh any slight advantage there may be in its use.

4.4.2 Antibiotics

A range of antibiotics is available in topical form. They are potentially hazardous and they are not always absorbed into the wound. There is considerable risk of sensitisation to the patient as well as the development of resistant organisms. Systemic antibiotics are the treatment of choice when treating infected wounds because the infection may be too deep for topical antibiotics to penetrate.

D'Arcy (1972) recommends that any antibiotic that is used systemically should not be applied to the skin. However, antibiotics that are not appropriate for systemic use may be developed for use on the skin or in wound care. This means that creams, gels, ointments or impregnated dressings containing gentamicin, tetracycline, fusidic acid or chlortetracycline hydrochloride should not be used as these antibiotics are used systemically. Neomycin is no longer used systemically but topical use may cause systemic side effects such as ototoxicity.

One preparation which would seem to be of benefit in wound care is mupirocin. Mupirocin is used predominantly for treating methicillin-resistant *Staphylococcus aureus* (MRSA) either in skin infections or for nasal colonisation. Several studies have demonstrated its efficacy in treating MRSA in burn wounds (Deng *et al.*, 1995; Rode *et al.*, 1989; Trilla & Miro,1995). However, Cookson (1998) warns of the potential dangers of resistance and cites a number of reported cases of mupirocin-resistant bacteria to support his arguments. He proposes that prolonged and widespread use of mupirocin should be stopped and a more judicious approach to its usage be adopted.

4.4.3 Honey

As was discussed earlier, honey has been used in wound care since ancient times and there has been a recent resurgence of interest in its use, particularly manuka honey (Flanagan, 2000). A review by Molan (1999) discussed the role of honey and considered that it had the following properties.

- Antibacterial action, as shown in laboratory studies and case studies, although, Kingsley (2001) did not find this in two case studies.
- Deodorising action, as demonstrated by Dunford and Hanano (2004) in a study of 40 patients with recalcitrant venous leg ulcers.
- Debriding action, as found by Ahmed *et al.* (2003).
- Anti-inflammatory action, as shown in histological studies.
- Stimulation of wound healing, as shown in several studies (Dunford & Hanano, 2004; Misirlioglu *et al.*, 2003; Subrahmanyam, 1998; Vandeputte & Van Waeyenberge, 2003;).
- Pain relief was not listed by Molan (1999) but was demonstrated by Dunford and Hanano in their study (Dunford & Hanano, 2004).

A systematic review by Moore *et al.* (2001) found that although honey appeared to be an effective treatment, many of the studies reviewed were of poor quality. There is a need for larger randomised controlled trials to determine the most effective use for honey. There is also an issue about frequency of dressing change, as Molan (1999) suggested that up to three times daily may be necessary initially. This is very labour intensive and may not be acceptable to the patient (Kingsley, 2001).

4.4.4 Saline 0.9%

This is the only completely safe cleansing agent and is the treatment of choice for use on most wounds. Manufacturers recommend that it is used in conjunction with many of the modern wound management products. Saline is presented in sachets, small plastic containers that allow the saline to be squirted onto the wound and also in aerosols. These last two presentations are more widely used in the community.

4.4.5 Tap water

Tap water is being used more frequently on a variety of wounds, in particular on areas already colonised such as wounds following rectal surgery or leg ulcers. Many patients may bath or shower prior to dressing change so there seems to be little point in then 'cleansing' the wound. However, the bath or shower should be thoroughly cleaned afterwards to avoid cross-infection. A recent systematic review found that using tap water to clean wounds did not differ from using sterile normal saline in respect of wound infection and healing rates (Fernandez *et al.*, 2002). This would therefore suggest that either saline or water can be used, selection being based on practicality and individual circumstances.

4.5 CLINICAL EFFECTIVENESS OF WOUND MANAGEMENT PRODUCTS

Originally dressings were seen merely as coverings that could provide some protection to the wound. The range of products currently available are much more sophisticated. There are so many products to choose from that it can cause considerable confusion. There is no single perfect dressing but an 'identikit' list of criteria can be established. A specific wound may not need all of the criteria listed. Selection can be assisted if the nurse has:

- assessed the wound and identified the specific objectives for the wound at that time.
- an understanding of what can be reasonably expected from a dressing.
- access to information regarding the characteristics and effectiveness of the range of dressings available.

The characteristics of a clinically effective wound management product are considered below. Dressings are generally considered in relation to their performance and their handling qualities. Performance relates to the ability to promote healing.

4.5.1 Providing an effective environment

The qualities that will promote an effective environment for healing were discussed in Chapter 3 under theories of wound management. They are:

- ability to maintain a moist environment.
- antibacterial properties.
- fluid-handling properties.

4.5.2 The handling qualities of an effective wound management product

These qualities can be listed as:

- easy to apply
- conformability
- easy to remove
- comfortable to 'wear'
- does not require frequent dressing change.

Easy to apply

A major advantage of many of the modern products is that they are very simple and quick to apply. Realistically, this has helped to promote their use with the nurses who regularly provide wound care.

Conformability

A dressing that conforms well to the shape of the wound is likely to assist in maintaining a moist environment and also provide an effective barrier for bacteria.

Easy to remove

If a dressing is easy to remove it is less likely to damage the newly formed tissue in the wound. It is also less likely to be painful for the patient.

Comfortable to 'wear'

Another advantage of many modern products is that they are comfortable for the patient when they are *in situ*. This means that the patient is more likely to want to comply with the treatment regime. In any case, there is no need for patients to suffer unnecessary pain or discomfort.

Does not require frequent dressing change

The majority of modern products can be left in place for several days, depending on the wound and, particularly, the amount of exudate. This not only saves nursing time and reduces costs but also reduces the amount of interference with the wound. Reduction in the frequency of dressing change helps to reduce the opportunities for a drop of temperature on the wound surface. This can potentially occur at each dressing change. Myers (1982) studied 420 patients and found that, after wound cleansing, it took 40 minutes before the wound regained its original temperature. Furthermore, he found that it took three hours for mitotic activity to return to its normal rate. Patients also find less frequent dressing changes beneficial. Some patients find dressing change an ordeal and others, especially community patients, an inconvenience which disrupts their life.

Comment

It should be recognised that no one dressing provides the optimum environment for the healing of all wounds. Equally, it may be necessary to use more than one type of dressing during the healing of a wound. Many dressings will fulfil some of the criteria and they should be selected following careful assessment of the wound (see Chapter 3).

4.6 MODERN WOUND MANAGEMENT PRODUCTS

In order to make sense of all the dressings that are available, they will be divided into different categories. Dressings can also be considered in terms of their suitability as a primary or secondary dressing on open wounds. In the UK, not all the dressings are freely available in the community as government restrictions control which dressings can be prescribed. This may considerably affect continuity and quality of care between hospital and community.

This section aims to describe the different categories of wound management products and some proprietary examples will be mentioned.

Absorbent pads

There are many versions of this type of dressing. Most are in the form of an absorbent core, which is covered by a sleeve of gauze or synthetic material. These dressings are not suitable as a primary dressing on open wounds but make an excellent secondary dressing, particularly when there is a heavy exudate. They are generally very cheap.

Absorbent cellulose dressings

Exu-dry™ and Mesorb™ are one-piece multilayer dressings that are highly absorbent and able to wick exudate away from the wound surface. They may be used in direct contact with the wound and are intended for use on heavily exuding wounds of all types.

Adhesive island dressings

These dressings consist of a central pad which is covered with a wider band of adhesive backing. They are lightweight and usually remain in position satisfactorily. There is little absorbent capacity in these dressings. They are widely used on postsurgical wounds, which are healing by first intention, but are not suitable for open wounds as a primary dressing.

Alginates

Alginate dressings contain calcium or sodium alginate, which is derived from seaweed. There are several types of alginate including Algisite M™, Algoster-il™, Curasorb™, Kaltostat™, Sorbalgon™, Sorbsan™ and Tegagen™. These dressings are interactive because as they react with the wound, their structure alters. As the dressing absorbs exudate, it changes from a fibrous structure to a gel. Some dressings allow removal in one piece, others have to be flushed from the wound. These dressings are available in a variety of formats: flat dressings, rope or ribbon, extra-absorbent versions and with an adhesive backing. They are appropriate for moderate or heavily exuding wounds and may require a secondary dressing. They should not be used on wounds with no or low exudate.

Antibacterials

Metrotop™ is a gel containing metronidazole. It reduces odour and anaerobic bacteria and is licensed for use as a deodoriser for fungating tumours. However, it has been used successfully on other wound types. Like all products of this type, it should not be used indiscriminately.

Antibiotics

See section 4.2.2.

Antiseptics

See section 4.2.1.

Barrier film dressings

Barrier film dressings have developed to protect the skin. Some films, such as Clinishield™ and Skin Prep™, were originally developed for use around stoma sites. Others, such as Cavilon™ and Comfeel Skin Care™, have been more specifically marketed for protecting the skin around a wound. The film is wiped on using an applicator such as an impregnated towel and dries to form a film barrier, protecting the skin from adhesives as well as moisture and resistant to urine and faeces.

Biosurgery

Biosurgery is another name for maggot or larval therapy. The often inadvertent use of maggots in wounds has been recognised for centuries. Morgan (1995) chronicled the use of maggots by Maya Indians through to the 1930s. He considered that it fell into disrepute with the advent of antibiotics and aseptic wound care and also noted the attendant aesthetic problems. However, larval therapy is enjoying a resurgence of popularity at present. Thomas *et al.* (1996) suggest this return in popularity might be in part because of the problems caused by resistant bacteria such as MRSA.

The larvae for biosurgery are packed in sterile containers directly from the supplier. They may be 'free range' within a small plastic container or sealed within a porous bag. Before applying the larvae, a hydrocolloid dressing should be applied around the wound to protect the skin from the proteolytic enzymes produced by the maggots (Sherman, 1997). Once placed in the wound, the free-range maggots are retained by means of a small net, taped in place; those in a bag are simply placed in the wound and held in place with tape. Once the larvae are removed from the wound, they are disposed of in the same way as all used dressings. They are used to debride necrotic, sloughy and infected tissue from a wound.

Cadexomer bead dressings

These dressings are composed of hydrophilic beads containing iodine. As they absorb exudate, the beads swell and the iodine is released slowly into the wound. They come in the form of a powder (Iodosorb™) and an ointment (Iodflex™). This dressing is intended for heavily exuding necrotic, sloughy or infected wounds. It should not be used for more than three months at a time and is not suitable for people with iodine sensitivity or thyroid problems.

Capillary wound dressings

Vacutex™ is the only dressing in this category. It is a non-interactive, three-layered dressing made from polyester filaments and polycotton fibres. It absorbs exudate into the middle layer and wicks it laterally in a capillary action. It may be cut to shape to fit a cavity and is suitable for all types of heavily exuding wounds.

Foams

Foam dressings are made from polyurethane. They are either available as a flat foam dressing, such as Allevyn™, Biatain™, Cutinova Hydro™, Lyofoam™ or Tielle™, or as a filler for cavity wounds, such as Allevyn Cavity Wound Dressing™. Allevyn, Lyofoam and Tielle come in a range of presentations such as shaped dressings, varying absorbent capacity, tracheostomy dressings and adhesive dressings. Allevyn Cavity Wound is a preformed foam stent, which comes in two shapes and two sizes in each. Cavi-Care™ is also a foam stent but it has to be mixed with a catalyst and then poured into the wound cavity where it sets in the shape of the wound. Foam dressings are best used on granulating or epithelialising wounds with some exudate.

Hydrocapillary and multilayered absorbent dressings

The dressings within this category all have a slightly different action, depending on their construction. They are Alione Hydrocapillary™, Transorbent™ and Versiva™. Alione™ has a non-adherent wound contact layer, a hydrocapillary pad that absorbs exudate and distributes it horizontally and an outer low-friction film. Transorbent™ is a multilayer dressing containing a film, foam and hydrogel. Versiva™ also comprises three layers: a wound contact layer of perforated hydrocolloid adhesive, a central absorbent layer of sodium carboxymethylcellulose fibres and an outer layer of polyurethane foam. These dressings can be left in place for several days. They are not suitable for dry wounds.

Hydrocolloids

Hydrocolloids are a development from stoma products. They are interactive dressings consisting of a hydrocolloid base made from cellulose, gelatins and pectins and a backing made from a polyurethane film or foam. The technology has progressed since the original hydrocolloid dressings were introduced and a second generation of products is now available which have greater absorbency and hold exudate more effectively within the dressing. Examples of hydrocolloid dressings include Comfeel Plus™, Cutinova Hydro™, Granuflex™ (known as Duoderm™ outside the UK) and Tegasorb™. Several come in a wide range of sizes and shapes and variations such as a thinner than standard dressing. No secondary dressing is necessary. Cutinova Hydro™ has a greater absorptive capacity than other hydrocolloids. Combiderm™ is another variation of hydrocolloid technology. It is composed of several layers including a thin hydrocolloid and an island pad containing polyacrylate granules which hold the exudate within the pad. Cutinova Cavity™ is suitable for cavity wounds; it is a flat sheet which can be folded or cut into a ribbon shape. Initially it should only fill half the cavity because it swells as it absorbs exudate and moulds to the shape of the cavity. It is suitable for moderate to heavily exuding cavity wounds.

Hydrocolloids can be used on a wide range of wounds but generally are most effective on the moderate to low exuding wounds.

Hydrofibres

Hydrofibre dressings are made from hydrocolloid fibres that gel in the presence of exudate. They are highly absorbent. Aquacel™ comes as a flat dressing in a range of sizes and also a ribbon for cavity wounds. They are not suitable for use over dry necrotic wounds.

Hydrogels

These dressings are made from insoluble polymers and have a high water content. The amorphous gel, such as Granugel™, Intrasite Gel™, Nu-Gel™ or Sterigel™, may be used on a wide variety of wounds. They have the ability to either absorb exudate or hydrate dry wounds such as necrotic eschar, thus encouraging debridement. They can be used on wounds with moderate to low exudate and in small cavities. The gel sheets such as 2nd Skin™ or Vigilon™ are best used on granulating moderate to low exuding wounds. They all require a secondary dressing.

Low-adherent dressings

These types of dressing are low adherent rather than non-adherent. They have little if any absorbent capacity and are best on wounds with little exudate. They may be used to 'carry' a dressing such as an amorphous hydrogel and mostly need to be used in combination with an absorbent pad. They do not provide a moist wound environment. Examples of this type of dressing are Melolin™, N-A Ultra™, Release™, Telfa™ and Tricotex™.

Low-adherent dressings (medicated)

Inadine™ is a low-adherent dressing that is impregnated with water-soluble povidone iodine. It is suitable for moderate to low exuding infected wounds or for prophylaxis in minor traumatic wounds. It is not suitable for patients with iodine sensitivity or thyroid problems. Activon Tulle™ is a low-adherent dressing impregnated with manuka honey.

Non-medicated and medicated tulles

Tulles are also called paraffin gauze and were originally known as tulle gras. They are made of open weave cotton or rayon impregnated with soft paraffin. Although the paraffin makes the dressing less adherent, it readily becomes incorporated into granulation tissue. A pattern can be seen on the wound surface when it is removed. It does not maintain a moist wound environment and has no absorbent capacity. It is widely used on minor burns and traumatic injuries. Examples are Jelonet™, Paranet™, Paratulle™ and Unitulle™. A secondary dressing is required with these dressings.

Some types of tulles are impregnated with either antiseptics or antibiotics. The commonest type of antiseptic is chlorhexidine which is present in Bactigras™, Chlorhexitulle™ and Serotulle™. These dressings are useful for superficial infected wounds. Two tulles are impregnated with antibiotics (Fucidin Intertulle™ and Sofra-Tulle™). The use of these dressings is not recommended because of the problems of sensitivity and resistance of bacteria.

Paste bandages

These are cotton bandages impregnated with medicated paste. The use of paste bandages has largely been superseded by more modern products but they are still used for leg ulceration, particularly when the surrounding skin is eczematous or inflamed. Whilst they are an effective form of treatment, many patients develop allergies to the contents of the paste so it is wise to patch test the patient before applying a bandage. There are several types of bandage with different pastes such as zinc paste with ichthammol or zinc paste with calamine. A secondary bandage is required.

Silicone wound dressings

Silicone products have a number of uses. Silicone gel sheets such as Cica-Care™, Silgel™ and Sil-K Film™ help with scar management as they are able to soften and flatten scars. Silicone N-A™ is similar to a low-adherent dressing as it is made from a knitted viscose material impregnated with silicone to allow easy removal and is virtually non-adherent. Mepitel™ is suitable for painful wounds or where there is macerated or fragile skin as it is very easy to remove. Exudate passes through the dressing to the secondary pad. The outer pad may be changed more frequently than the Mepitel, which can be left in place for up to ten days.

Silver and charcoal dressings

These dressings incorporate silver into their structure and some also contain activated charcoal cloth. Silver is an effective antibacterial and charcoal has been found to be effective in absorbing the chemicals released from malodorous wounds. Infected, necrotic or fungating wounds may have a very unpleasant odour. Actisorb Plus 25™ or Actisorb Plus 220™ are both in the form of a charcoal pad impregnated with silver; they are used with a primary dressing and require a covering pad. Arglaes™ contains alginate powder and a mixture of inorganic polymer and ionic silver. As the alginate gels, the silver is gradually released. Aquacel Ag™ acts in a similar fashion. Acticoat™, Acticoat 7™ and Contreet Ag™ are made from polyethylene or polyurethane coated with silver. Dressings such as Carbonet™, Clinisorb™ or Lyofoam C™ are a combination of dressing and charcoal. Most of these dressings require a secondary dressing.

TenderWet

TenderWet™ is a multilayer dressing with a central core of polyacrylate, which is activated by soaking the dressing with an appropriate volume of Ringer's solution. The Ringer's solution is delivered to the wound surface for up to 12 hours and helps to soften necrotic tissue. It is able to absorb exudate but should be changed daily.

Vapour-permeable films

There is a wide range of these film dressings available. They provide a moist healing environment but have no absorbency. They should not be used on infected wounds. The method of application varies according to make. Most require a certain amount of skill and practice in application. Examples include Bioclusive™, Cutifilm™, Mefilm™, Opraflex™, Opsite™ and Tegaderm™.

Vapour-permeable membranes

Tegapore™ allows exudate to pass through the dressing and can be left in place for several weeks whilst the outer dressings are changed. It is non-adherent and will protect delicate skin.

4.7 ADVANCED TECHNOLOGIES

As with any other aspect of healthcare, new developments in wound care are regularly announced. Sometimes they are variations on an older form of treatment and sometimes they are new developments. This section seeks to identify these innovations and consider the evidence to support their use.

4.7.1 Growth factors

Growth factors have been used for some time in wound care. In the USA, the use of growth factors was primarily via the establishment of wound care centres that provided a comprehensive programme of full assessment and planned care. Many of the patients treated in these centres have leg or foot ulcers such as demonstrated in a randomised controlled trial undertaken by Knighton *et al.* (1990). They found a significantly higher rate of healing in those treated with growth factor solution compared with a blinded placebo.

The use of growth factors has not had the results that were initially expected. Spencer *et al.* (1996) suggested that whilst the results of clinical trials have so far been disappointing, the interest in the use of growth factors has led to a greater understanding of the physiological make-up of different types of chronic wound. Falanga (2000) suggested that part of the reason for this apparent failure may be because the concept of wound bed preparation (WBP) was imperfectly understood at the time of many of the trials and there was a failure to prepare the wound adequately before applying the growth factor. It is interesting to note that the only growth factor product licensed in both the UK and the USA is becaplermin (Regranex™) (platelet-derived growth factor), specifically for diabetic foot ulcers. It has been long understood that sharp debridement of neuropathic diabetic foot ulcers is an essential aspect of good practice (Brem *et al.*, 2004). Ladin (2000) suggested that there is a direct correlation between debridement prior to becaplermin application and healing rates.

It is not just the preparation of the wound that needs to be considered; the method of delivery of a growth factor to the wound surface may also affect the outcome (Robson *et al.*, 1998). There is increasing interest in the idea of using gene transfer as a delivery system. Skin gene therapy has the potential to facilitate delivery of a number of different growth factors (Guarini, 20003). Galeano *et al.* (2003) have demonstrated that it is possible to deliver a virus vector-mediated vascular endothelial growth factor (VEGF) gene transfer to a burn wound, using an animal model. This model of delivery has considerable potential and, combined with WBP, may reinvigorate the use of growth factors. However, there is still some way to go before this can become a clinical reality.

4.7.2 Protease-modulating wound management products

As discussed in Chapter 1, excessive levels of proteases such as matrix metalloproteinases (MMPs) have been shown to be a factor in delayed healing of chronic wounds. Relatively recent additions to the range of dressings are two products designed to reduce the harmful effects of MMPs: Promogran™ and Dermax™. These products are dissimilar in their structure and do not act in the same way. Promogran™ is made from collagen and oxidised regenerated cellulose and is able to bind MMPs, thus negating their harmful effects. Dermax™ is made from ethylene vinyl acetate mesh fabric impregnated with oak bark extract that downregulates MMP production, thus promoting healing. As yet, there is limited published evidence for their use.

Veves et al. (2002) undertook a randomised study comparing Promogran™ with standard care in the USA (moistened gauze) in 276 patients with diabetic foot ulcers. Overall, there was no statistical difference between the two groups at 12 weeks. However, there was borderline significance in favour of Promogran™ in a subset of patients with ulcers that had been present less than six months. Vin et al. (2002) randomly allocated 73 patients with venous leg ulcers to either Promogran™ or Adaptic™ (a low-adherent dressing impregnated with petrolatum emulsion) and followed their progress for 12 weeks. Although more ulcers healed with Promogran™ than with Adaptic™, this did not achieve significance. There was, however, a significant reduction in ulcer size in the Promogran™ group. A cost modelling study was undertaken by Ghatnekar et al. (2002) to determine the cost-effectiveness of Promogran™ for treating diabetic foot ulcers, using costs from France, Germany, Switzerland and the UK. Based on the assumption that within the first three months of treatment, 26% of ulcers were treated with Promogran™ and 20.7% were treated with standard practice, the authors calculated both recurring and non-recurring costs. They estimated that there was potential for cost savings in each country, there being considerable variation due to overall treatment costs.

To date, there is only a small pilot study showing the clinical use of Dermax™ in the public domain. Karim et al. (2002) studied the impact of using Dermax™ on four non-healing chronic wounds over six weeks. They found an increase in fibroblast activity and a decline in the levels of MMP2. Further clinical trials are in progress and the results are required before the value of this product can be clearly determined.

4.7.3 Hyaluronan-based products

Hyaluronan is an important component of the extracellular matrix and it plays a role in regulating the inflammatory response, stimulation of cell proliferation and angiogenesis and also epithelialisation (Taddeucci et al., 2004). Hyalofill-F™ is a non-woven fleece dressing made from HYAFF, an esterified benzyl ester of hyaluronic acid. There are as yet limited studies of its efficacy.

Boyce et al. (1997) undertook a randomised study of pilonidal sinus wounds comparing Hyalofill-F™ placed under a foam stent with the foam stent alone. An interim analysis was undertaken after 41 patients had been recruited that showed a dramatic reduction in wound size in the Hyalofill-F™ group during the first two weeks. Unfortunately, no statistical analysis was undertaken and there have been no further reports on this study.

Hollander *et al.* (2000) undertook two case studies to evaluate the use of Hyalofill-F™ in patients with traumatic wounds with healing difficulties and found a rapid reduction in wound size within two weeks. They called for further randomised studies to determine the most effective use of this product. Vazquez *et al.* (2003) undertook a non-comparative pilot study of 36 patients with diabetic foot ulcers to provide data for a future randomised, controlled trial. They achieved a 75% healing rate within the 20-week study period. The mean healing time for this group was 10.0 ± 4.8 weeks. Unsurprisingly, they found that superficial ulcers healed more quickly than deep ulcers.

Two studies have been reported of the use of Hyalofill-F™ in the treatment of venous leg ulcers. Colletta *et al.* (2003) undertook a non-comparative pilot study of non-healing venous ulcers, using the dressing in combination with compression bandages. The 19 ulcers were followed for eight weeks. They found that four ulcers healed completely with a mean healing time of 24.5 days. The mean percentage reduction of the remaining ulcers was 53% during the study period. The research team noticed a rapid reduction in ulcer size during the first two weeks of treatment. Taddeucci *et al.* (2004) compared Hyalofill-F™ with paraffin gauze (standard treatment in Italy) for the treatment of 24 venous ulcers. At eight weeks, they found a significant reduction in ulcer size and rate of epithelialisation in the experimental group. There was also a significant reduction in maceration in this group. Overall, the research team considered that the product had been shown to be effective in treating chronic venous ulcers.

This product looks to be a useful tool but larger studies are needed to determine its most effective use.

4.7.4 Hyperbaric oxygen

Hyperbaric oxygen chambers have been used for many years in recompression of divers with the bends or decompression illness. More recently, they have also been used for non-healing wounds. Hyperbaric oxygen (HBO) treatment has been defined as "the patient breathing in 100% oxygen intermittently at a point higher than sea level pressure" (British Medical Association Board of Science and Education, 1993). It is delivered by placing a patient inside a pressure chamber, which may be designed for one or more people. The length of time over which treatments are given varies according to the condition being treated.

There have been two systematic reviews of the use of HBO therapy for chronic wounds. Kranke *et al.* (2004) undertook a Cochrane review of five randomised studies using HBO. Four of the studies were of diabetic foot ulcers (a total of 147 patients). The authors were able to pool the results of three studies and found a reduction in the risk of major amputation with HBO therapy compared to controls. A numbers needed to treat analysis showed that four patients would need to be treated in order to prevent one amputation in the long term. Kranke *et al.* (2004) also reviewed a study of 16 venous ulcer patients. Although there was a significant reduction in ulcer size in the HBO group, the numbers are very small. They conclude that overall, the reviewed studies were of poor quality and inadequately reported. There seems to be a benefit for diabetic foot ulcers but there is a need for adequately powered, randomised studies that include an economic evaluation.

Wang *et al.* (2003) undertook a more inclusive review that included randomised, controlled trials, cohort studies and case series of at least five patients. They found a total of 57 studies involving more than 2000 patients. The authors considered that HBO could potentially provide improved outcomes for non-healing diabetic foot ulcers, compromised skin grafts, wounds damaged by radiotherapy and gas gangrene. Wang *et al.* (2003) also concluded that the quality of the studies that they reviewed was poor and that there is insufficient evidence to provide guidance on when it would be appropriate to commence HBO or which patients would benefit most. Kalani *et al.* (2002) followed 38 diabetic foot ulcer patients for three years to monitor long-term outcomes of using HBO and found improved outcomes in the HBO group, but also expressed a desire for more studies to be undertaken to clearly determine the role of HBO within the wound management armamentarium.

It is obvious that there is only a limited case for the use of hyperbaric oxygen at present. However, for most nurses the argument is academic as they are not likely to have access to such equipment.

4.7.5 Topical negative pressure

Topical negative pressure (TNP) therapy or vacuum-assisted closure (VAC) is a device which applies a universal negative pressure to a wound, encouraging blood flow and faster granulation (Baxandall, 1996). It comprises a foam sponge to fit into the wound, tubing to connect the foam to the pump via a canister to collect exudate. The sponge is covered with a film dressing to create an airtight seal (Fig. 4.1). Pressure can be applied continuously or intermittently.

Argenta pioneered the development of TNP therapy. He described successful outcomes in 296 of 300 cases of chronic, acute and subacute wounds

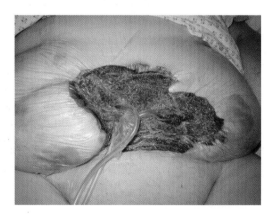

Fig. 4.1 VAC therapy *in situ*.

(Argenta & Morykwas, 1997). Subsequently, there have been numerous reports of its use, many of which have been case series or case studies. Some of the benefits of TNP can be described as follows.

- Reduction of tissue oedema. Although this is particularly difficult to measure, Banwell (1999) suggests that this action could be very useful in the management of crush injuries or burns.
- Reduction of bacterial load. There are mixed reports of the impact of TNP on bacterial colonisation. Morykwas *et al.* (1997) found a significant reduction in bacterial counts in the animal model. Banwell (1999) reported the same outcome, whereas Moues *et al.* (2004) and Weed *et al.* (2004) found a variable outcome with reduction of some bacteria and an increase in others. However, both the latter studies still reported good healing rates. There are also consistent reports of beneficial outcomes in infected wounds such as for deep sternal wound infection following open heart surgery (Gustaffson *et al.*, 2003; Luckraz *et al.*, 2003).
- Management of chronic wound fluid. TNP can be a useful method of collecting and managing wound exudate. Banwell (1999) suggested that TNP may be able to reduce the levels of MMPs within the wound.
- Removal of slough and promotion of granulation tissue. TNP has been demonstrated to be effective in removal of slough (Gustaffson *et al.*, 2003; Loree *et al.*, 2004; Luckraz *et al.*, 2003).
- Promotion of wound healing. Numerous cohort or uncontrolled studies have concluded that TNP is effective. However, a Cochrane review (Evans & Land, 2004) was only able to identify two small randomised, controlled trials of chronic wounds with a total of 34 patients up until November 2002. These studies showed weak evidence of efficacy but the numbers are too small for any firm conclusions to be drawn.
- Improved take in skin grafts. Blackburn *et al.* (1998) reported using VAC therapy prior to skin grafting of large complex open wounds and found that they were able to get a minimum of a 95% take.
- Cost effectiveness of TNP. The unit costs of using TNP are high but a review by Neubauer and Ujlaky (2003) investigated the treatment costs using data derived from three studies and concluded that TNP has the potential to make cost savings of up to $9000 per patient through a faster healing time. However, they also emphasise the need for further prospective studies in order for firm conclusions to be obtained.

TNP therapy is gradually being used more widely, especially as a portable version is now available. However, it can potentially be harmful if used inappropriately and skill is needed in its application. Birchall *et al.* (2002) describe how one acute trust developed a centralised system for the use of TNP, along with guidelines to ensure appropriate use and a competency-based education programme for nurses. The whole system was both clinically- and cost-effective as well as being more efficient.

4.7.6 Tissue culture

Tissue culture describes the process whereby a small full-thickness section of skin is harvested from a patient or donor and then cultured in the laboratory to form large sheets of cells (cultured keratinocytes). The sheets of cells are then grafted onto a granulating wound completely free of any necrotic material. Autologous tissue (that taken from the patient) has been found to be more effective than allogenic tissue (that taken from a donor). However, it can take more than a month to prepare (Kakibuchi *et al.*, 1996). Tissue culture has become well established since the early 1980s when the first clinical reports of its use appeared. Kumagai *et al.* (1997) followed up 38 patients who had received autologous cultured keratinocyte grafts for over two years. They concluded that cultured tissue has site specificity even after grafting and therefore, where possible, the maxim "closer is best", which is applied to conventional skin grafting, should also be used for tissue cultures.

Wright *et al.* (1998b) describe the use of a polyurethane foam dressing as a carrier for cultured keratinocytes. They found it to be a useful vehicle but there was slow proliferation of cells. They suggest that cells should be expanded using the standard methods and then seeded onto the dressing. Myers *et al.* (1997) tested a hyaluronic membrane delivery system for cultured keratinocytes on an animal model and found that it gave a superior keratinocyte take. The researchers suggest that this system requires further investigation and clinical evaluation. Caravaggi *et al.* (2003) used a similar product in the treatment of diabetic foot ulcers, comparing it with paraffin gauze (standard treatment in Italy). The results from 79 patients showed greater numbers of healed ulcers in the experimental group but this difference failed to reach statistical significance, possibly because the study was underpowered. The ulcers were subdivided into those on the plantar surface or dorsum. There were a significantly higher number of healed ulcers in the experimental group on the dorsum of the foot but the precise significance of this is uncertain.

Generally, cultured keratinocytes have been used by plastic surgeons particularly for treating burn patients. However, they have also been used for treating leg ulcers that have not responded to other forms of treatment. In reviewing this, Kakibuchi *et al.* (1996) consider that it has not been an unqualified success as grafts have only shown a 10–20% take. Tissue culture is an important therapy for burn patients and it may have potential for a wider use, but needs some further development.

4.7.7 Tissue engineering

Tissue engineering takes tissue culture a step forward. It uses human dermal fibroblasts and cultures them on a biosynthetic scaffold. The fibroblasts proliferate and secrete proteins and growth factors, resulting in the generation of a three-dimensional human dermis that can then be used to graft over wound sites. Two brands are currently available, Apligraf™ (also known as Graftskin) and Dermagraft™, and they can be described as cultured human skin equivalent (HSE).

Falanga *et al.* (1998) studied the effect of using a HSE (Apligraf™) on patients with venous ulcers in a multicentre trial. A total of 240 patients were randomised to HSE and compression or compression therapy alone. They found a significantly faster healing rate in the HSE group. In those patients ($n = 120$) whose ulcer had been open for more than a year, HSE was significantly more effective in achieving healing. Falanga and Sabolinski (1999) investigated the results from this last group of patients in more detail. They found that 47% of those treated with HSE were healed by six months compared with 19% of controls. They suggest that HSE is particularly useful in the treatment of ulcers of long duration. Omar *et al.* (2004) undertook a pilot study using Dermagraft™ for venous ulcers. Eighteen patients were randomised to either the HSE and compression or compression alone and followed up for 12 weeks. Five patients in the HSE group and one of the controls were healed at 12 weeks, but this did not achieve significance. However, there was a significant reduction in ulcer size and in the linear rate of healing in the HSE group.

Brem *et al.* (2001) discussed the success of two centres in the use of HSE (Apligraf™) for 33 patients with 54 venous ulcers that had been present for more than a year. They considered that their results were better than those reported in an earlier trial (Falanga *et al.*, 1998; Falanga & Sabolinski, 1999) as they were able to achieve healing rates of 70% in six months. The authors suggest that this was due to improved wound bed preparation, particularly in the use of antiseptics to reduce wound exudate prior to commencement of HSE therapy. They also meshed the HSE prior to application to allow excessive exudate to escape. Schonfeld *et al.* (2001) undertook an economic analysis of the use of HSE (Apligraf™) in hard-to-heal venous ulcers using a semi-Markov model. They calculated that as ulcers would heal faster using HSE compared with compression alone, the overall treatment costs were lower ($20 141 compared with $27 493 over a 12-month period).

HSE has also been used to treat diabetic foot ulcers. Gentkow *et al.* (1996) carried out a randomised, controlled, single-blinded trial of 50 patients with diabetic foot ulcers. Patients were allocated to four groups: three different dosages of HSE (Dermagraft™) or a control group. They found that all three of the treatment regimens were significantly better than the control. Furthermore, after 14 months' follow-up there were no recurrences in the HSE patients. The authors considered this fact to be significant, quoting recurrence rates from other studies of 19.6–46% in times less than 12 months. Hanft and Surprenant (2002) compared HSE (Dermagraft™) with moistened gauze in 28 patients with diabetic foot ulcers. They found that there was a significant difference in the healing rate in the HSE group by week 12 and in the overall rate of healing. A larger multicentre randomised study of 245 diabetic foot ulcers compared Dermagraft™ with conventional therapy (Marston *et al.*, 2003). A significantly higher number of patients in the HSE group were healed by 12 weeks. This group also experienced significantly fewer ulcer-related adverse events. Veves *et al.* (2001) reported a multicentre study of 208 neuropathic diabetic foot ulcers comparing HSE (Apligraf™) with moistened gauze. All patients had surgical debridement prior to treatment and adequate foot off-loading. There were significantly more ulcers healed in the HSE group at 12 weeks and the median time to healing was 65 days compared with 90 days for the controls ($p = 0.0026$).

Newton *et al.* (2002) studied the microvascular blood flow in seven full-thickness diabetic foot ulcers before and after application of Dermagraft™. They found that by eight weeks, there was a 72% increase of blood flow in five of the seven ulcers and that they were healed by 12 weeks. The other two ulcers reduced in size by 25%.

Allenet *et al.* (2000) used a Markov model to undertake an economic evaluation of the costs of using HSE (Dermagraft™) compared with standard treatment for diabetic foot ulcers over a 52-week period. The overall treatment costs were lower for the HSE because of a faster healing rate (53 522FF compared with 56 687FF). Redekop *et al.* (2003) undertook a similar exercise comparing Apligraf™ with general wound care for diabetic foot ulcers. They found that there was a 12% reduction in costs using HSE.

It would seem that the use of HSE has considerable potential in the treatment of wounds that have failed to heal with other methods. Although the economic evaluations described above indicate that cost savings can be made using HSE, it should be remembered that this is only the case in those wounds that are not healing. Other methods should be used first, before considering HSE.

4.8 ALTERNATIVE THERAPIES AND WOUND MANAGEMENT

Alternative or complementary therapies have been defined as those therapies that usually lie outside the official health sector (WHO, 1983). Trevelyn and Booth (1994) divided them into three categories in relation to their potential links to nursing (see Box 4.1). Although there is much written in the literature

---

Box 4.1   Categories of alternative therapies related to nursing.

Category 1: can be incorporated into nursing care

- Massage
- Reflexology
- Aromatherapy
- Therapeutic touch

Category 2: can be used to some extent by nurses with relevant training

- Homeopathy
- Herbal medicine

Category 3: not usually practised as part of nursing care

- Acupuncture
- Osteopathy
- Chiropractic

regarding these therapies, there is a paucity of research evidence to demonstrate their place in patient care. Gates (1994) and Vickers (1997) have discussed this problem and suggested the need for a critical appraisal of the literature on the subject.

One such review has been undertaken by Finch (1997), who appraised the therapy of therapeutic touch, healing by laying on of hands, in relation to wound healing. Its use in nursing was introduced in the USA in the 1970s. It is based on the principle that human beings are energy fields and illness is the result of an imbalance in the energy field. Therapeutic touch focuses on redirecting the energy to restore balance. Finch reviewed five studies of therapeutic touch and wound healing carried out on healthy volunteers by the same researcher. She concluded that therapeutic touch was unreliable and generally ineffective when used to treat wounds. A Cochrane review by O'Mathuna and Ashford (2004) considered the use of therapeutic touch in healing acute wounds. They concluded that there was insufficient evidence to show whether it had a role in healing acute wounds. However, it has been shown to be beneficial in treating anxiety (see Chapter 2).

Aromatherapy involves the use of essential oils that are applied to the skin. A variety of oils can be used, depending on the effect required. Unfortunately, there are a number of inconsistencies found in the literature with a variety of contradictory properties being given to the same oil (Vickers, 1997). A study by Kite *et al.* (1998) suggests that aromatherapy is effective in reducing anxiety and stress. They assessed 58 cancer patients using a HAD score before and after six sessions of aromatherapy and found a significant reduction in anxiety and depression at the end of the course of treatment. Asquith (1999) undertook a review of the literature and reported a number of case studies that found lavender and tea tree oils beneficial in healing a variety of wounds. Asquith also identified studies that improved other aspects of patient care such as sleep patterns. She concluded that there was little evidence to show a direct benefit to wound healing.

There is no doubt that some patients find alternative therapies helpful. Whether these types of therapies have a role in wound healing remains questionable. There is a real need for the development of high-quality research methodologies to explore the multifaceted nature of these treatments.

REFERENCES

Ahmed, A.K., Hoekstra, M.J., Hage, J.J., Karim, R.B. (2003) Honey-medicated dressing: transformation of an ancient remedy into a modern therapy. *Annals of Plastic Surgery*, **50** (2), 143–137.

Allenet, B., Paree, F., Lebrun, T. *et al.* (2000) Cost-effectiveness modelling of Dermagraft for the treatment of diabetic foot ulcers in the French context. *Diabetes and Metabolism*, **26** (2), 125–132.

Anderson, I. (2003) Should potassium permanganate be used in wounds? *Nursing Times*, **99** (31) (suppl), 19.

Argenta, L.C., Morykwas, M.J. (1997) Vacuum-assisted closure: a new method for wound control and treatment: clinical experience. *Annals of Plastic Surgery*, **38** (6), 563–576.

Asquith, S. (1999) The use of aromatherapy in wound care. *Journal of Wound Care*, **8** (6), 318–320.

Banwell, P. (1999) Topical negative pressure therapy in wound care. *Journal of Wound Care*, **8** (2), 79–84.

Baxandall, T. (1996) Healing cavity wounds with negative pressure. *Nursing Standard*, **11** (6), 49–51.

Becker, G.D. (1986) Identification and management of the patient at high risk of wound infection. *Head and Neck Surgery*, **8**, 205–210.

Bennett, L.L., Rosenblum, R.S., Perlov, C., Davidson, J.M., Barton, R.M., Nannet, L.B. (2001) An in vivo comparison of topical agents in wound repair. *Plastic and Reconstructive Surgery*, **108** (3), 675–685.

Birchall, L., Street, L., Clift, H. (2002) Developing a trust-wide centralised approach to the use of TNP. *Journal of Wound Care*, **11** (8), 311–314.

Bishop, W.J. (1959) *A History of Surgical Dressings.* Robinson and Sons Ltd, Chesterfield.

Blackburn, J.H., Boemi, L., Hall, W.W. *et al.* (1998) Negative-pressure dressings as a bolster for skin grafts. *Annals of Plastic Surgery*, **40** (5), 453–457.

Bloomfield, S.F., Sizer, T.J. (1985) Eusol BPC and other hypochlorite formulations used in hospitals. *Pharmaceutical Journal*, **253**, 153–157.

Bond, C.J. (1915) The application of strong antiseptics to wounds. *British Medical Journal*, **March 6**, 405–406.

Borgognoni, T. (1955) *The Surgery of Theodoric* vol 1. Translated from the Latin by Campbell, E., Colton, J. Appleton-Century-Crofts, New York.

Boyce, D.E., Miller, L., Moore, K., Harding, K.G. (1997) An open comparative randomised parallel-group clinical trial to evaluate the performance of HYAFF™ wound dressing in the management of pilonidal sinus excision wounds: an interim analysis, in (eds) Leaper, D.J., Cherry, G.W., Dealey, C., Lawrence, J.C., Turner, T.D., *Proceedings of the 6th European Conference on Advances in Wound Management.* Macmillan Magazines Ltd, London.

Brem, H., Balledux, J., Sukkarieh, T., Carson, P., Falanga, V. (2001) Healing of venous leg ulcers of long duration with a bilayered living skin substitute: results from a general surgery and dermatology department. *Dermatologic Surgery*, **27** (11), 915–919.

Brem, H., Sheehan, P., Boulton, A.J.M. (2004) Protocol for treatment of diabetic foot ulcers. *American Journal of Surgery*, **187** (5) (suppl), 1S–10S.

Brennan, S.S., Leaper, D.J. (1985) The effect of antiseptics on the healing wound: a study using the rabbit ear chamber. *British Journal of Surgery*, **72** (10), 780–782.

Brennan, S.S., Foster, M.E., Leaper, D.J. (1986) Antiseptic toxicity in wounds healing by second intention. *Journal of Hospital Infection*, **8** (3), 263–267.

British Medical Association Board of Science and Education (1993) *Clinical Hyperbaric Medicine Facilities in the UK.* British Medical Association, London.

Caravaggi, C., Clerici, G., De Giglio, R. *et al.* (2003) HYAFF 11-based autologous dermal and epidermal grafts in the treatment of noninfected diabetic plantar and dorsal foot ulcers. *Diabetes Care*, **26** (10), 2853–2859.

Carneiro, P.M., Nyawawa, E.T. (2003) Topical phenytoin versus EUSOL in the treatment of non-malignant leg ulcers. *East African Medical Journal*, **80** (3), 124–129.

Colletta, V., Dioguardi, D., Di Lonardo, A., Maggio, G., Torasso, F. (2003) A trial to assess the efficacy and tolerability of Hyalofill-F in non-healing venous leg ulcers. *Journal of Wound Care*, **12** (9), 357–361.

Cookson, B. (1998) The emergence of mupirocin resistance: a challenge to infection control and antibiotic prescribing practice. *Journal of Antimicrobial Chemotherapy.* **41** (1), 11–18.

Daltrey, D.C., Cunliffe, W.J. (1981) A double-blind study of the effects of Benzol peroxide 20% and Eusol and liquid paraffin on the microbial flora of leg ulcers. *Acta Dermato-Venereologica,* **61**, 575–577.

D'Arcy, P.F. (1972) Drugs on the skin: a clinical and pharmaceutical problem. *Pharmaceutical Journal,* **209**, 491–492.

Dealey, C. (2002) Wound healing in Moorish Spain. *EWMA Journal,* **2** (1), 32–34.

Dealey, C. (2003) Wound healing in medieval and renaissance Italy: was it art or science? *EWMA Journal,* **3** (1), 15–17.

Dealey, C. (2004) The contribution of French surgeons to wound healing in medieval and renaissance Europe. *EWMA Journal,* **4** (1), 33–35.

Deng, S., Sang, J., Cao, L. (1995) The effects of mupirocin on burn wounds with staphylococcus aureus infection. *Chung Hua Cheng Hsing Shao Shang Wai Ko Tsa Chih,* **11** (1), 45–48.

Dobrzanski, S., Duncan, S.E., Harkiss, A., Ball, A., Robertson, D. (1983) Topical applications in pressure sore therapy. *British Journal of Pharmaceutical Practice,* **5** (5), 10.

Duin, N., Sutcliffe, J. (1992) *A History of Medicine.* Simon and Schuster, London.

Dunford, C.E., Hanano, R. (2004) Acceptability to patients of a honey dressing for non-healing venous ulcers. *Journal of Wound Care,* **13** (5), 193–197.

Evans, D., Land, L. (2001) Topical negative pressure for treating chronic wounds (Cochrane review). *Cochrane Library,* Issue 1. Update Software, Oxford.

Falanga, V. (2000) Classification for wound bed preparation and stimulation of chronic wounds. *Wound Repair and Regeneration,* **8** (5), 347–352.

Falanga, V., Sabolinski, M. (1999) A bilayered living skin construct (Apligraf) accelerates complete closure of hard-to-heal venous ulcers. *Wound Repair and Regeneration,* **7** (4), 201–207.

Falanga, V., Marolis, D., Alvarez, O. *et al.* (1998) Rapid healing of venous ulcers and lack of clinical rejection with an allogeneic cultured human skin equivalent. *Archives of Dermatology,* **134**, 293–300.

Fernandez, R., Griffiths, R., Ussia, C. (2002) Water for wound cleansing. *Cochrane Database Systematic Review.* 4: CD003861.

Finch, A. (1997) Therapeutic touch and wound healing. *Journal of Wound Care,* **6** (10), 501–504.

Flanagan, M. (2000) Honey and the management of infected wounds. *Journal of Wound Care,* **9** (6), 287.

Forrest, R.D. (1982) Early history of wound treatment. *Journal of the Royal Society of Medicine,* **75**, 198–205.

Foster, L., Moore, P. (1997) The application of a cellulose-based fibre dressing in surgical wounds. *Journal of Wound Care,* **6** (10), 469–473.

Galeano, M., Deodato, B., Altavilla, D. *et al.* (2003) Effect of recombinant adeno-associated virus vector-mediated vascular endothelial growth factor gene transfer on wound healing after burn injury. *Critical Care Medicine,* **31** (4), 1017–1025.

Gates, B. (1994) The use of complementary and alternative therapies in health care: a selective review of the literature and dicussion of the implications for nurse practitioners and health-care managers. *Journal of Clinical Nursing,* **3** (1), 43–47.

Gentkow, G.D., Iswaki, S.D., Hershon, K.S. *et al.* (1996) Use of Dermagraft, a cultured human dermis, to treat diabetic foot ulcers. *Diabetes Care,* **19** (4), 350–354.

Gerster, A.G. (1910) Surgical manners and customs in the times of Henry de Mondeville. *Proceedings of the Charaka Club*, **3**, 70–90.

Ghatnekar, O., Willis, M., Persson, U. (2002) Cost-effectiveness of treating deep diabetic foot ulcers with Promogran in four European countries. *Journal of Wound Care*, **11** (2), 70–74.

Guarini, S. (2003) New gene therapy for the treatment of burn wounds. *Critical Care Medicine*, **31** (4), 1280–1281.

Gustafsson, R.I., Sjogren, J., Ingemansson, R. (2003) Deep sternal wound infection: a sternal-sparing technique with vacuum-assisted closure therapy. *Annals of Thoracic Surgery*, **76** (6), 2048–2053.

Guthrie, D. (1945) *A History of Medicine*. Thomas Nelson, London.

Hanft, J.R., Surprenant, M.S. (2002) Healing of chronic foot ulcers in diabetic patients treated with human fibroblast-derived dermis. *Journal of Foot and Ankle Injury*, **41** (5), 291–299.

Heister, L. (1768) A *General System of Surgery in Three Parts*, 6th edn. Translated into English by Heister L. Whiston, London.

Helling, T.S., Daon, E. (1998) In Flanders fields: the Great War, Antoine Deparge and the resurgence of debridement. *Annals of Surgery*, **228** (2), 173–181.

Herzog, W. (1915) German experiences. The dangers of tincture of iodine as a first-aid dressing. *British Medical Journal*, **March 6**, 441–442.

Hollander, D., Schmandra, T., Windolf, J. (2000) Using an esterified hyaluronan fleece to promote healing in difficult-to-treat wounds. *Journal of Wound Care*, **9** (10), 463–466.

Humzah, M.D., Marshall, J., Breach, N.M. (1996) Eusol: the plastic surgeon's choice? *Journal of the Royal College of Surgeons of Edinburgh*, **41**, 269–270.

Johnson, A. (1987) Wound care, packing cavity wounds. *Nursing Times*, **83** (36), 59–62.

Johnson, P.C. (1989) Guy de Chauliac and the Grand Surgery. *Surgery, Gynaecology and Obstetrics*, **169**, 172–176.

Kakibuchi, M., Hosokawa, K., Fujikawa, M., Yoshikawa, K. (1996) The use of cultured epidermal cell sheets in skin grafting. *Journal of Wound Care*, **5** (10), 487–490.

Kalani, M., Jorneskog, G., Naderi, N., Lind, F., Brismar, K. (2002) Hyperbaric oxygen (HBO) therapy in treatment of diabetic foot ulcers: long term follow-up. *Journal of Diabetes and its Complications*, **16**, 153–158.

Kanal, H. (1975) *Encyclopaedia of Islamic Medicine*. General Egyptian Book Organisation, Cairo.

Karim, R.B., Ahmed, A.K.J., Brito, B.L.R. (2002) *Balancing MMPs in chronic wounds: a pilot study with Dermax*. Paper presented at the Dutch Association for Plastic Surgery Meeting, Aalst, Belgium, November 23.

Kearney, J.N., Arain, T., Holland, K.T. (1988) Antimicrobial properties of antiseptic impregnated dressings. *Journal of Hospital Infection*, **11** (1), 68–76.

Kingsley, A. (2001) The use of honey in the treatment of infected wounds: case studies. *British Journal of Nursing*, **10** (22) (suppl), S13–S20.

Kirkpatrick, J.J.R., Naylor, I.L. (1997) Ulcer management in medieval England. *Journal of Wound Care*, **6** (7), 350–352.

Kite, S.M., Maher, E.J., Anderson, K. *et al.* (1998) Development of an aromatherapy service at a cancer centre. *Palliative Medicine*, **12** (3), 171–180.

Knighton, D.R., Ciresi, K., Fiegal, V.D., Schumerth, S., Butler, E., Cerrs, F. (1990) Stimulation of repair in chronic non-healing cutaneous ulcers using platelet-derived wound healing formula. *Surgery, Gynaecology and Obstetrics*, **170**, 56–60.

Kranke, P., Bennett, M., Roeckl-Wiedmann, I., Debus, S. (2004) Hyperbaric oxygen therapy for chronic wounds. *Cochrane Database for Systematic Reviews* 2: CD004123.

Kumagai, N., Oshima, H., Tanabe, M., Ishida, H., Uchikoshi, T. (1997) Favourable donor site for epidermal cultivation for the treatment of burn scars with autologous cultured epithelium. *Annals of Plastic Surgery*, **38** (5), 506–513.

Ladin, D. (2000) Becaplermin gel (PDGF-BB) as topical wound therapy. Plastic Surgery Educational Foundation DATA Committee. *Plastic and Reconstructive Surgery*, **105** (3), 1230–1231.

Lansdown, A.B.G. (2004) A review of the use of silver in wound care: facts and fallacies. *British Journal of Nursing*, **13** (6) (suppl), S6–S19.

Lawrence, J.C. (1987) A century after Gamgee. *Burns*, **13** (1), 77–79.

Levine, J.M. (1992) Historical Notes on Pressure Ulcers: The Cure of Ambrose Paré. *Decubites*, **5**(2), 23–26.

Lineaweaver, W., Howard, R., Soucy, D. *et al.* (1985) Topical antimicrobial toxicity. *Archives of Surgery*, **120**, 267–270.

Linker, R.W., Womack, N. (1969) *Ten Books of Surgery by Ambroise Paré*. University of Georgia Press, Athens, GA.

Loree, S., Dompmartin, A., Penven, K., Harel, D., Leroy, D. (2004) Is vacuum assisted closure a valid technique for debriding leg ulcers? *Journal of Wound Care*, **13** (6), 249–252.

Luckraz, H., Murphy, F., Bryant, S., Charman, S.C., Ritchie, A.J. (2003) Vacuum-assisted closure as a treatment modality for infections after cardiac surgery. *Journal of Thoracic and Cardiovascular Surgery*, **125** (2), 301–305.

Marston, W.A., Hanft, J., Norwood, P., Pollack, R. (2003) The efficacy and safety of Dermagraft in improving the healing of diabetic foot ulcers. *Diabetes Care*, **26** (6), 1701–1705.

Mayo-Robson, A.W. (1915) Hints on war surgery. *British Journal of Dermatology*, **July 24**, 136.

McLure, A.R., Gordon J. (1992) In-vitro evaluation of povidone-iodine and chlorhexidine against methicillin resistant Staphylococcus aureus. *Journal of Hospital Infection*, **21**, 291–299.

Meade, R.H. (1968) *An Introduction to the History of General Surgery*. W.B. Saunders Philadelphia, PA.

Mengistu, Y., Erge, W., Bellete, B. (1999) In vitro susceptibility of gram-negative bacterial isolates to chlorhexidine gluconate. *East African Medical Journal*, **76** (5), 243–246.

Merchant, J. (1988) Aseptic technique reconsidered. *Care, Science and Practice*, 6 (3), 74–77.

Michel, D., Zach, G.A. (1997) Antiseptic efficacy of disinfecting solutions in suspension test in vitro against methicillin-resistant Staphylococcus aureus, Pseudomonas aeruginosa and Escherichia coli in pressure sore wounds after spinal cord injury. *Dermatology*, **195** (suppl 2), 36–41.

Millward, J. (1989) Assessment of wound management in a Care of the Elderly unit. *Care, Science and Practice*, **7** (2), 47–49.

Misirlioglu, A., Eroglu, S., Karacaoglan, N., Akan, M., Akoz, T., Yildirim, S. (2003) The use of honey as an adjunct in the healing of split-thickness skin graft donor site. *Dermatologic Surgery*, **29** (2), 168–172.

Molan, P.C. (1999) The role of honey in the management of wounds. *Journal of Wound Care*, **8** (8), 415–418.

Moore, O.A., Smith, L.A., Campbell, F., Seers, K., McQuay, H.J., Moore, R.A. (2001) Systematic review of the use of honey as a wound dressing. *BMC Complementary and Alternative Medicine*, **1** (1), 2.

Morgan, D. (1993) Is there still a role for antiseptics? *Journal of Tissue Viability*, **3** (3), 80–84.

Morgan, D. (1995) Myiasis: the rise and fall of maggot therapy. *Journal of Tissue Viability*, **5** (2), 43–51.

Morykwas, M.J., Argenta, L.C., Shelton-Brown, E.I., McGuirt, W. (1997) Vacuum-assisted closure: a new method for wound control and treatment: animal studies and basic foundation. *Annals of Plastic Surgery*, **38**, 553–562.

Moues, C.M., Vos, M.C., van den Bemd, G.J., Stijen, T., Hovius, S.E. (2004) Bacterial load in relation to vacuum-assisted closure: a prospective, randomised trial. *Wound Repair and Regeneration*, **12** (1), 11–17.

Murray, Y. (1988) An investigation into the care of wounds in a health authority. *Care, Science and Practice*, **6** (4), 97–102.

Myers, J.A. (1982) Modern plastic surgical dressings. *Health and Social Services Journal*, **92**, 336–337.

Myers, S.R., Grady, J., Soranzo, C. *et al.* (1997) A hyaluronic acid membrane delivery system for cultured keratinocytes: clinical "take" rates in the porcine keratodermal model. *Journal of Burn Care Rehabilitation*, **18**, 214–222.

Neubauer, G., Ujlaky, R. (2003) The cost-effectiveness of topical negative pressure versus other wound-healing therapies. *Journal of Wound Care*, **12** (10), 392–393.

Newton, D.J., Khan, F., Belch, J.J., Mitchell, M.R., Leese, G.P. (2002) Blood flow changes in diabetic foot ulcers treated with dermal replacement therapy. *Journal of Foot and Ankle Surgery*, **41** (4), 233–237.

Omar, A.A., Mavor, A.I.D., Jones, A.M., Homer-Vanniasinkam, S. (2004) Treatment of venous leg ulcers with Dermagraft™. *European Journal of Endovascular Surgery*, **27**, 666–672.

O'Mathuna, D.P., Ashford, R.L. (2004) Therapeutic touch for healing acute wounds (Cochrane Review). Cochrane Library, Issue 2. John Wiley, Chichester.

O'Toole, E.A., Goel, M., Woodley, D.T. (1996) Hydrogen peroxide inhibits human keratinocyte migration. *Dermatology Surgery*, **22** (6), 525–529.

Paterson, L.M. (1988) Military surgery: knights, sergeants and Ramon of Avignon's version of Chirugia of Roger of Salerno, in (eds) Harper-Bus, C., Harvey, R., *The Ideals and Practice of Medieval Knighthood*. The Bodell Press, Woodbridge, Suffork.

Popp, A.J. (1995) Crossroads at Salerno: Eldridge Campbell and the writings of Teodorico Borgognoni on wound healing. *Journal of Neurosurgery*, **83**, 174–179.

Redekop, W.K., McDonnell, J., Verboom, P., Lovas, K., Kalo, Z. (2003) The cost effectiveness of Apligraf in the treatment of diabetic foot ulcers. *Pharmacoeconomics*, **21** (16), 1171–1183.

Rees, J.E. (2003) Where have all the bubbles gone? An ode to hydrogen peroxide, the champagne of all wound cleaners. *Accident and Emergency Nursing*, **11**, 82–84.

Reynolds, J.E.F. (ed.) (1982) *Martindale: The Extra Pharmacopoeia*, 28th edn. Pharmaceutical Press, London.

Robson, M.C., Mustoe, T.A., Hunt, T.K. (1998) The future of recombinant growth factors in wound healing. *American Journal of Surgery*, **176** (suppl 2A), 80S–82S.

Rode, H., Hanslo, D., de Wet, P.M., Millar, A.J., Cywes, S. (1989) Efficacy of mupirocin in methicillin-resistant staphylococcus aureus burn wound infection. *Antimicrobial Agents and Chemotherapy*, **33** (8), 1358–1361.

Russell, A.D., Hugo, W.B., Ayliffe, G.A.J. (1982) *Principles and Practice of Disinfection, Preservation and Sterilisation*. Blackwell Scientific Publications, London.

Schonfeld, W.H., Villa, K.F., Fastenau, J.M., Mazonson, P.D., Falanga, V. (2001) An economic assessment of Apligraf (Graftskin) for the treatment of hard-to-heal venous leg ulcers. *Wound Repair and Regeneration*, **8** (4), 251–257.

Schulz, G.S., Sibbald, R.G., Falanga, V. *et al.* (2003) Wound bed preparation: a systematic approach to wound management. *Wound Repair and Regeneration*, **11** (2) (suppl), S1–S28.

Sherman, R.A. (1997) A new dressing design for use with maggot therapy. *Plastic and Reconstructive Surgery*, **100** (2), 451–456.

Selvaggi, G., Monstrey, S., Van Landuyt, K., Hamdi, M., Blondeel, P. (2003) The role of iodine in antisepsis and wound management: a reappraisal. *Acta Chirurgica Belgica*, **103** (3), 241–247.

Sinclair, R.D., Ryan, T.J. (1993) A great war for antiseptics. *Wound Management*, **4** (1), 16–18.

Sleigh, J.W., Linter, S.P.K. (1985) Hazards of hydrogen peroxide. *British Medical Journal*, **291**, 1706.

Spencer, M.J., Herrick, S.E., Shah, M. *et al.* (1996) Growth factor therapy: redressing the balance, in (eds) Cherry, G.W., Gottrup, F., Lawrence, J.C., Moffatt, C.J., Turner, T.D., *Proceedings of the 5th European Conference on Advances in Wound Management.* Macmillan Magazines Ltd, London.

Subrahmanyam, M. (1998) A prospective randomised clinical and histological study of superficial burn wound healing with honey and silver sulphadiazine. *Burns*, **24** (2), 157–161.

Taddeucci, P., Pianigiani, E., Colletta, V., Torasso, F., Andreassi, L., Andreassi, A. (2004) An evaluation of Hyalofill-F plus compression bandaging in the treatment of chronic venous ulcers. *Journal of Wound Care*, **13** (5), 202–204.

Tatnall, F.M., Leigh, I.M., Gibson, J.R. (1990) Comparative study of antiseptic toxicity on basal keratinocytes, transformed human keratinocytes and fibroblasts. *Skin Pharmacology*, **3** (3), 157–163.

Thomas, S. (1990) Eusol revisited. *Dressing Times*, **3** (1), 3–4.

Thomas, S., Jones, M., Shutler, S., Jones, S. (1996) Using larvae in modern wound management. *Journal of Wound Care*, **5** (2), 60–69.

Thomlinson, D. (1987) To clean or not to clean. *Nursing Times*, **83** (9), 71–75.

Tredget, E.E., Shankowsky, H.A., Groeneveld, A., Burrell, R. (1998) A matched-pair, randomised study evaluating the efficacy and safety of Acticoat™ silver coated dressing for the treatment of burn wounds. *Journal of Burn Care and Rehabilitation*, **19** (6), 531–537.

Trevelyn, J. (1997) Spirit of the beehive. *Nursing Times*, **93** (7), 72–74.

Trevelyn, J., Booth, B. (1994) *Complementary Medicine for Nurses, Midwives and Health Visitors*, Macmillan Press, London.

Trilla, A., Miro, J.M. (1995) Identifying high risk patients for staphylococcus aureus infections: skin and soft tissue infections. *Journal of Chemotherapy*, **7** (suppl 3), 37–43.

Turner, T.D. (1986) Recent advances in wound management products, in (eds) Turner, T.D., Schmidt, R.J., Harding, K.G., *Advances in Wound Management.* John Wiley, Chichester.

Vandeputte, J., Van Waeyenberge (2003) Clinical evaluation of L-Mesitran™ – a honey-based ointment. *EWMA Journal*, **3** (2), 8–11.

Vazquez, J.R., Short, B., Findlow, A.H., Nixon, B.P., Boulton, A.J.M., Armstrong, D.G. (2003) Outcomes of hyaluronan therapy in diabetic foot wounds. *Diabetes Research and Clinical Practice*, **59**, 123–127.

Veves, A., Falanga, V., Armstrong, D.G., Sabolinski, M.L. (2001) Graftskin, a human skin equivalent, is effective in the management of noninfected neuropathic diabetic foot ulcers: a prospective multicentre clinical trial. *Diabetes Care*, **24** (2), 290–295.

Veves, A., Sheehan, P., Pham, H.T. (2002) A randomised, controlled trial of Promogran (a collagen/oxidised regenerated cellulose dressing) vs standard treatment in the management of diabetic foot ulcers. *Archives of Surgery*, **137** (7), 822–827.

Vickers, A. (1997) Yes, but how do we know it's true? Knowledge claims in massage and aromatherapy. *Complementary Therapy in Nursing and Midwifery*, **3** (3), 63–65.

Vin, F., Teot, L., Meaume, S. (2002) The healing properties of Promogran in venous leg ulcers. *Journal of Wound Care*, **11** (9), 335–341.

Walsh, M., Ford, P. (1989) *Nursing Rituals, Research and Rational Actions*. Heinneman Nursing, Oxford.

Wang, C., Schwaitzberg, S., Berliner, E., Zarin, D.A., Lau, J. (2003) Hyperbaric oxygen for treating wounds: a systematic review of the literature. *Archives of Surgery*, **138** (3), 272–279.

Weed, T., Ratcliff, C., Drake, D.B. (2004) Quantifying bacterial bioburden during negative pressure therapy: does the wound VAC enhance bacterial clearance? *Annals of Plastic Surgery*, **52** (3), 276–280.

World Health Organisation (WHO) (1983) *Traditional Medicine and Health-Care Coverage*. World health Organisation, Geneva.

Wright, J.B., Lam, K., Burrell, R.E. (1998a) Wound management in an era of increasing bacterial antibiotic resistance: a role for topical silver treatment. *American Journal of Infection Control*, **26** (6), 572–577.

Wright, K.A., Nadire, K.B., Busto, P., Tubo, R., McPherson, J.M., Wentworth, B.M. (1998b) Alternative delivery of keratinocytes using polyurethane membrane and the implications for its use in the treatment of full-thickness burn injury. *Burns*, **24** (1), 7–17.

Zhou, L.H., Nahm, W.K., Badiavas, E., Yufit, T., Falanga, V. (2002) Slow-release iodine preparation and wound healing: in vitro effects consistent with lack of in vitro toxicity in human chronic wounds. *British Journal of Dermatology*, **146**, 365–374.

Zimmerman, L.M., Veith, I. (1961) *Great Ideas in the History of Surgery*. Williams and Wilkins, Baltimore, MD.

Chapter 5
The Management of Patients with Chronic Wounds

5.1 INTRODUCTION

Fowler (1990) defined a chronic wound as one where there is tissue deficit as the result of long-standing injury or insult or frequent recurrence. Despite medical or nursing care, they do not heal easily. They are more likely to occur in the elderly or those with multisystem problems. This section will consider the care of patients with pressure ulcers, leg ulcers, diabetic foot ulcers and fungating wounds.

Chronic wounds cause much discomfort and pain for the many people who have to suffer them. A multidisciplinary approach is needed for their management and prevention. Nurses can play an important role in the team as they usually have the most contact with the patient. An essential part of this role is communication and co-operation across the disciplines. Healing is not possible for all chronic wounds and in those cases, the goal is to assist the patient to achieve the maximum independence and function possible.

It cannot be denied that the treatment of chronic wounds is costly. Harding (1998) suggests that chronic wounds cost the National Health Service (NHS) about £1 bn a year. The Department of Health calculates the costs for inpatient treatments by category. Although there is no specific category for chronic wounds, they fit within the category of 'skin ulcers'. The costs for skin ulcers for the year 2000 were nearly £4.5 million and the average length of stay was 21 days. In comparison, inpatient treatment for diabetes was just under £2.5 million. These figures are very limited as they only include costs for inpatients with skin ulcer as a primary diagnosis and they do not include community costs, which can be considerable as many of these patients are primarily cared for in the community.

5.2 THE PREVENTION AND MANAGEMENT OF PRESSURE ULCERS

Pressure ulcers are also called pressure sores, bed sores and decubitus ulcers. A pressure ulcer can be described as localised damage to the skin caused by disruption of the blood supply to the area, usually as a result of pressure, shear or friction or a combination of any of these. There has not been a national survey of pressure ulcer prevalence in the UK but a series of surveys by O'Dea (1999) of hospital patients in 35 acute care hospitals, carried out between 1992 and

1998, provides some information. O'Dea found a gradual decline in pressure ulcer prevalence rates from 18.6% in 1992 to 10% in 1997–1998. The fifth national survey in the USA was undertaken in 356 acute care hospitals in 1999 (Amlung *et al.*, 2001). The researchers found a pressure ulcer prevalence of 14.8%, an increase on previous surveys. They also found a nosocomial rate of 7.1%. Kaltenthaler *et al.* (2001) compared prevalence and incidence data of surveys undertaken in the UK, USA and Canada and found large variations in methods, patient groups and prevalence, making comparisons difficult. They noted one unexpected finding – none of the studies undertaken during the period 1976–1997 had a prevalence rate below 5%. They suggested that there may be a point beyond which it is difficult to reduce prevalence rates further.

Prevalence surveys have been undertaken in a number of other countries, with variable results. Bours *et al.* (2002) report on a national survey in the Netherlands that showed a prevalence rate of 23.1% whereas a national survey in Iceland found a prevalence rate of 8.9% (Thoroddsen, 1999). A survey across 18 rural hospitals in Australia identified a rate of 6% (Pearson *et al.*, 2000) and in Sweden a similar survey identified 3.75% of patients with pressure ulcers (Lingren *et al.*, 2000). It is difficult to draw conclusions from this wide range of prevalence rates, mostly because of the variation in methods. However, the fact that they have been carried out at all demonstrates the increasing interest in the topic.

For many years pressure ulcers were seen as a failure of care, in particular as the result of bad nursing. Florence Nightingale (1861) considered that good nursing could prevent them whereas a very influential French doctor called Jean-Martin Charcot (1825–1893) believed that doctors could do nothing about pressure ulcers. As a result, pressure ulcers became a very emotive issue and were only discussed by doctors as 'a nursing problem' and by nurses with comments like 'we do not have pressure ulcers here'.

This attitude is changing. A document published by the Department of Health stated that pressure ulcers should be considered a key indicator of the quality of care provided by a hospital (DoH, 1993). There is a much greater awareness that all healthcare professionals need to be involved in pressure ulcer prevention (Culley, 1998). A number of multidisciplinary societies have been formed, such as the Tissue Viability Society and the European Pressure Ulcer Advisory Panel, with the intent of expanding knowledge and supporting good practice and there are now NICE guidelines available. As all topics for guideline development have to be agreed by the Secretary of State for Health, this indicates the level of interest in the Department of Health.

5.2.1 The cost of pressure ulcers

A recent cost-model for pressure ulcers undertaken in the Netherlands calculated that the cost of treatment ranged from $362 m to $2.8 bn and potentially used 1% of the total Dutch healthcare budget (Severens *et al.*, 2002). Bennett *et al.* (2004) also used a cost-model to calculate the cost of treating pressure ulcers in the UK. They found the costs to be even greater than those in the Netherlands, as they ranged from £1.4 bn to £2.1 bn annually, which represented about 4% of NHS expenditure. It is less easy to measure the cost to either the individual or the state in terms of loss of earnings and state support and no figures are currently available to determine the overall cost.

Other studies have addressed the measurement of costs in other ways. Allman *et al.* (1999) measured hospital costs and length of stay in patients developing pressure ulcers in a university teaching hospital. After adjusting the costs for admission characteristics and hospital complications, they found that the mean cost of patients who developed pressure ulcers was $1877 greater than those who did not and their length of stay was 4.0 days longer. Lapsley and Vogels (1996) looked at the cost of pressure ulcers in patients who had undergone surgery either for hip replacement or coronary artery bypass graft. They found a significantly longer stay for those patients who developed pressure ulcers compared with those who did not. Stordeur *et al.* (1998) also studied patients undergoing cardiovascular surgery. They found that total length of stay was longer by a mean of six days for those who developed pressure ulcers.

A classic study by Hibbs (1988) calculated that the cost of treating one patient with a deep sacral pressure ulcer was £25 905.58. This patient was in hospital for 180 days. A further calculation looked at the opportunity costs, which describe what has been foregone because of specific circumstances. For example, because of the extended stay in hospital of this patient, the opportunity to carry out 16 routine hip or knee replacements was lost. Similar calculations can also be made looking at standard days and standard costs. A critique of this work was undertaken by two economists, nine years later (Brookes & Thompson, 1997). They support Hibbs' approach and regret that there have been few economic appraisals in relation to pressure sore prevention.

Another cost that has to be taken into consideration is that of litigation. Tingle (1997) described a number of legal cases where the patient or their families were awarded damages ranging from £3500 to £12 500. More recently, McKeeney (2002) described two cases in which the settlements were £32 000 and £14 000. In all of these cases there is a chronicle of incompetence and negligent care. In some instances the pressure ulcer directly contributed to the patient's death. Allied to this, there is often inadequate assessment and poor documentation. Compliance with clinical guidelines could, potentially, reduce the level of litigation, as discussed by Goebel and Goebel (1999) in an analysis of the situation in the USA. However, not all patients wish to comply with a guideline-derived treatment plan (McKeeney, 2002). Patients have a right to refuse treatment if they wish but it is incumbent upon the nurse to clearly explain the possible risks and record the matter in detail.

5.2.2 The aetiology of pressure ulcers

Pressure ulcers are caused by a combination of external factors and factors within the patient.

Extrinsic factors

There are three extrinsic factors that can cause pressure ulcers either on their own or in any combination of the three. They are pressure, shear and friction.

Pressure is the most important factor in pressure ulcer development. When the soft tissue of the body is compressed between a bony prominence and a hard surface, causing pressures greater than capillary pressure, localised ischaemia occurs. The normal body response to such pressure is to shift position so the pressure is redistributed. When pressure is relieved a red area appears over the bony prominence. This is called reactive hyperaemia and is the result of a temporarily increased blood supply to the area, removing waste products and bringing oxygen and nutrients. It is a normal physiological response.

Capillary pressure is generally described as being approximately 32 mmHg, based on the research of Landis (1931). His research was carried out on young, healthy students. He found the average arteriolar pressure was 32 mmHg but the average pressure in the venules was 12 mmHg. There is also a certain amount of tissue tension that resists deformation. It is not uncommon for interface pressures of around 30–40 mmHg to be seen as 'safe' but this is not always correct. Ageing causes a reduction in the numbers of elastic fibres in the tissues, resulting in reduced tissue tension. In situations where the blood pressure is artificially lowered, such as during some types of surgery, capillary pressure is also likely to be lower. In these circumstances, very little pressure is required to cause capillary occlusion. Ek et al. (1987) found that a pressure of only 11 mmHg was necessary to cause capillary occlusion in some hemiplegic patients.

If unrelieved pressure persists for a long period of time, tissue necrosis will follow. Prolonged pressure causes distortion of the soft tissues and results in destruction of tissue close to the bone. A cone-shaped ulcer is created, with the widest part of the cone close to the bone and the narrowest on the body surface. Thus, the visible ulcer fails to reveal the true extent of tissue damage. The bony prominences that are most vulnerable to pressure ulcer development are sometimes referred to as the pressure areas. They include the sacrum, ischial tuberosities, trochanters, heels and elbows (see Fig. 5.1).

Some authors have discussed the possibility that pressure damage actually results from repeated ischaemia-reperfusion injury (Houwing et al., 2000; Mustoe, 2004). In simple terms, this suggests that the precipitating factor in pressure ulcer development is repeated periods of ischaemia followed by repeated periods of reperfusion that trigger a series of cellular events. These events result in a lack of tissue perfusion (no-reflow phenomenon) that occurs in reperfusion injury. Mustoe (2004) suggests that the elderly (or their aged cells) are less able to cope with this situation than those younger, so that repeated ischaemia-reperfusion injury results in a cycle of inflammation and protease and oxidant injury leading to tissue necrosis. Two research groups have been able to demonstrate this cycle of events using an animal model (Houwing et al., 2000; Peirce et al., 2000).

Gebhardt (1995) argues that pressure is rarely applied uniformly and that the subsequent distortion leads to shearing. Shear forces can deform and disrupt tissue and so damage the blood vessels. Shearing may occur if the patient slides down the bed. The skeleton and tissues nearest to it move but the skin on the buttocks remains still. One of the main culprits of shearing is the backrest of

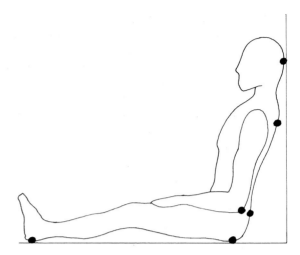

Fig. 5.1   The bony prominences.

the bed which encourages sliding. Chairs that fail to maintain a good posture may also cause shearing. Friction occurs when two surfaces rub together. The commonest cause is when the patient is dragged rather than lifted across the bed which causes the top layers of epithelial cells to be scraped off. Moisture, which exacerbates the effect of friction, may be found on a patient's skin as a result of excessive sweating or urinary incontinence.

Intrinsic factors

The human body is frequently subjected to some or all of the extrinsic factors but does not automatically develop pressure ulcers. The determining factor(s) come from within the patient.

General health is important as the body can withstand greater external pressure in health than when sick. Bliss (1990) suggested that the acutely ill are particularly vulnerable. Although the reasons for this are not certain, Bliss listed some precipitating factors including pain, low blood pressure, heart failure, the use of sedatives, vasomotor failure, peripheral vasoconstriction due to shock and others. Margolis *et al.* (2003) studied 75 168 older adults on the UK General Practitioner Research Database and identified those with pressure ulcers (1.61%). They found a number of medical conditions that were significantly associated with pressure ulcers: Alzheimer's disease, congestive heart failure, chronic obstructive pulmonary disease, cerebral vascular accident, diabetes mellitus, deep venous thrombosis, hip fracture, hip surgery, limb paralysis, lower limb oedema, malignancy, malnutrition, osteoporosis, Parkinson's disease, rheumatoid arthritis and urinary tract infections. It is interesting to note that many of these conditions are also on the list put forward by Bliss (1990), based on her extensive clinical experience.

Age is a major factor in the development of pressure ulcers, as shown by early studies such as those of David *et al.* (1983), Nyquist and Hawthorn (1987) and also Thoroddsen (1999). Bergstrom *et al.* (1996) studied a sample of 843 patients in a variety of care settings over a period of four weeks for the incidence of pressure ulcers. They found that those who developed pressure ulcers were significantly older than those who did not.

As people age, their skin becomes thinner and less elastic. In part, this is because the collagen in the dermis reduces in quantity and quality. Collagen provides a buffer that helps to prevent disruption of the microcirculation (Krouskop, 1983). There may be wasting of the overall body mass, resulting in loose folds of skin. There is also an increased likelihood of chronic illness or disease developing, many of which may also predispose to pressure ulcer development. Once an ulcer occurs it is much harder to heal in an older person than a young one (see Chapter 2).

Reduced mobility can affect the ability to relieve pressure effectively, if at all. It also predisposes to shearing and friction if the patient is confined to bed or chair. General prevalence surveys, such as those of David *et al.* (1983), Nyquist and Hawthorn (1987) and Bergstrom *et al.* (1996), found reduced mobility to be a factor for many patients with pressure ulcers. In their study of 109 long-term care facilities, Horn *et al.* (2002) also found reduced mobility to be a significant factor for those who developed pressure ulcers. In a similar study of 2015 patients in long-term care facilities, Baumgarten *et al.* (2003a) also found immobility to be a factor. A classic study by Versluysen (1986) studied 100 patients over the age of 60 years with a fractured femur and found an incidence of 66%. Much attention has subsequently been paid to the management of this group of patients and a study by Baumgarten *et al.* (2003b) of elderly patients with hip facture has a pressure ulcer incidence rate of 8.8%.

Exton-Smith and Sherwin (1961) studied the number of movements made by 50 elderly patients during the night. A strong relationship was found between those with reduced movement and the development of pressure ulcers. Reduced movement during sleep may be associated with a variety of drugs such as hypnotics, anxiolytics, antidepressants, opioid analgesics and antihistamines. Berlowitz and Wilking (1989) studied a variety of factors in patients with pressure ulcers and patients developing pressure ulcers and found that reduced mobility was significantly associated with pressure ulcers in both groups. Brandeis *et al.* (1994) also found reduced mobility to be a significant factor in a study involving nursing home patients.

Another aspect of reduced mobility is that of the patient undergoing major surgery. Operations may last many hours whilst the patient lies immobile on the operating table. Mobility may be reduced in the immediate postoperative period because of the effects of the anaesthetic, pain, analgesia, infusions or drains. Today very sophisticated surgery is carried out, often on the older patient. The risks of pressure ulcer development associated with such surgery are consequently increased. Schoonhoven *et al.* (2002a) observed 208 patients undergoing surgery lasting at least four hours and found that 44 (21.2%) developed pressure ulcers within two days of surgery. The research team also identified possible risk indicators in these surgical patients and found that the only predictor of pressure ulcer development was length of surgery (Schoonhoven *et al.*, 2002b). This outcome replicates the finding of Aronovitch (1999) who found that the incidence of pressure damage increased with the length of surgery.

Neurological deficit may be associated with reduced mobility, such as in a patient with paraplegia, but this is not always so. The diabetic may suffer from neuropathy without loss of mobility. Neurological deficit may be associated with strokes, multiple sclerosis, diabetes and spinal cord injury or degeneration. Loss of sensation means the patient is unaware of the need to relieve pressure, even if he is able to do so. Dealey (1991a) found that neurological deficit was a common factor in those patients with pressure ulcers in a survey of a teaching hospital. Kabagambe *et al.* (1994) compared ten patients with spinal cord injury with 11 healthy subjects. They found an impaired reactive hyperaemia response in those with spinal cord injury.

Reduced nutritional status impairs the elasticity of the skin. In the long term, it will lead to anaemia and a reduction of oxygen to the tissues. Poor nutrition has long been considered to be a factor in pressure ulcer development although research results are inconsistent (Langer *et al.*, 2003; Mathus-Vliegen, 2001). Some studies, such as those of Berlowitz and Wilking (1989), Brandeis *et al.* (1994) and Williams *et al.* (2000), found impaired nutritional intake to be a factor in pressure ulcer development. Guenter *et al.* (2000) found that newly hospitalised patients with grade 3 or 4 pressure ulcers had malnutrition. The factors that may lead to malnutrition are discussed in Chapter 2.

Body weight should also be considered. Very emaciated patients have no 'padding' over bony prominences and so have less protection against pressure. On the other hand, very obese patients are difficult to move. Unless great care is taken, they may be dragged rather than lifted in the bed. Another problem of the obese patient is that moisture from sweating may become trapped between the rolls of fat, causing maceration. Both of these types of patient may also have a poor nutritional status.

Incontinence of urine can contribute to maceration of the skin and thus increase the risk of friction. Constant washing because of either urinary or faecal incontinence removes natural body oils, drying the skin. Urinary incontinence may be caused by the use of diuretics or sedatives. Diarrhoea may cause incontinence in the elderly or immobile patient and is a side effect of some antibiotics. There is no clear evidence as to whether incontinence is a risk factor for pressure ulcer development or not. Baumgarten *et al.* (2003a) found faecal incontinence to be a risk factor whereas Reed *et al.* (2003) did not. Other studies have found both urinary and faecal incontinence to be risk factors (Ferrell *et al.*, 2000; Schue & Langemo, 1999).

Poor blood supply to the periphery lowers the local capillary pressure and causes malnutrition in the tissues. It may be caused by disease, such as heart disease, peripheral vascular disease or diabetes. Bergstrom *et al.* (1996) found cardiovascular disease to be a significant predictor of pressure ulcer development. Drugs, such as beta-blockers and inotropic sympathomimetics, may cause peripheral vasoconstriction. These drugs may be used following cardiac surgery when the patient is already suffering from reduced mobility. Blood flow may also be affected during surgery. Sanada *et al.* (1997) measured blood flow during surgery in the skin over the iliac crest and sacrum. They found a 500% increase in flow in those patients who did not develop pressure sores but a drop in flow in those who later developed pressure sores. Spittle *et al.* (2001) measured the incidence of pressure ulcers in patients who had undergone lower limb amputations for either ischaemia or neuroischaemia and found an incidence rate of 55% in those who had had major amputations and 20% in minor amputees. They suggest that the presence of peripheral vascular disease may have been a risk factor for these patients.

External factors

Dealey (1997) cited a number of external factors that can exacerbate the factors discussed above. They include:

- inappropriate positioning, which may increase pressure or shear.
- restrictions to movement, such as lying for long periods on a trolley.
- lying for long periods in one position on hard surfaces, such as the X-ray table.
- poor lifting and handling techniques which increase the risk of friction and shear.
- poor hygiene that leaves the skin surface moist from urine, faeces or sweat.
- drugs such as sedatives that make the patient drowsy and less likely to move.

5.2.3 Prevention of pressure ulcers

Whilst it is a truism, as far as pressure ulcers are concerned, prevention is better than cure. Waterlow (1988) suggested that 95% of all pressure ulcers could be prevented. Although this concept was based on opinion, it has been supported by a study undertaken in Japan (Haglsawa & Barbenel, 1999) that observed the outcome of providing preventive care for at-risk patients admitted to an internal medicine ward. The researchers found an incidence rate of 4.4% in the 240 patients they studied. They suggest that this may approach the lowest rate achievable in very ill patients.

In response to the development of evidence-based guidelines, most hospital and primary care trusts use them as a framework from which a local policy may be developed. The most recent pressure ulcer prevention guidelines are those published by the National Institute for Clinical Excellence (NICE, 2003). The guidelines can be divided into sections on risk assessment, pressure ulcer prevention, education and training and they will be used to provide a framework for this next section. They are also summarised in a useful poster that can be downloaded from www.nice.org.uk.

Identify individuals vulnerable to or at elevated risk of pressure ulcers

Too often, risk assessment is just seen as using a risk calculator to determine the patient's score and then following a 'recipe' of care. The first part of the assessment guidance is listed in Box 5.1 and describes some of the issues about

---

Box 5.1   NICE Clinical Guideline 7: pressure ulcer prevention. Assessment of patients to determine risk of pressure ulcer development.*

- Assessing an individual's risk of developing pressure ulcers should involve both informal and formal assessment procedures.
- Risk assessment should be carried out by personnel who have undergone appropriate training to recognise the risk factors that contribute to the development of pressure ulcers and know how to initiate and maintain correct and suitable preventive measures.
- The timing of risk assessment should be based on each individual case. However, it should take place within six hours of the start of admission to the episode of care.
- If an individual is not considered to be vulnerable to or at elevated risk of pressure ulcers on initial assessment, reassessment should occur if there is a change in an individual's condition that increases risk.
- All formal assessments of risk should be documented/recorded and made accessible to all members of the interdisciplinary team.

*(reproduced from the NICE Clinical Guideline 7: pressure ulcer prevention (2003), with permission)

---

the type, timing and documentation relating to assessment. Assessment should include identifying risk factors such as: reduced mobility, sensory impairment, acute illness, level of consciousness, extremes of age, vascular disease, severe chronic or terminal illness, previous history of pressure damage, malnutrition and dehydration (NICE, 2003). The guidelines also state that risk assessment tools or risk calculators should only be used as an *aide mémoire* and should not replace clinical judgement.

There are a number of risk calculators available. The earliest that was developed was the Norton Score (Norton *et al.*, 1975). Probably the most widely used within UK hospitals is the Waterlow Score (Waterlow, 1985) which considers a wider range of variables than the Norton. The scoring is also reversed so that the higher the score, the higher the risk. It has the advantage of dividing the degree of risk into categories: at risk, high risk and very high risk. These can be useful when considering the use of appropriate support systems. Waterlow included suggestions for preventive measures on the reverse of the card. The Braden Scale (Bergstrom *et al.*, 1985) is widely used in the USA and elsewhere. It has been demonstrated to have greater sensitivity and specificity than other scales but only if used by registered nurses (Bergstrom *et al.*, 1987).

Risk calculators have been judged according to their sensitivity and specificity. Sensitivity relates to the percentage of patients predicted to develop pressure ulcers, who have gone on to develop them. Specificity is defined as the percentage of patients deemed not to be at risk who do not develop pressure ulcers (Anthony, 1996). Bridel (1993) found that the Waterlow Score had a high sensitivity but a lower specificity whereas the reverse was true for the Braden Scale. However, the effect of nursing care may be responsible, rather than failure of the calculator. Deeks (1996) suggests that where sensitivity and specificity appear to be poor, it is often in settings where effective prevention methods are being used.

Schoonhoven *et al.* (2002b) compared the Norton, Braden and Waterlow scores for 1229 patients admitted to one of two acute hospitals and found that none of them was able to satisfactorily predict all patients who developed pressure ulcers. They suggest that this is because the components of the calculators are based on clinical observation rather than prognostic research. Papanikolaou *et al.* (2002) undertook secondary analysis of data collected for a prospective study of 213 inpatients and determined that a modified version of the Waterlow Score was more accurate than the original but only in the case of the specific patient group on whom it was tested. The researchers suggest that larger studies of high-quality data are necessary in order to finally determine more accurately the most relevant factors to include in a risk calculator.

Despite the criticisms that can be made of the risk calculators, there is benefit in using a systematic method of assessing and identifying patients at risk of pressure ulcer development. Flanagan (1997) stresses the importance of regular assessment of patients rather than just doing one initial assessment. It should also be noted that once a patient is identified as being at risk, appropriate preventive action must follow. Failure to do so would be a failure in the duty of care that all nurses have to their patients.

Skin inspection

There is a natural resilience in skin that enables the healthy individual to overcome many of the problems of friction or shear met in everyday life. It makes sense to utilise these properties and to enhance them where possible. Skin assessment should be undertaken daily for the at-risk patient. The NICE guidelines on skin inspection can be seen in Box 5.2. Where possible, the patient and/or carer should be involved in this process. Any alterations in skin status should be recorded immediately. Unqualified staff should be alerted to the need to inform a qualified nurse as a change in the plan of care may be required.

Skin assessment is important in two ways. It provides baseline data of the initial skin status at the beginning of a care episode and it provides ongoing information of the effectiveness of the prevention plan. Skin inspection should encompass the following.

- Assessment of the bony prominences, remembering that emaciated patients may develop sores in uncommon areas, e.g. ribs.
- Skin status should be identified – areas of dryness, fragility, erythema or maceration are all vulnerable to tissue damage.
- Skin colour – dark skin is more difficult to assess for early signs of tissue damage; watch for dryness, cracking or induration.

Pressure ulcer prevention

Positioning

Relief of pressure is the main strategy used in the prevention of pressure ulcers. The commonest method is that of repositioning the patient. Clark (1998) undertook a systematic review of the literature to determine the evidence

---

Box 5.2   NICE Clinical Guideline 7: pressure ulcer prevention. Skin inspection.*

- Skin inspection should occur regularly and the frequency determined in response to changes in the individual's condition in relation to either deterioration or recovery.
- Skin inspection should be based on an assessment of the most vulnerable areas of risk for each patient. These are typically: heels; sacrum; ischial tuberosities; parts of the body affected by antiembolic stockings; femoral trochanters; parts of the body where pressure, friction or shear is exerted in the course of an individual's daily living activities; parts of the body where there are external forces exerted by equipment and/or clothing; elbows; temporal region of the skull; shoulders; back of head and toes. Other areas should be inspected as necessitated by the patient's condition.
- Individuals who are willing and able should be encouraged, following education, to inspect their own skin.
- Individuals who are wheelchair users should use a mirror to inspect the areas that they cannot see easily or get others to inspect them.
- Healthcare professionals should be aware of the following signs, which may indicate incipient pressure ulcer development: persistent erythema; non-blanching hyperaemia previously identified as non-blanching erythema; blisters; discolouration; localised heat; localised oedema; and localised induration. In those with darkly pigmented skin: purplish/bluish localised areas of skin; localised heat that, if tissue becomes damaged, is replaced by coolness; localised oedema; and localised induration.
- Skin changes should be documented/recorded immediately.

*(reproduced from the NICE Clinical Guideline 7: pressure ulcer prevention (2003), with permission)

---

demonstrating the effectiveness of repositioning as preventive strategy. He concluded that not only was there little evidence to determine the appropriate frequency of repositioning, there was little evidence to show its effectiveness in preventing pressure ulcers, despite it being an internationally used nursing strategy. More recently, Defloor *et al.* (2005) undertook a study to measure the effectiveness of a range of turning regimes on two types of mattress. They were: turning every two hours or every four hours on a standard hospital mattress, and turning every four hours or every six hours on a viscoelastic polyurethane foam mattress. They found a significantly lower incidence of pressure ulcers in the group that received the pressure-reducing mattress and four-hourly turning compared with two-hourly turning on a standard mattress.

An alternative to traditional side-to-side turning of patients is the 30° tilt. This method of positioning patients was developed in a younger disabled unit (Preston, 1988). The position is achieved by placing pillows in such a manner that the patient is tilted as shown in Figure 5.2. Once in position, there is no pressure on the sacrum or heels. The interface pressure on the buttock is around 25 mmHg. Colin *et al.* (1996a) compared the effect of the 90° lateral position with the 30° tilt and found significant hypoxaemia over the trochanter in the former position but none in the latter.

In the 30° tilt, patients can be left for increasingly longer periods without turning, although careful observation must be made of all vulnerable areas. Once patients have become accustomed to using the 30° tilt, they may be left

The 30° tilt is a useful method for positioning patients who are difficult to turn or are not able to lie on their side. Patients may be safely left for long periods in this position but the pressure areas should be carefully monitored to establish an appropriate time for each patient.

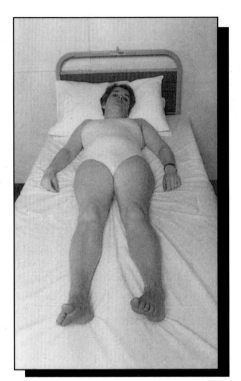

1 Place the patient in the centre of the bed with sufficient pillows to support the head and neck.

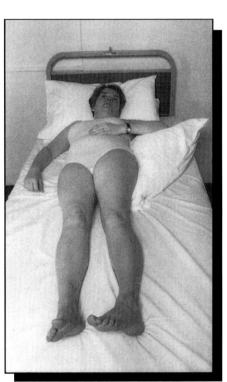

2 Place a pillow at an angle under one buttock; thus tilting the pelvis by 30°. Check with a flattened hand that the sacrum is just clear of the mattress.

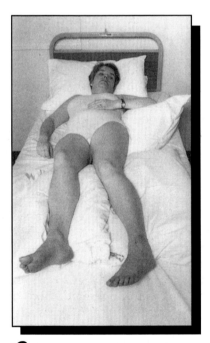

3 Place a pillow lengthways under each leg so that the heels are lifted clear of the bed.

The patient may be turned by removing the pillow under the buttock and placing it under the other buttock.

This can be done by two nurses rolling the patient slightly. No lifting is necessary.

Fig. 5.2 The 30° tilt position.

for up to eight hours without turning. Not only does this allow a patient to have an undisturbed night's sleep but also it is of great benefit for use in the community. This method of positioning is not suitable for all patients, as shown by Young (2004) who randomised 46 elderly acutely ill patients to either 30° or 90° lying. She found that many of the patients were unable to maintain the 30° position and questioned the value of the widespread advice to use it. It seems reasonable to conclude that further evidence is needed to determine when it may best be used. In the meantime, nurses should know how to use the position but should recognise that it probably has limited value for the acutely ill, conscious patient.

The use of correct positioning and repositioning techniques, as well as appropriate methods for transferring patients from one surface to another, will reduce both friction and shear forces. Incorrect positions in either bed or chair can cause patients to slide. Regular moving of patients puts nurses at risk of back injury. The European Community directive on the moving and handling of heavy loads states that all healthcare institutions must have a policy for manual handling and staff should have regular training on correct methods of moving patients. Hoists, slides and other aids for moving patients should be available. The RCN (2003) code of practice suggests that manual handling should be eliminated in all but exceptional or life-threatening situations. All nurses have a responsibility to take reasonable care for their own safety and that of patients and colleagues.

Seating

● *Chairs* ●

Most of the research in relation to pressure-redistributing equipment has involved mattresses and beds rather than seating and yet sitting vulnerable patients in armchairs is part of the routine rehabilitation process for many (McCafferty *et al.*, 2000). In many instances, hospital armchairs have been purchased without any reference to clinical staff or the varied needs of patients (Collins, 1999; McCafferty *et al.*, 2000). Once ill patients start to sit out of bed, they are perceived to be 'mobile' and so may be left in a chair for long periods of time without being moved. The NICE guidelines suggest that patients at risk of pressure ulcer development should not be sat in a chair for more than two hours at a time (NICE, 2003).

Many hospital armchairs are in a poor state and fail to give any pressure relief or maintain a good posture (Dealey *et al.*, 1991). Chairs should be checked and replaced or repaired in the same way as mattresses. Many chairs have a reclining back of between 15° and 40° that puts the patient in a semi-reclining posture. This may make it more difficult for the patient to stand. Ideally, a chair should have a recline of not more than 10°, enabling the patient to move more freely. Although cushions may be added to chairs to improve pressure relief, they should not make the chair so high that the patient's feet cannot touch the floor. Collins (1999) undertook a comparative study of an armchair with an integral pressure-relieving cushion and standard hospital armchairs. She found a significantly lower incidence of pressure ulcers in the experimental group compared with the control group. Conventional seating is not suitable for everyone. Some patients have severe seating problems due to contractures, deformity or infirmity. Specialised seating must be considered for these people.

● Cushions ●

Most of the research on cushions has been on those for use in wheelchairs. Wheelchairs have a canvas base, which Rithalia (1989) found exerted pressures in the region of 226 mmHg. It is essential that a cushion should always be used in a wheelchair. For those people who become wheelchair bound because of disability, special assessment should be made to identify the cushion most suited to the specific needs of the patient (NICE, 2003). Many physiotherapists and occupational therapists have developed specialist skills in assessment. There are many cushions available but there is insufficient evidence to demonstrate whether any cushion outperforms the others and so no specific recommendation can be made (NICE, 2003).

● Use of aids ●

The NICE guidelines specifically state that water-filled gloves and doughnut-type devices should not be used (NICE, 2003).

Pressure-relieving devices (beds, mattresses and overlays)

In 1995, an Effective Health Care Bulletin (1995) on pressure ulcer prevention recommended that pressure-relieving foam mattresses should be used for at-risk patients rather than the standard mattress. Since then many hospitals have replaced worn-out standard hospital mattresses with this type of mattress. In the NICE guidelines, this type of mattress is seen as a minimum provision for those at risk of pressure ulcer development (NICE, 2003).

There is an ever-increasing range of pressure-redistributing equipment available for use. They range from overlays to highly sophisticated beds and can be divided into high-tech and low-tech categories (Cullum *et al.*, 2001a). Low-tech devices conform to the shape of the body, thus 'spreading the load' and reducing the pressure over bony prominences, whereas high-tech devices are dynamic systems with various modes of action. Examples of both high- and low-tech devices are given in Box 5.3.

The NICE guidelines suggest that selection of a device should be based on a holistic assessment that includes:

- identified levels of risk.
- skin assessment.
- patient comfort.
- general health state.
- lifestyle and physical and mental abilities.
- critical care needs.
- acceptability of the proposed device to both patient and carer.

Box 5.3   Examples of high-tech and low-tech pressure redistributing devices.

Low-tech
High-spec foam (overlay, mattress)
Gel (overlay, mattress)
Fluid (overlay, mattress)
Fibre (overlay)
Air (overlay, mattress)

High-tech
Alternating air (overlay, mattress, bed)
Low air loss (overlay, mattress, bed)
Air fluidised (mattress, bed)
Turning beds (manual controls, motorised)

Whilst a risk assessment calculator may form part of the assessment, equipment selection should not be based on the score alone (NICE, 2003).

The Effective Health Care Bulletin (1995) examined the evidence regarding the range of product types available and considered that it was not possible to recommend any one product as a best buy. Sadly, this situation is unchanged and the current NICE guidelines are still unable to make specific recommendations. However, the guidelines do acknowledge that there is professional consensus that high-tech devices should be used:

- as a first-line preventive strategy for those patients seen to be at high risk of pressure ulcer development.
- if the patient's previous history in relation to pressure ulcer prevention or current clinical condition indicates that a high-tech device would be more suitable.
- if there are indications of pressure damage when on a low-tech device.

Jay (1997) suggested that cost, patient comfort, clinician satisfaction, safety and reliability and logistical factors need to be taken into consideration as well as efficacy.

● *Additions to the bed* ●

Pressure relief can be enhanced by the use of simple measures. The use of bed cradles can lift the weight of the bed clothes off the patient. Backrests are widely used but it should be remembered that they cause the patient to slide down the bed, risking damage by shearing. Strategic placing of pillows can relieve pressure on bony prominences such as heels, malleoli and knees.

● *Other hospital equipment* ●

Vulnerable patients may spend time lying or sitting on very hard surfaces such as operating tables, X-ray tables, trolleys and some types of wheelchair. Very little consideration has been given to the need to provide some sort of pressure relief in these circumstances. Versluysen (1986) undertook a study of 100 consecutive elderly patients admitted with a fractured femur. The interface pressures were measured on the casualty trolleys and operating tables. The casualty trolleys with a 5 cm deep foam mattress showed pressures of 56–60 mmHg at the sacrum and 150–160 mmHg at the heels. The operating table had interface pressures of 75–80 mmHg at the sacrum and 60–120 mmHg at the heels. NICE (2003) states that all patients undergoing surgery who are identified as being at risk of pressure ulcer development should be placed on a high-specification foam theatre mattress or similar.

● *Organisation of delivery of devices* ●

It is not practical for every clinical area to maintain their own stock of pressure-redistributing devices and many hospital and primary care trusts have some form of equipment store to ensure effective provision and use of devices. NICE (2003) states that there should be a co-ordinated approach to the acquisition, allocation and management of equipment and that prevention strategies or policies should have a specified standard time between assessment and allocation of equipment. NICE also provides guidance on auditing the use of equipment (NICE, 2003).

Every patient at risk of pressure ulcer development should have an individualised written plan of care. It is important to document all assessments and the care given. This will enable staff to monitor the effectiveness of the plan and to identify any early signs of tissue damage. It should also ensure effective use of equipment as patients may be moved to less sophisticated equipment when they no longer have need of the high-tech equipment or vice versa.

Additional prevention strategies not mentioned in the NICE guidelines
● *Skin care* ●

Traditionally, skin care involved rubbing patients' pressure areas at regular intervals. A variety of lotions and potions were used. A review of the literature by Buss *et al.* (1997) considered the effects of massage or rubbing on pressure sore prevention. They concluded that this practice could not be recommended. When the practice of rubbing was discontinued most nurses developed a reluctance to use any type of cream over the pressure areas. Whilst this is generally appropriate, there may be exceptions in the case of very dry or very moist skin. Emollients should be considered when caring for patients with very dry skin, either in the bath or an emollient cream. Creams should be applied gently to the affected area. If the skin is moist, the source of the moisture should be identified and dealt with if possible. A barrier cream may be needed to protect the skin from the harmful effects of moisture.

Frequent cleansing using soap and water for incontinent patients can cause excessive drying of the skin. Dealey and Keogh (1998) found a significant improvement in skin status using a cleanser and barrier cream compared to soap and water in elderly incontinent patients at risk of pressure sore development. Cooper and Gray (2001) undertook a similar study comparing soap and water with a combination cleanser and emollient in 93 elderly nursing home residents. They found borderline significance ($p = 0.05$) in favour of the combination cleanser and emollient. Use of these types of products provides better protection for the skin than soap and water.

● *Nutrition* ●

If nutritional assessment suggested that a patient had reduced nutritional status then an appropriate plan of care must be developed. Chapter 2 discusses this in more detail.

● *Mobility* ●

As has already been noted, pressure ulcers may be associated with acute illness. As the patient's general condition improves, so their levels of mobility and activity should increase. Some patients may require considerable rehabilitation to optimise their mobility levels. It is important that patients achieve as great a level of mobility and activity as is practical for each individual which has the additional benefit of enabling an individual to relieve pressure by movement.

● *Education and training* ●

There is little point in developing a policy for pressure ulcer prevention if no attempt is made to provide relevant education for healthcare professionals and assistants, patients and carers. A number of authors have described the beneficial outcomes of educational programmes. O'Brien *et al.* (2000) found a reduction in the biannual prevalence rate following an educational programme. Regan *et al.* (1995) and Danchaivijitr *et al.* (1995) found a reduction in pressure ulcer incidence following the introduction of a prevention programme supported by staff education. All healthcare professionals should receive education and training on pressure ulcer risk assessment and prevention (NICE, 2003). Box 5.4 lists the topics identified within the NICE guideline that should be included in an education programme. However, it is not just healthcare professionals who need education. Patients and carers also require information and this should be provided both verbally and in a written format. Information for patients and carers that is written in appropriate language can be obtained from www.nice.org.uk.

Summary

The various aspects of pressure ulcer prevention can be summarised as follows.

● Assessment: identify those at risk, assess and monitor the skin, especially bony prominences, identify continence problems.
● Plan appropriate preventive measures.
● Evaluate outcomes by maintaining vigilant skin assessment.
● Monitor all support systems, establishing replacement or maintenance programmes where appropriate.
● Ensure that staff have an adequate knowledge of the causes and prevention of pressure ulcers.

Box 5.4 NICE Clinical Guideline 7: pressure ulcer prevention. Recommended education programme content.*

- Risk factors for pressure ulcer development
- Pathophysiology of pressure ulcer development
- The limitations and potential applications of risk assessment tools
- Skin assessment
- Skin care
- Selection of pressure-relieving equipment
- Use of pressure-relieving equipment
- Methods of documenting risk assessments and prevention activities
- Positioning to minimise risk
- Shear and friction damage, including the correct use of manual handling devices
- Roles and responsibilities of interdisciplinary team members in pressure ulcer management
- Policies and procedures regarding transferring individuals between care settings
- Providing education and information to patients

*(reproduced from the NICE Clinical Guideline 7: pressure ulcer prevention (2003), with permission)

- Establish a teaching programme for long-term at-risk patients and their carers.
- Monitor outcomes of prevention strategies by measuring the prevalence and incidence of pressure ulcers.
- Audit the quality of care by utilising the benchmarking system known as the *Essence of Care* (DoH, 2003). Birchall *et al.* (2004) found it a useful tool after it had been adapted to meet local needs.

5.2.4 Management of pressure ulcers

If a pressure ulcer occurs, preventive measures should still be continued. The precise cause of the ulcer and the effectiveness of any prevention plan must be evaluated. Any necessary changes must be made, such as using a different support system or increasing proteins and vitamins in the diet. The European Pressure Ulcer Advisory Panel (EPUAP) has developed guidelines for the treatment of pressure ulcers (EPUAP, 1999) The guideline includes assessment, assessing complications, managing tissue loads, use of pressure ulcer prevention devices and wound management. Managing tissue loads and use of devices has been discussed in the previous section and the principles of wound management can be found in Chapter 3. The rest of the guideline will be used as a framework for this section.

Assessing the pressure ulcer

The EPUAP guideline states that pressure ulcers should be assessed for location, grade, size, wound bed, exudate, pain and status of surrounding skin. Also any undermining or sinus formation should be identified (EPUAP, 1999).

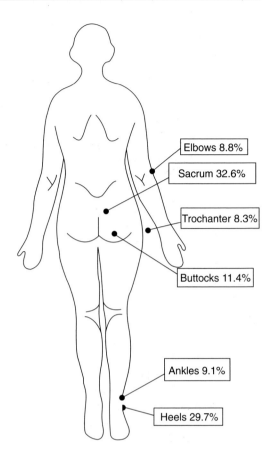

Fig. 5.3   The common position of pressure ulcers (based on Clark *et al.*, 2003).

The location of pressure ulcers

Some bony prominences are more prone to pressure ulcers than others. Clark *et al.* (2003) reported a pressure ulcer prevalence survey of nearly 6000 patients in five European countries and noted the position of the 1630 ulcers. Figure 5.3 shows the range of positions with the percentages found in each. There are some specific aspects of care that need to be considered.

- *Sacrum* – dressings must be chosen with care, as many tend to ruckle up as the patient moves. Chair sitting must be strictly regulated as to type of chair and length of time seated in it.
- *Buttocks* – as for sacrum.
- *Heels* – ideally dressings must not be too bulky as this may impede mobility. Dressings may need to be 'tailored' in order to fit correctly around the heel. If footwear is being worn, care must be taken to ensure that it is not too tight or this will exert pressure on the foot. Ensure there is adequate pressure relief when in bed.
- *Trochanters* – some dressings may ruckle up so select carefully.

- *Elbows* – these pressure ulcers are usually caused by friction from moving about the bed. Consider ways of reducing friction – use of a monkey pole, pads or semipermeable film dressings.
- *Trunk* – ulcers here are uncommon; try and identify source of pressure and remove or modify it.

Grading of pressure ulcers

The use of a recognised system of grading pressure ulcers can be helpful, as it provides an objective description and gives a more accurate picture of the amount of tissue damage than comments such as 'a deep ulcer'. It should be used in conjunction with other descriptive tools such as measuring or tracing the ulcer and describing its appearance. The EPUAP uses the following grading system.

- *Grade 1* – non-blanchable erythema of intact skin. Discolouration of the skin, warmth, oedema and induration may be used as indicators, especially for dark skin.
- *Grade 2* – partial-thickness skin loss involving epidermis and/or dermis. The ulcer is superficial and may be seen as a blister, abrasion or crater.
- *Grade 3* – full-thickness skin loss involving damage to or necrosis of subcutaneous tissue that may extend down to but not through underlying fascia.
- *Grade 4* – extensive destruction, tissue necrosis or damage to muscle, bone or supporting structures with or without full-thickness skin loss.

Figure 5.4 shows examples of each of these grades of pressure ulcer.

There are a number of issues that need to be considered when utilising any grading system: accurate identification of grade 1 ulcers, incontinence lesions, reverse grading and interrater reliability.

Grade 1 pressure ulcers are often found to account for approximately 50% of all ulcers in prevalence surveys (Halfens *et al.*, 2001). However, there are problems with both over- and underreporting. Overreporting may occur if nurses fail to differentiate between blanching and non-blanching erythema. Alternatively, underreporting may occur because of the difficulties in identifying erythema on dark skin (Scanlon & Stubbs, 2004). Attempts have been made to provide additional descriptors to the definition, as can be seen above. However, there is a need to undertake further research to identify a truly accurate method of assessment that overcomes skin colour.

Incontinence lesions are sometimes mistaken for pressure ulcers (Defloor & Schoonhoven, 2004). Incontinence can cause erythema, excoriation and maceration of the skin and thus an incontinence lesion may have a similar appearance to a grade 2 or 3 pressure ulcer. Care should be taken to determine the precise position of any lesion/ulcer in incontinent patients. If a lesion is not over a bony prominence, it is more likely to be due to incontinence than pressure.

Reverse grading is the practice of describing a healing pressure ulcer as moving from a grade 4, through grade 3 and then to grade 2 as the grade 4 cavity heals and becomes shallower. The American National Pressure Ulcer Advisory Panel (NPUAP) debated this topic and produced a position statement that can be found at www.npuap.org. This states that as pressure ulcers heal,

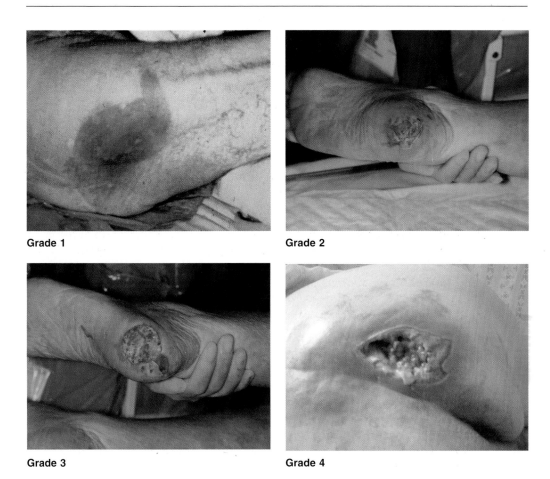

Grade 1

Grade 2

Grade 3

Grade 4

Fig. 5.4   Pressure ulcer grades.

they fill with granulation tissue that is not the same as the tissue it replaces; therefore reverse staging should not be used. A grade 4 pressure ulcer should therefore be described as a healing grade 4 ulcer.

Interrater reliability is the term used to describe the frequency with which different individuals achieve the same score; in this case, the same grade when grading pressure ulcers. The level of interrater reliability of different grading systems has been tested by using either photographs of pressure ulcers (Defloor & Schoonhoven, 2004; Russell & Reynolds, 2001) or actual patients with pressure ulcers (Pedley, 2004) and asking healthcare professionals to determine the grades. The methods and findings of these studies vary, making it difficult to compare the findings and ascertain the most effective scoring system.

Wound bed

Wound bed has been discussed in detail in Chapter 3. The same principles can be applied to pressure ulcers. A pressure ulcer should be assessed for its appearance as well as its grade. For example, grades 3 and 4 ulcers can be necrotic, infected, sloughy or granulating in appearance. Accurate assessment is necessary in order to select a suitable wound management product.

Patient assessment

The EPUAP guidelines suggest that pressure ulcers need to be assessed in the context of the patient's overall condition (EPUAP, 1999) This has been discussed in detail in Chapter 2.

Assessing complications

The EPUAP guidelines identify nutrition, pain and psychosocial factors as potential areas of complication; again, these factors have been discussed in Chapter 2.

Selection of wound management products

A variety of wound management products can be used when treating pressure ulcers. The range of wound management products available is discussed in Chapter 4. At present, there is insufficient evidence to determine which dressing is the most appropriate for each grade of pressure ulcer (Bradley et al., 1999). It is, of course, entirely possible that such prescriptive wound care would never be appropriate and that a range of products is needed in order to address individual situations. Many of the studies compare two products and find little or no difference in performance. This may be because there truly is no difference or because the sample size is too small to detect any differences. Some examples of clinical trials are given below.

Colin et al. (1997) compared a film dressing with a thin hydrocolloid dressing for the management of grade 1 and 2 pressure ulcers ($n = 40$). They found no difference in healing rates but there was a significantly greater reduction in wound size in the film group compared to the thin hydrocolloid group. Teot et al. (1998a) compared two thin hydrocolloids on grade 1 and 2 pressure ulcers and found no differences in outcome ($n = 41$). Both film and thin hydrocolloid dressings would seem to be suitable for this grade of ulcer.

Several studies have considered appropriate products for grade 2–4 pressure ulcers. Teot et al. (1998b) compared a hydrofibre dressing with a traditional tulle dressing ($n = 62$). The hydrofibre dressing produced a better healing rate and a greater reduction in wound size. However, these results were not significant. Sopata (1997) compared a gel dressing with an adhesive foam dressing and found no differences in performance between the two ($n = 34$). Seeley et al. (1998) found no difference in healing rates in a comparison of a hydrocolloid and an adhesive hydrocellular foam dressing ($n = 40$). A similar study in the UK of the same dressings produced the same results ($n = 61$) (Bale et al., 1997). However, the researchers found a high drop-out rate (26%), unrelated to the dressings, mainly due to patient discharge or death. They proposed that future study designs should include larger patient numbers. Thomas et al. (1997) compared a hydropolymer foam dressing with a hydrocolloid dressing ($n = 99$) and found no differences in outcome.

Several researchers have investigated the management of sloughy or necrotic pressure sores. Colin *et al.* (1996b) compared a hydrogel with a dextranomer paste ($n = 135$). They found a significant reduction in wound size at 21 days in the hydrogel group. The hydrogel treatment costs were also significantly lower than those of the dextranomer paste. The other studies compared two different hydrogels and found no difference in healing rates (Bale *et al.*, 1998; Bale & Crook, 1998; Young *et al.*, 1997). Hydrogels are effective products for managing sloughy pressure sores but there is no evidence to indicate which is best.

The use of plastic surgery

The healing time of a large cavity pressure ulcer can be considerably reduced by plastic surgery. However, this is not appropriate for all patients. Their condition may be too poor or the ulcer may be healing rapidly. Sorensen *et al.* (2004) suggest that only a small proportion of patients are suitable candidates, generally those with spinal cord injury and deep grade 3 or 4 ulcers. Khoo and Bailey (1990) have described the principles of reconstructive surgery. Underlying infected bone also indicates a need for surgery. The first stage of reconstruction is debridement followed by either simple closure or use of a flap. If a wound is heavily colonised, it is best to undertake reconstruction in two separate stages, so that there is an opportunity to reduce the bacterial count (Sorensen *et al.*, 2004).

The major problem with reconstruction surgery is the high rate of recurrence. Tavakoli *et al.* (1999) found a recurrence rate of 62% when monitoring outcomes over an eight-year period. However, Kierney *et al.* (1998) found that such rates could be reduced by working collaboratively with colleagues in the Department of Physical Medicine and Rehabilitation. In a longitudinal study of 158 patients, they found a recurrence rate of 25%. They considered their success was related to improved patient selection combined with a protocol for rehabiliation following surgical repair.

5.3 THE MANAGEMENT OF LEG ULCERS

Leg ulcers are a very common type of chronic wound that has been recognised for many years. Those following the Hippocratic view, that disease was the result of imbalance of the four bodily humours, believed that a leg ulcer allowed the bad humours to leach out. In some areas, this belief still persists – the ulcer lets the 'bad' out and if it heals, the person will die. Hopefully, this type of old wives' tale will gradually disappear.

Until recently there was little interest amongst doctors in the treatment of this condition. Their views seemed to coincide with that of an eighteenth-century physician who described the care of leg ulcers as 'an unpleasant and inglorious task where much labour must be bestowed and little honour gained' (Loudon,

1982). Modern developments in wound management have revitalised those caring for patients with leg ulcers.

5.3.1 The epidemiology of leg ulcers

Briggs and Closs (2003) undertook a review of leg ulcer prevalence surveys performed before March 2003, and the various methods used. Using the most reliable estimates from studies undertaken in Europe, Australia and the USA, they concluded that the prevalence of open ulcers is around 0.11–0.18%. They also found that those suffering from recurrent leg ulceration were about 1–2% of the population. These figures should not be extrapolated to other parts of the world where the prevalence rates may be entirely different.

Moffatt *et al.* (2004) have undertaken a leg ulcer prevalence survey in a large, inner London borough and found a prevalence rate of 0.45/1000 population. They compared their findings with two earlier UK surveys (Callam *et al.*, 1985; Cornwall *et al.*, 1986) that had found prevalences of 1.48/1000 population and 1.79/1000 population. The authors suggested that this reduction could partly be explained by the improvements in leg ulcer care in the last 15–20 years, although the large numbers of patients from ethnic minority groups may also have influenced the outcome.

One of the problematic features of leg ulcers is the length of time they can take to heal and the frequency of recurrence. Baker and Stacey (1994) found that 24% had had their ulcers open for more than a year, 35% for more than five years and 20% of leg ulcer suffers had had ten or more episodes of ulceration. They also noted that 45% of the leg ulcer population were so immobile as to be housebound. The more recent survey by Moffatt *et al.* (2004) found 55% of patients had had their ulcers for more than a year and 35% had had them for more than 18 months.

5.3.2 The cost of leg ulcers

As has already been shown, leg ulcers can be a long-standing and recurrent problem. Inevitably, they are also very expensive. The majority are cared for in the community and so require home visits or to be taken to clinics; the worst cases may be admitted to hospital. Gruen *et al.* (1996) analysed the cost of hospitalisation for leg ulcer patients over a two-year period and found that patients were admitted for a mean of 44.2 days at a total cost of A\$2 750 000. What was even worse was that less than 50% of patients ($n = 119$) had any documented improvement on discharge. Tennvall *et al.* (2004) calculated the cost of treating venous ulcers in Sweden based on existing epidemiological data. They found the annual cost to be €73 million. Kumar *et al.* (2004) undertook a similar study in New Mexico, USA, using retrospective data from the Medicaid health insurance system. They found the cost of treating venous ulcers for a five-year period was \$588 413 but gave no indication of the number of ulcers treated.

Several centres have established community leg ulcer clinics and costed the outcomes. Ellison *et al.* (2002) undertook a study to compare the cost and outcomes of leg ulcer care provision in two large health authorities. They found that in one health authority there was a 65% reduction in costs with the introduction of the clinics. Even so, 156 patients cost £212707.84 to treat over a three-month period in 1999.

None of the studies quoted above considers the cost to the patient but several other researchers have investigated this cost. Persoon *et al.* (2004) undertook a review of the literature to determine the impact of leg ulceration on daily life. They included 37 studies, with both qualitative and quantitative methodologies. The common problem identified in all studies was pain and a number also identified disturbed sleep associated with pain; for example, Hofman *et al.* (1997) interviewed 94 patients with venous ulcers and found that 64% had severe pain, 38.3% had continuous pain and 63.8% were woken by pain. Another problem identified by the reviewers is impaired mobility. Some of the qualitative studies also found that heavily exuding malodorous ulcers resulted in limitations in patients' work and leisure activities and often resulted in poor self-esteem and social isolation. The reviewers conclude that leg ulceration has a major impact on the life of the sufferer.

5.3.3 The causes of leg ulcers

There are a variety of causes of leg ulcers, the commonest being venous disease and arterial disease. O'Brien *et al.* (2000) surveyed a health district in Ireland and found that 81% of ulcers were venous in origin and 16.3% were due to arterial disease.

Increasingly, more complex aetiologies are being identified, perhaps because of increasing age and also improved management of the straightforward cases. A recent survey within London found uncomplicated venous ulceration was still the commonest cause (43%), but 35% of the ulcers in the survey had complex aetiologies: lymphoedema (42%), mixed venous and diabetes (35%) and rheumatoid arthritis (26%) (Moffatt *et al.*, 2004).

5.3.4 Venous ulceration

Aetiology

Chronic venous insufficiency is the main cause of venous leg ulcers. Initially, thrombosis or varicosity causes damage to the valves in the veins of the leg. The deep vein is surrounded by muscle. When the leg is exercised, the calf muscle contracts and squeezes the veins, encouraging the flow of blood along the vein. This is often referred to as the calf muscle pump.

Normally blood flows from the superficial veins to the deep veins via a series of perforator vessels. The valves in the vessels ensure that blood moves from the capillary bed towards the heart. If some of the valves become damaged then blood can flow in either direction. The backflow of blood towards the capillary bed leads to venous hypertension. As a result, the capillaries become distorted and more permeable. Larger molecules than normal are able to escape into the extravascular space, for example fibrinogen and red blood cells. The haemo-globin is first released from the red blood cells and then broken down, causing eczema and a brown staining in the gaiter area. Ultimately there is fibrosis of the underlying tissues, giving the leg a 'woody' feeling. This condition is called lipodermatosclerosis. The slightest trauma to the leg and an ulcer will develop. Common examples of trauma are knocking the leg on the corner of a piece of furniture or a fall, injuring the lower leg.

The lymphatic system may also be affected. The lymphatics are responsible for removing protein, fat, cells and excess fluid from the tissues. Ryan (1987) has described how the superficial lymphatics in the dermis disappear. This results in waste products accumulating in the tissues, which can cause fibrosis and further oedema.

Management

Assessment

Full assessment of the patient is essential as many factors can delay the healing of chronic wounds (see Chapter 2). A medical assessment may be necessary to ensure accurate diagnosis. The leg ulcer guidelines developed by the Royal College of Nursing (RCN, 1998) suggest a number of factors that may be speci-fically indicative of venous ulceration and those that are indicative of other aetiologies. They can be seen in Box 5.5. Other factors that may need to be particularly considered include nutritional status, mobility, sleeping, pain, psychological effects of leg ulceration and the patient's understanding of the disease process. A comprehensive assessment of the affected leg must be made, as it is important to rule out arterial disease. The treatments for these two types of ulcer are not compatible.

Box 5.5 Factors to include in assessment of patients with leg ulceration (based on RCN, 1998).

Factors indicative of venous ulceration
Family history
Varicose veins
Proven DVT in affected leg
Phlebitis in affected leg
Suspected DVT
Surgery/fractures to the leg
Episodes of chest pain, haemoptysis, history of pulmonary embolus

Factors indicative of non-venous ulceration
Family history of non-venous ulcers
Heart disease, stroke, TIA
Diabetes mellitus
Ischaemic rest pain
Cigarette smoking
Rheumatoid arthritis
Peripheral vascular disease/intermittent claudication

First, look at the legs. The characteristic staining of lipodermatosclerosis is usually clearly seen in the gaiter area. Ankle flare may also be present; this is distension of the network of small veins situated just below the medial malleolus. Oedema may be present but can also be found in arterial ulceration. Theoretically, the leg and foot should feel warm to touch but if the weather is cold, this may not be the case. The skin surrounding the ulcer may be fragile and eczematous.

Typically, venous ulcers are found on or near the medial malleolus. They tend to be shallow and develop slowly over a period of time. It should also be noted that pain will be increased if there is any infection in the ulcer. The ulcer appearance should be assessed as in Chapter 3. Many venous ulcers have a heavy exudate. Figure 5.5 shows a typical venous ulcer with staining in the gaiter area.

Differential diagnosis between venous and arterial ulcers can be achieved by assessing the blood supply to the leg, ideally by means of Doppler ultrasound. This procedure should be undertaken by healthcare professionals who have received relevant training. Doppler ultrasound is used to compare the blood pressure in the lower leg to the brachial pressure. It is usually presented in the form of a ratio, the ankle brachial pressure index (ABPI), which is calculated by the following formula:

$$\frac{\text{Ankle systolic pressure}}{\text{Brachial systolic pressure}} = \text{Ankle brachial pressure index}$$

An ABPI of 0.9 or above indicates a normal arterial supply to the leg. If it is below 0.9 then some ischaemia is present. Compression therapy should not be used if the ABPI is below 0.8. If there is any doubt about the presence of arterial disease, further medical opinion should be sought.

Planning

There are three aspects to the management of venous ulcers: improving the drainage of the leg, skin care and the use of appropriate wound management products. Any one of these alone will not be truly effective without the others.

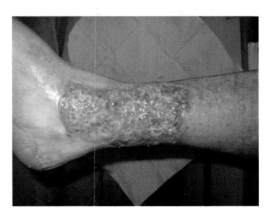

Fig. 5.5   An example of a venous ulcer.

● *Drainage of the legs* ●

The drainage of the legs can be improved in several ways: exercise, compression and elevation. The use of exercise stimulates the calf muscle pump, promoting drainage. Allen (1983) recommends that patients should walk as much as they are able and, if standing still, they should move from one foot to the other. He also suggests that frequent ankle exercises should be performed when sitting. Obviously exercise should be tailored to the abilities of the patient. Regular encouragement will be needed to ensure patients persist with their exercises.

Compression works with exercise to aid drainage from the superficial veins. It should be graduated so that there is a higher pressure at the ankle than at the calf. It can be achieved by the use of either bandages or stockings. Bandages are probably easiest to use in the early stages when the dressings may be rather bulky. Some remain *in situ* day and night whilst others may be removed at night. Reapplying bandages is best done before rising when the leg has the least amount of oedema.

The commonest type of compression bandage used in the UK is elastic, whereas in the rest of Europe inelastic or short-stretch bandages are used. In many instances, three or four different types of bandage are used to achieve a multilayer system comprising three or four layers. This may involve orthopaedic padding, crepe, elastic bandage and a cohesive layer (four-layer) or orthopaedic padding, crepe and high compression bandage (three-layer). The benefit of the orthopaedic padding is that it helps to absorb excess exudate and can provide extra padding over bony prominences.

A system called Unna's boot (a non-compliant plaster-type bandage) is used in North America.

Clark (2003) described the British Standard 7505 for bandages. Elastic compression bandages are defined as type 3 and divided into four categories:

● 3A providing up to 20 mmHg pressure.
● 3B providing 21–30 mmHg pressure.
● 3C providing 31–40 mmHg pressure.
● 3D providing 41–60 mmHg pressure.

All the above measurements are based on the sub-bandage pressure achieved when applying the bandage to a leg with a 23 cm ankle and with a 50% overlap in the bandage layers. In a normal-shaped leg, if the bandage is applied with constant tension and overlap, the pressure will automatically become lower as the bandage is applied up the leg (Clark, 2003). This concept is based on Laplace's Law and has been described in detail by Thomas (2003).

Inelastic or short-stretch bandages provide a rigid layer over the limb that does not 'give' when the wearer is mobilising, thereby providing increased compression during walking. They are applied in a combination of figure of eight and spirals and achieve a multilayered effect. The pressures tend to drop during periods of immobility and the bandages become loose as oedema reduces. This bandage is not suitable for immobile patients.

The level of compression needed for venous ulceration is around 40 mmHg (Stemmer, 1969). Therefore, the high compression bandages are generally suitable. However, these pressures are dependent on the size of the limb. A large limb, swollen with oedema, would require a higher compression bandage than a thinner limb in order to achieve an adequate level of compression. There is also a need to ensure protection over bony prominences as there is the potential risk of pressure damage, especially if the bandage is poorly applied.

A systematic review of clinical trials of compression bandaging found that multilayered bandage systems were more effective than single-layer and high compression better than low compression (Cullum *et al.*, 2001b). There were no clear differences to dermine the most effective type of high compression. Since this review a number of studies have been published that provide further evidence. Two studies compared the four-layer bandage system with a short-stretch bandage and both found that the four-layer system gave a faster healing rate (Iglesias *et al.*, 2004; Ukat *et al.*, 2003). The research teams also found the four-layer system was less expensive to use, mostly because the short-stretch bandages needed to be reapplied more frequently than the four-layer system. One study compared a three-layer paste bandage system with four-layer and found the paste system gave a significantly faster healing rate (Meyer *et al.*, 2003). A small study by Polignano *et al.* (2004) compared the four-layer system with Unna's boot and found no difference in healing rates. Overall, the multilayered systems such as the four-layer bandage would seem to provide the most effective compression.

Unfortunately, not all patients can tolerate high compression bandage systems and a pragmatic approach to the problem may be necessary. Tubular bandages may be better tolerated by some patients and can be used to provide some compression. There is a shaped tubular bandage that can be most useful as it is relatively easy to apply. This type of compression may be the easiest to pull on for someone with arthritic hands. Bale and Harding (2003) studied 28 patients unable to tolerate high compression and found that using three layers of graduated tubular bandage was effective in healing ($n = 14$) or reducing the ulcer. The tubular bandage was applied in gradually reduced lengths: layer 1 = toe to knee; layer 2 = toe to calf; layer 3 = toe to malleolus. The authors concluded that whilst using this type of bandage system cannot be recommended for routine care, it is a possible alternative for those unable to tolerate therapeutic compression. It should be noted that the straight variety of tubular bandage does not give appropriate compression as pressure is higher at the calf than the ankle.

Another method of applying compression that can be used, particularly if oedema is present, is pneumatic compression. It may be applied once or twice a day for periods of up to an hour. Initially the time should be shorter and gradually increased. Whilst this may be a useful form of treatment, it is difficult in the community where there is limited access to such equipment. The use of pneumatic compression should be seen as an addition to the treatment regime rather than an alternative. A Cochrane review found limited evidence of the benefits of pneumatic compression and concluded that further research is required to determine whether it increases healing rates (Mani *et al.*, 2004).

Elevation of the legs allows gravity to aid venous return. However, many people tend to place their feet on a low stool, which is of no benefit whatsoever. To be effective, the feet should be higher than the heart. If there is an acute exacerbation of the ulcer with oedema and heavy exudate, it may be worth admitting the patient to hospital to allow a short period of bedrest. Bedrest with elevation of the foot of the bed can significantly reduce oedema and improve venous return but it should not be considered as a long-term measure because the ulcer will merely break down again once the patient is up and about. It may also seriously affect the mobility of older patients. A more practical method is to raise the foot of the bed at home so that the legs are elevated at night. This may be achieved by the use of bricks or blocks of wood.

● *Skin care* ●

Management of the ulcer involves cleansing and a suitable topical application. Consideration must be given to the presence of eczema, scaling on the legs around the ulcer, any allergies to treatment and wound infection. Cleansing is an important factor as many patients may have been told in the past that they must never get their ulcer wet. As a result, they may not have had a bath for years. Footbaths are very useful as they allow the patient the opportunity to give the affected leg a good soak. Plain tap water is suitable for most patients. Attention needs to be paid to the adequate cleansing of the footbath after use in order to prevent cross-infection.

One skin complication associated with 37–44% of venous ulcers is gravitational or varicose eczema (Patel *et al.*, 2001). It presents as skin excoriations with a diffuse edge, dryness, scaling and weeping and the patients may complain of itching, burning or stinging (Patel *et al.*, 2001). Quartey-Papafio (1999) discussed the importance of being able to differentiate between gravitational eczema and cellulitis and suggested that the most important sign in gravitational eczema is the presence of scaling or crusting. Potassium permanganate 1:10000 solution may be used for heavily weeping eczema for short periods, in conjunction with a steroid cream. Otherwise, emollients and topical steroids may be used and care taken to avoid any irritants that may aggravate the eczema.

When taking an initial history, any reported allergies should be noted. Many long-term leg ulcer sufferers develop allergies to their treatment. Cameron (1998) reviewed the problems of allergic contact dermatitis or contact sensitivity. Substances which have been found to cause sensitivities include lanolin, neomycin, framycetin, emulsifiers such as cetyl alcohol, rubber, parabens and colophony. Cameron recommends avoiding the use of any products containing potential irritants. Bland emollients such as a 50/50 mixture of soft white paraffin and liquid paraffin should be applied following cleansing of the leg. This can be massaged gently into the skin, helping to lift the skin scales that rapidly build up on the leg. Machet *et al.* (2004) reviewed changes in sensitivities reported in France since 1990 and found an 8.5% increase in sensitivity rates. There was a slight decrease in sensitivity to lanolin and a marked increase in sensitivity to balsam of Peru.

● *Wound management* ●

Management of the ulcer depends on the assessment and the factors previously discussed. Selection of suitable dressings is discussed in Chapter 4. There have been of number of clinical trials of modern products on leg ulcers, many of which have been of small size or inconclusive. Overall, there is insufficient evidence to recommend one product over another. Alginates, foams, hydrocolloids, hydrogels and low-adherent dressings may be particularly effective. Marston and Vowden (2003) suggest that dressing selection should be based on the status of the ulcer and surrounding skin. It should be remembered that whilst the ulcer may be new to the nurse, the patient could have lived with it for some time. There may be a credibility gap as the patient starts yet another course of treatment which will 'definitely resolve the problem'.

Paste bandages have been widely used in the treatment of leg ulcers in the past, although less frequently now. They are cotton bandages impregnated with different types of paste according to the manufacturer. They are particularly useful for sore, eczematous legs as they are soothing and will also lift off some of the scales that tend to form around the ulcer. Paste bandages do not provide compression but they enhance the effect of the compression bandages used over the top. Paste bandages have to be applied in such a way as to allow for any swelling of the leg. This may be achieved by making a pleat on each turn at the front of the leg. An alternative method is to overlap each turn and cut the bandage. Paste bandages can be left in place for up to a week.

Skin grafts are used in some centres to promote faster healing. Either mesh grafts or pinch grafts may be used but the former requires hospital admission. Grafting should be used in conjunction with compression therapy. A Cochrane review assessed the benefits of skin grafts, including tissue culture and tissue-engineered products (artificial skin) (Jones & Nelson, 2001). The authors concluded that there was limited evidence of the benefits of using artificial skin and further research is needed. Margolis *et al.* (2000) suggested using a simple prognostic model to identify those patients who would not heal with a simple dressing plus compression bandaging within 24 weeks. Those identified could be considered for more sophisticated treatment, such as artificial skin.

Evaluation

Regular assessment of the ulcer may be done by the use of tracings or photographs which are essential to monitor the progress of the ulcer. If there appears to be no progress over a period of 2–3 months, the ulcer should be reassessed and any ischaemia or infection ruled out. Patient assessment will identify any relevant factors such as loss of appetite. Skin care should be continued as the skin is likely to remain scaly.

Below-knee compression stockings are widely used as the ulcer improves and after healing. Some manufacturers also produce compression socks for men that look like ordinary socks. For many patients, socks and stockings are easier to apply than bandages. Jones and Nelson (1998) have reviewed the use of compression stockings.

The British Standards Institute has specified three classes of stockings available on prescription which provide different ranges of compression at the ankle.

- Class I has pressures of 14–18 mmHg.
- Class II has pressures of 18–24 mmHg.
- Class III has pressures of 25–35 mmHg.

It is very important that the patient should be correctly fitted for stockings. Class II may be appropriate for many patients. If Class III stockings are required but the patient is unable or unwilling to pull them on, it may be better to use two layers of Class I stockings. Fentem (1986) has shown that this would provide the same level of compression. A systematic review of the use of compression hosiery for preventing ulcer recurrence found only two trials to report (Nelson *et al.*, 2004). The reviewers noted that both studies found that not wearing compression was strongly associated with leg ulcer recurrence, although this is circumstantial evidence as this condition was not being tested in either trial.

Some authors have discussed the benefits of surgery to correct venous reflux. Ghauri *et al.* (1998) found that the introduction of superficial venous surgery reduced one-year recurrence rates from 23% to 9% within a vascular-led specialist clinic service. They followed this with a randomised, controlled trial that found that surgery plus compression was significantly more effective than compression alone (Barwell *et al.*, 2004).

Patients still need to be seen regularly once the ulcer is healed in order to provide encouragement and to ensure that the preventive care is understood. They should also be given information on how to get further help if the ulcer recurs. The sooner that appropriate care can be given, the sooner the ulcer will heal. Poore *et al.* (2002) monitored the impact of a healed ulcer clinic over a two-year period. Of the 110 patients studied, 14 patients did not attend after the first year, 75 (78%) remained healed and 21 (22%) had recurrence. The authors examined the medical records to determine the actual length of time the healed ulcers had remained healed. The commonest length of time was three years (32%) with a range of 1.5 to 19 years.

Prevention is obviously better than cure. Ruckley *et al.* (2002) undertook a cross-sectional survey of adults aged 18–64 years randomly selected from 12 general practices. They found a 9.4% prevalence of chronic venous insufficiency in men and 6.6% in women. However, the rate rose steeply with age to 21.2% in men and 12% in women over 50 years. The research team suggests that as about a third of the subjects had damage to the superficial veins, it would be worth advocating surgical treatment to prevent leg ulceration developing at a later date.

5.3.5 Arterial ulcers

Aetiology

Arterial ulcers are the result of inadequate tissue perfusion to the feet or legs. This is due to complete or partial blockage of the arterial supply to the legs and the underlying condition is often referred to as peripheral vascular disease. This is a general term used to encompass disease which reduces the blood supply to the periphery. The commonest disease is arteriosclerosis in which the artery walls become thickened. It is usually found in combination with atherosclerosis, the formation of plaques on the inner lining of the vessels. The lumen of the vessels gradually narrows, causing ischaemia in the surrounding tissue and ultimately resulting in necrosis. This type of arterial insufficiency is most commonly found in men over the age of 50.

Buerger's disease is another type of disease affecting the peripheral arteries. Inflammation of the vessels results in thrombus formation and occlusion of the vessels. It is associated with heavy smoking and is found most commonly in men between the ages of 20 and 35 years. Ulceration associated with necrosis and gangrene may develop.

Management

Assessment

Assessment of the patient may reveal pain particularly associated with walking which is relieved by resting; this is called intermittent claudication. Pain may also occur at night when the patient is in bed and can be relieved by hanging the legs down. Past medical history may reveal known peripheral vascular disease or arterial surgery. A past or present history of smoking should also be noted.

When the legs are examined they may feel cold to touch and have a shiny, hairless appearance. The toe nails may be thickened and opaque. The legs become white when elevated and a reddish/blue colour when dependent. Pedal pulses are diminished or absent. Doppler examination will reveal the presence of ischaemia with an ABPI below 0.9. If the patient has intermittent claudication, the ABPI is likely to be between 0.5 and 0.9. Rest pain and an ABPI below 0.5 are indicative of critical ischaemia. The patient should be referred to a vascular surgeon.

Arterial ulcers may occur anywhere on the leg or foot but are most commonly found on the foot. The ulcer has a punched-out appearance and may be deep, involving muscles or tendons. Necrosis is often present and there is often far less exudate than in venous leg ulcers (see Fig. 5.6). Table 5.1 compares venous and arterial ulcers (Dealey, 1991b).

Planning

Arterial ulcers are notoriously difficult to heal and arterial surgery to improve the blood supply may be necessary before an ulcer will heal. Early referral for reconstructive surgery is ideal. Ray *et al.* (1995) found that percutaneous transluminal angioplasty was effective in promoting healing in all those with ulcers in their study ($n = 14$). The standard surgical procedure is a bypass graft. Sieggreen and Kline (2004) discussed the advantages and disadvantages of both bypass grafts and percutaneous procedures and concluded that appropriate patient selection is the key to successful outcomes. Unfortunately, for some patients, despite treatment, there is considerable risk of the onset of gan-

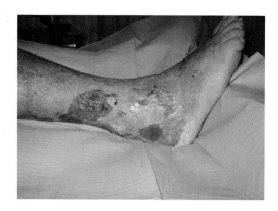

Fig. 5.6   An arterial ulcer

Table 5.1   A comparison of venous and arterial ulcers.

Sign/symptom	Venous ulcer	Arterial ulcer
Site	On/near medial malleolus	May be on toes, foot, heel or lateral aspect of leg
Development	Develops slowly	Develops rapidly
Appearance of ulcer	Shallow margin; deep tissues not affected	Often deep with involvement of tendons or muscles
Appearance of leg	Brown, varicose staining, and eczema, warm to touch	Shiny skin, cold to touch, white on elevation, may become blue when dependent
Oedema	Present – usually worse at end of day	Only present if patient immobile – stasis oedema
Pain	Level and time of pain varies	Very painful – worse at night. Relieved by hanging leg over side of bed
Medical history	DVT, phlebitis, varicose veins	Peripheral vascular disease, ischaemic heart disease,
ABPI	0.9 and above	Below 0.9

grene and even septicaemia, and amputation of the limb may be the only solution.

If a patient has severe resting pain, good pain control is an essential part of the management. The patient should also be encouraged to give up smoking as failure to do so will further compromise the blood supply to the leg. Gentle exercise will help to encourage the development of a collateral supply to the limb, thus improving tissue perfusion. The limbs should be kept warm as cold may precipitate pain.

The major aim of ulcer management is to remove necrotic tissue and to prevent infection. Selection of appropriate wound management products depends on the ulcer appearance, the amount of exudate and the position of the ulcer (see Chapter 4). A Cochrane review found only one small trial of a topical agent for arterial ulcers and concluded that there was insufficient evidence to determine whether the choice of dressing affects the healing of arterial ulcers (Nelson & Bradley, 2003).

Any dressing needs to be effectively retained and yet not so bulky as to restrict mobility unduly. Areas such as the toes are not at all easy to dress. Bandages are often needed to hold the dressing in place. Compression bandages should not be used on arterial ulcers. Comfortable retention bandages such as cotton conforming bandages are suitable. Lightweight tubular bandages can be very useful, particularly on toes. It is important to ensure that, whatever bandage is used, it does not constrict the blood supply.

Evaluation

The progress of both the patient and the ulcer should be evaluated. The effectiveness of pain control can be ascertained using a pain ruler (see Chapter 2). When monitoring the progress of the ulcer, attention should be paid to any indications of infection.

5.3.6 Ulcers of mixed aetiology

Some patients will have both an arterial and a venous component to their ulcer. It is important to define the predominant factor, so that appropriate treatment may be given.

Management

Assessment

Doppler assessment and assessment of the leg will provide an indication of the mixed aetiology. A full assessment in a vascular laboratory may be of benefit.

Planning

If the main factor is venous, moderate graduated compression should be worn during the day. The degree of compression should be based on patient tolerance. The International Leg Ulcer Advisory Board has provided a care pathway that gives guidance on the levels of compression that should be used for different levels of arterial insufficiency in a mixed ulcer as well as for venous ulcers (Stacey *et al.*, 2002). Figure 5.7 shows this section of the pathway. Most patients will need to remove the compression garment at night when elevation of the legs is likely to increase ischaemic pain. Butcher (2002) suggests that short-stretch bandages may be particularly useful, as they do not exert pressure when the limb is resting. Bowering (1998) achieved reduced compression by omitting the elastic third-layer bandage from the four-layer system and achieved 67% healing. Arthur and Lewis (2000) used reduced compression on 24 mixed aetiology ulcers and achieved 74% healing ($n = 19$). However, it must also be noted that two patients were unable to continue this therapy as their limbs became

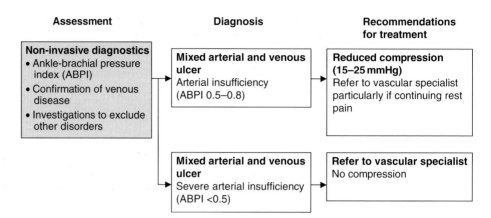

Fig. 5.7 Guidance on levels of compression for mixed aetiology ulcers from the treatment pathway developed by the International Leg Ulcer Advisory Board (adapted from Stacey *et al.*, 2002).

too ischaemic. Care and careful monitoring must be exercised if using compression for these patients. When arterial disease predominates, a vascular opinion must be sought. However, exercise and short periods of limb elevation can be encouraged, within the limits of patient toleration.

Evaluation

If healing is very slow, further advice from a vascular surgeon should be obtained. Butcher (2002) emphasised the importance of regular reassessment to monitor any changes in the level of arterial insufficiency. The RCN leg ulcer guidelines suggest that this should be every three months (RCN, 1998).

5.3.7 Malignant leg ulcers

A small number of leg ulcers may be malignant or become malignant. Voisard *et al.* (2001) reported on patients attending a vascular clinic between 1991 and 1999 where they found six cases of squamous cell carcinoma and four with Marjolin's ulcer. The authors observed that they did not see any existing leg ulcers become malignant in their series. Yang *et al.* (1996) monitored patients attending a specialist leg ulcer clinic and found 43 patients with 55 malignant lesions, an incidence of 4.4%. In this group 75% were basal cell carcinoma and 25% squamous cell carcinoma. They concluded that malignant changes are common in chronic leg ulcers. Over a 12-month period, Taylor (1998) found 12 patients in a cohort of less than 200 patients attending a community leg ulcer clinic.

Hayes and Dodds (2003) discussed the identification and diagnosis of malignant ulcers and suggested that there are a number of clinical signs of malignancy.

- Irregular nodular appearance on the wound surface.
- A raised or rolled edge.

- Raised granulation tissue on the ulcer bed with firm surrounding skin.
- Islets of epithelialisation that do not persist.
- Apparently healthy granulation tissue that is exuberant, translucent, shining and rolls over the wound margins.

Yang *et al.* (1996) suggest that any ulcer that fails to heal when treated appropriately should rouse suspicion. Walsh (2002) discussed the importance of taking a biopsy from atypical ulcers or non-healing ulcers and of early referral for specialist advice.

Treatment of malignant ulcers is by excision and skin grafting when caught at a reasonably early stage. Amputation may be necessary for large ulcers. Although only a small percentage of leg ulcers are malignant, it is important for nurses to be aware of the possibility and alert to the need to obtain biopsies of any atypical ulcers.

5.3.8 Leg ulceration in rheumatoid arthritis

It has been noted that patients with rheumatoid arthritis (RA) are more vulnerable to leg ulceration and that the aetiology is frequently multifactorial (McRorie, 2000). In their leg ulcer survey, Moffatt *et al.* (2004) found that 35% of ulcers were multifactorial and of these, 26% were associated with rheumatoid arthritis. This indicates a significant minority of patients who require careful assessment and management.

Oien *et al.* (2001) studied 20 patients with chronic leg ulcers and RA in order to determine the ulcer aetiology. They found that three patients had vasculitis as well as both venous and arterial components; five had both vasculitis and venous disease; two had vasculitis and diabetes; seven had venous disease alone; one had vasculitis alone; one had arterial disease alone; one had neither vasculitis nor venous or arterial problems. The research team also noted that the ulcers were very painful.

Management

Assessment

A specialist rheumatology assessment as well as a vascular assessment is required for these patients. McRorie (2000) also suggests that nutritional assessment and assessment of footwear should be undertaken.

Planning

Management of these patients is complex and depends on the underlying aetiologies. Compression can be used with caution where venous disease is the dominant factor, particularly if peripheral oedema is present. A small study of 15 patients by Hafner *et al.* (2000) found that vein or arterial surgery was effective in achieving healing in 9/15 patients and markedly improving the ulcers of 5/15. They suggest a prospective trial was needed to confirm these results. Oien *et al.* (2001) used pinch grafts to treat the patients in their study group. They achieved healing in 8/20 patients, the ulcers in these patients being much smaller (range 0.4–13.2 cm^2) than the unhealed ulcers (range 6.7–356.6 cm^2). They also found a significant reduction in pain in 18/20 patients following the pinch grafting.

Evaluation

Regular monitoring of these patients is essential, especially as arterial disease may be accelerated in patients with RA (McRorie, 2000).

5.4 DIABETIC FOOT ULCERS

Ulceration of the foot is a serious complication of diabetes mellitus, which can lead to disability and possible amputation of the affected limb. Jeffcoate and Harding (2003) reviewed current data on surveys of foot ulcers and noted that 5.3% (type 2 diabetes) and 7.4% (type 1 and 2 combined) have either an active ulcer or have previously had an ulcer. The lifetime risk for people with diabetes developing an ulcer is about 15%. The incidence of major amputation is 0.5–5.0 per 1000 people with diabetes and the perioperative mortality rates associated with amputation have been found to range from 9% to 15% (Jeffcoate & Harding, 2003).

Girod *et al.* (2003) evaluated the direct and indirect costs of treating foot ulcers in diabetic patients. They monitored the cost of 239 patients cared for by 80 physicians and found the average monthly cost was €2287.96. This gives a total monthly cost for treating the 239 patients of €546 822.44.

5.4.1 Aetiology

The underlying causes of diabetic ulcers are peripheral neuropathy and peripheral vascular disease. Infection is an ever-present risk for the diabetic and can exacerbate the development of ulceration and increase the risk of amputation.

Peripheral neuropathy affects the peripheral sensory, motor and autonomic nerves of the leg. This has a twofold effect of causing a loss of sensation and compromising the biomechanics of the foot. Muscle atrophy in the foot, particularly over the arch of the foot, causes a transfer of body weight and reactive callus formation on the plantar surface. Ultimately, deformities of the foot, such as claw toes or Charcot foot, may occur along with alterations in gait. Walters *et al.* (1993) found foot ulceration was significantly associated with foot deformity. Poorly fitting shoes or a foreign body within the shoe can cause undetected injury, resulting in ulcer formation. The patient may be completely unaware of the ulcer for some time.

Vascular disease in diabetics primarily affects the smaller arterioles within the foot. Intermittent claudication is unlikely, as larger arteries are not usually occluded. As with all types of vascular disease, it is exacerbated by smoking. Gangrene of the toes can be caused by thrombosis in the artery supplying the affected digit. Pressure from poorly fitting shoes is the commonest cause of ischaemic ulceration.

Microvascular dilation plays a significant role in the healing of minor wounds. The ability of these vessels to dilate can be measured by using a laser Doppler to test the response to heat. A study by Sandeman *et al.* (1991) measured the ability to respond to heat by vasodilation in insulin-dependent (ID) diabetics, non-insulin dependent (NID) diabetics and a control group of healthy individuals. A significantly worse response was found in the NID diabetics than in the other two groups.

5.4.2 Prevention

Given the grave implications of ulceration, prevention is very important. The main methods used in prevention are patient education and adequate monitoring of the patient by the healthcare team. Litchfield and Ramkissoon (1996) monitored the outcome of providing an educational footcare video for diabetics. They found that whilst most patients were aware of the need for good footcare, there was a lack of compliance with the recommended care. NICE has produced guidelines for the prevention and management of foot problems in diabetics (NICE, 2004). The guidelines include guidance on the content of any education programmes to be targeted at those with low risk of developing foot ulcers, those at high risk and those with foot ulcers. The guidelines also state that effective prevention and care involves a partnership between patients and professionals (NICE, 2004).

Regular monitoring of diabetic feet is essential and should occur at least annually. Assessment should include testing of foot sensation, palpation of foot pulses, inspection for any foot deformity and inspection of footwear (NICE, 2004). Assessment allows the classification of foot risk as follows:

- low current risk (normal sensation, palpable pulses).
- increased risk (neuropathy or absent pulses or other risk factor).
- high risk (neuropathy or absent pulses plus deformity or skin changes or previous ulcer).
- ulcerated foot (NICE, 2004).

Once patients have been identified as being at risk, they should be made aware of their responsibilities for prevention of foot problems. Feet should be washed daily and dried carefully. They should be inspected for any red areas or swelling and cracked or broken skin. Toe nails should be cut straight across. Socks should be changed daily and not wrinkle. Shoes should be well fitting. They should be checked before wearing for any foreign bodies. New shoes should be properly fitted and feet carefully observed for signs of rubbing. Patients should not wear sandals or go barefoot. Those with poor vision may need assistance. Those who smoke should be encouraged to stop.

At each attendance at the diabetic clinic, the patient should have a full foot check. This may involve the doctor, diabetic nurse specialist and chiropodist/podiatrist. Treatment of callus formation and management of any fungal infections is usually carried out by the chiropodist/podiatrist. If the patient has any deformity of the feet it may be helpful for the orthotist to assess for suitable footwear. If the patient has other pathology requiring treatment, other health professionals should be vigilant in identifying any potential foot problems.

5.4.3 Management

Ideally, the care of patients with diabetic foot ulcers should be within the context of a multidisciplinary footcare team comprising podiatrists, orthotists, nurses and diabetologists, all of whom should have specialist expertise in this area.

Assessment

When assessing the patient, there may be an indication of the type of ulcer. A history of pain associated with the ulcer, for example, almost certainly indicates ischaemia. Deformities of gait are indicative of neuropathy. Assessment of the diabetic state is important because of the increased risk of infection in the presence of hyperglycaemia.

Assessment of the leg and foot will provide objective evidence of the presence of either ischaemia or neuropathy or both. Table 5.2 indicates the differences between the two types of ulcers. However, both pathologies may be present in many patients. A survey of diabetic foot ulcer management in secondary healthcare found that 33% were neuropathic, 40% were neuroischaemic and 20% were ischaemic (Jude *et al.*, 2003). Vascular assessment using Doppler

Table 5.2 A comparison of signs of peripheral neuropathy and peripheral vascular disease in the diabetic foot.

Sign/symptom	Neuropathic ulcer	Ischaemic ulcer
Deformity of the foot	Present as claw toe, hammer toe, Charcot foot or other	Not present
Skin temperature of foot	Warm	Cold
Colour of foot	Normal	White when elevated or cyanotic
Toe nails	Atrophic	Atrophic
Pedal pulses	Present	ABPI below 0.9 (false high readings if small vessels calcified)
Pain	Present in some – associated with numbness and diminished sensation	Present, relieved by hanging legs down
Callus formation	Present, especially on plantar surface	Not present
Ulcer site	Commonly on plantar surface of foot	Commonly on toes and the edges of the foot

ultrasound can help to determine the level of ischaemia. However, it is important to be aware of the potential for a falsely elevated ABPI because of calcification of the arteries. If this is suspected, the patient should be referred for more intensive vascular assessment. An important aspect of assessment is to identify the precipitating factor. Careful assessment of footwear and the precise position of the ulcer can provide clues. It is essential to identify the cause of the ulcer or further ulceration may occur.

Neuropathic ulcers may be surrounded by callus and have a punched-out appearance (see Fig. 5.8). Ischaemic ulcers are usually covered by necrotic tissue. Neither type of ulcer generally has much exudate. The ulcer should be carefully observed for any indication of infection.

Wagner (1981) devised a scale for assessing diabetic ulcers.

- Grade 0 – at-risk foot.
- Grade 1 – superficial ulcer, not clinically infected.
- Grade 2 – deeper ulcer, often infected, no osteomyelitis.
- Grade 3 – deeper ulcer, abscess formation, osteomyelitis.
- Grade 4 – localised gangrene (toe, forefoot or heel).
- Grade 5 – gangrene of whole foot.

Ulcers graded 0–3 tend to be predominantly neuropathic, whereas in those graded 4 or 5 ischaemia is the main factor.

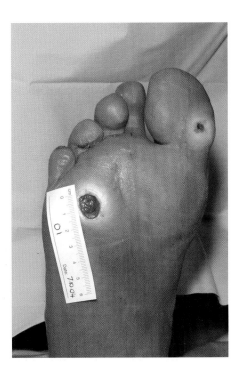

Fig. 5.8 A neuropathic ulcer.

Planning

Adequate control of the diabetic state is the primary goal when managing patients with foot ulceration. Pain control may also be necessary. Management of the ulcer depends on the causative factors. On the whole, neuropathic ulcers should be referred to the chiropodist/podiatrist as the callus needs to be removed before the ulcer can heal. Pressure must also be removed from the ulcer and this can be achieved in several ways such as use of extra-depth insoles, Scotchcast boot, Aircast boot, Total Contact Cast or even the use of crutches. Ischaemic ulcers may be resistant to treatment. Necrotic tissue must be debrided by use of appropriate wound management products (as discussed in Chapter 3). Any infection should be treated with systemic antibiotics and the application of suitable dressings (see Chapter 4). Compression bandages should not be used but, if necessary, a simple retention bandage can be used to hold the dressing in place.

Some patients may benefit from revascularisation and should have a prompt referral for a vascular opinion (NICE, 2004). Faries *et al.* (2004) discussed the role of arterial reconstruction and noted that in centres of excellence, 70% of surgical bypass grafts will still be patent after five years and the associated five-year limb salvage rate was greater than 80%.

Evaluation

Measurement of the ulcer by tracing may not provide adequate information as the surface area may not appear to alter greatly. A photographic record may be of more value. Careful assessment for any indication of infection should be made at each dressing change. Failure to respond to treatment can result in osteomyelitis. Surgical treatment is necessary to eradicate the infection. The NICE guidelines state that patients should be referred to a multidisciplinary foot clinic within 24 hours if there is a new ulcer, new swelling or new discolouration of the foot (NICE, 2004).

Once the ulcer is healed, preventive measures need to be instigated.

5.5 FUNGATING WOUNDS

Malignant fungating wounds are particularly difficult wounds to manage. They are distressing for both the sufferer and the nurse. A major problem is that there has been very little research into the management of this type of lesion. It is interesting to note that what little research there is has predominantly been undertaken within the UK (Schiech, 2002). A postal survey (Thomas, 1992) has provided some information about current practice in radiotherapy centres across the UK. Thomas noted that several respondents commented on the lack of published data and the generally unscientific approach to the management of fungating wounds. Little has changed in the years since that survey was undertaken. It is undoubtedly a difficult area to research but it is an important area to tackle, not least in order to improve the quality of life for these patients.

5.5.1 Aetiology and incidence

Fungating lesions occur when a cancerous mass invades the epithelium, thus ulcerating through to the body surface. It has been estimated that between 5% and 10% of patients with metastatic cancer will develop a fungating wound (Haisfield-Wolfe & Rund, 1997). It most commonly occurs with cancer of the breast but may also be found in cancers of the skin, head and neck, vulva and bladder (Dowsett, 2002). Fungating wounds not only develop at the site of the primary tumour but if the nodes of the groin or axilla are affected, ulceration may also occur at that site.

Fungating lesions are often associated with neglect; that is, the patient delays seeking medical help. This is commonly seen in patients with breast cancers. A typical example is the lady who 'ignores' her breast lump for several years and only seeks help when her family notice the offensive odour.

5.5.2 Management of fungating wounds

Management of the patient

This is a vital part of the management of these wounds. Many factors within the patient can affect the progress of the wound. Naylor (2001) discussed the issue of wound pain for patients with fungating wounds and the need to address the psychological, social and spiritual aspects of pain. Chapter 2 discusses patient care in greater detail.

Management of the wound

Chapter 3 covers the general principles of wound management. This section will address the specific problems related to fungating wounds.

Assessment

When assessing the wound, the following factors need to be considered.

- Fungating lesions are often necrotic, sloughy or infected.
- There are usually copious amounts of exudate, which may have an offensive odour.
- Many of these wounds become malodorous as a result of bacterial invasion. This causes distress to the patient, relatives and visitors and may be very difficult to control.
- The position of the wound obviously depends on the type of cancer. However, it may spread along the trunk or limbs, sometimes in the form of isolated nodules. Applying a dressing to protect such a spread-out lesion can be very difficult and requires considerable nursing skill.
- Capillary bleeding may occur as the cancer increases in size and erodes blood vessels. It may be sufficiently heavy or frequent as to cause anaemia. Removal of the old dressing must be done with great care in order to avoid loosening any clots.

- Lymphoedema may be present with cancers of the breast, cervix or vulva. This is a chronic swelling of the adjacent limb(s) due to a failure of lymph drainage. It may be associated with loss of function of the affected limb. (See also section 5.6.)

Planning

It is essential to identify patient problems rather than nurse problems. Whilst in many instances they may be the same, they are not always. In her studies, Grocott (1998, 2000) reported the impact of fungating wounds on the patients, quoting patients using words such as 'revulsion' and describing the constant washing of soiled clothing and bedclothes. She concluded that an efficient dressing system that would cope with the exudate was essential to allow patients to cope with their disease (Grocott, 2000).

Once the specific problems have been identified, the treatment options have to be planned in the light of the patient's condition. If the expected outcome is very poor, then totally palliative care with the minimum need to dress the wound must be the treatment of choice. For others, a more aggressive approach can be used. A course of radiotherapy may be prescribed to help reduce the size of the lesion. It should be remembered that many patients find dressing change a major ordeal that leaves them feeling very tired.

As previously noted, copious exudate is a problem that concerns patients. Very absorbent dressings are necessary to provide comfort and dryness for the patient. Alginates and hydrocellular foams can be effective in controlling exudate. Grocott (1997, 1998) has undertaken a longitudinal multiple case study design to monitor the outcomes when using different dressings to manage exudate. She considered that the factor of greatest importance is fitting conformable dressing materials to the wound, thus reducing the risk of leakage. Dressing bulk can be reduced by the use of outer dressings with high moisture vapour transfer rates.

Odour causes great distress to patients. It is mostly due to bacterial invasion, although exuding necrotic wounds may also be offensive. A wound swab will identify the invading bacteria, so that appropriate systemic antibiotics can be prescribed. Topical agents can also be used. Clark (2002) reviewed the use of metronidazole for malodorous wounds and concluded that there was a lack of evidence to determine the best method of delivery, the dose and the optimum length of treatment. However, it is widely used to reduce odour. Silver sulphadiazine cream can be used for *Pseudomonas aeruginosa* infections. Honey and other types of silver dressings may be useful for odour reduction.

If the odour cannot be reduced or whilst action is being taken to reduce odour, other steps can be taken. The aim is to mask the smell which can be achieved in a variety of ways. Activated charcoal dressings can be effective in absorbing odour (Lawrence *et al.*, 1993) and are often used in conjunction with other dressings. Air fresheners can help and stoma therapists can give advice on the use of deodorant solutions used by ostomists.

When aggressive treatment is suitable, wound debridement is an option. Removal of necrotic or sloughy tissue can reduce odour and exudate. The quickest method is surgical debridement which must be done by a skilled surgeon because of the distorted anatomy and the risk of capillary bleeding. Surgical debridement is not a suitable option for patients with a history of capillary bleeding into the wound. A variety of wound management products can be used, depending on the amount of exudate. Alginates can be used on heavily exuding wounds. When there is moderate to low exudate, an amorphous hydrogel and occasionally hydrocolloids can be used. The position, size and spread of the lesion can affect dressing choice.

Capillary bleeding can be frightening for both the patient and the nurse. When there is a history of capillary bleeding, great care should be taken when removing the old dressing. If the dressing is adherent, it should be soaked with saline before removal is attempted. It may also be necessary to remove the dressing slowly in stages. It is better to take a long time to remove a dressing than to start bleeding which is difficult to control.

Adrenaline can be applied directly to the wound to control profuse bleeding. However, it should be used with caution, under medical supervision. Alginate dressings are useful when there is oozing and can be removed easily by washing away with saline. If there is persistent bleeding, the haemoglobin should be checked regularly. Blood transfusions may be necessary to treat anaemia.

If the lesion is being treated with radiotherapy, attention must be given to dressing selection. A variety of dressings have been found to be suitable: charcoal dressings, alginates and an amorphous hydrogel. Dressing retention may be a problem. Ideally, the dressing should not be too bulky because it makes the wearing of clothes difficult and the patient becomes very self-conscious. Bandages and tubular net and tubular gauze are probably the most versatile means of dressing retention. Tape should be used with care as the skin may become sore with repeated dressing change. If the patient is undergoing a course of radiotherapy to the lesion, it may be necessary for the outer dressing to be removed for treatment. Again, the skin may become sore. 'Garments' made from tubular net allow easy access to the wound and will not further damage the skin.

Evaluation

Evaluation of the management of fungating wounds should always consider whether the predetermined goals have been attained. Good documentation can be used to maintain a record of effective care, thus providing guidelines for the management of other patients. Managing a fungating wound and providing care for the patient require considerable nursing skills. More research is needed in order to be able to identify the most effective care.

5.6 LYMPHOEDEMA

Lymphoedema occurs when there is absence, obliteration or obstruction of the lymph vessels, which results in accumulation of fluid distal to the damage as the transporting capacity of the system is reduced. Although associated with cancer, lymphoedema can be either primary or secondary. To date, no cause of primary lymphoedema has been identified (BLS, 2001). Secondary lymphoedema is primarily seen to be a consequence of cancer or cancer treatment but it may also be caused by low-grade infection or inflammation, trauma or filariasis (Board & Harlow, 2002a). Filariasis is a parasitic invasion of the lymph system, enabled by mosquitoes, and is estimated to affect more than 120 million people worldwide (WHO, 2001).

5.6.1 Lymphoedema management

Although there is much greater awareness of lymphoedema management than there used to be, some patients with lymphoedema may have been told that nothing can be done to reduce the swelling. This is not true. Whilst it is not possible to cure lymphoedema, it can be controlled. Ideally, patients should be referred to a specialist treatment centre to ensure the most effective care. Within Europe, especially Germany, Austria and the UK, there are a number of centres available that offer this treatment (Board & Harlow, 2002b).

Assessment

Board and Harlow (2002a) list the clinical features that need to be considered as part of an assessment.

- *Identify the cause* of the lymphoedema and any associated medical conditions, in conjunction with the medical team.
- *Oedema* – assess the extent of the oedema. Does it affect one or more limbs? Has it spread to the trunk? Measure limb size by taking measurements every 4 cm along both the affected and the unaffected limb.
- *Skin status* – the skin may become dry, scaly and rough or it may be taut and shiny. Eventually skinfolds and crevices occur because of the severe oedema and will result in hyperkeratosis.
- *Acute inflammatory episodes* – the presence of lymphoedema makes an individual more vulnerable to infection from small breaks in the skin. Cellulitis can spread rapidly through the affected limb (Mortimer, 2001).
- *Lymphorrhoea* – the leakage of lymph through small breaks in the skin; this can be seen as fluid constantly trickling down the affected limb.
- *Mobility* – has the oedema affected movements of the limb? What impact has this had on activities of daily living? Is there associated pain with the heaviness of the limb?

Management

Board and Harlow (2002b) suggest that treatment should be offered in three categories: intensive, in order to reduce moderate or severe oedema; maintenance, to provide long-term control of oedema; and palliative, to alleviate symptoms in the final stage of life. Any treatment plan needs to be developed in partnership with the patient and it may also need to involve family members. Treatment comprises skin care, compression, massage and exercise.

Skin care is a vital aspect. Williams and Venables (1996) describe the need for daily washing and careful drying, especially between the digits. Emollient creams should be applied to prevent the skin drying out and cracking and the development of hyperkeratosis. Care should be taken to prevent the swollen limb getting burnt by the sun. Cuts and scratches can be a source of infection and should be treated with antiseptic cream. Gloves should be worn for protection when working in the kitchen or garden. Jeffs (1993) has reviewed the effects of infection in lymphoedema. She suggests that Streptococcus is generally the causative organism. The infection should be treated with appropriate antibiotics.

Compression can be provided by means of multilayer bandages or compression hosiery, such as a sleeve (Board & Harlow, 2002b). In the initial stages of treatment, bandages assist in reducing limb size. In severe cases the digits as well as the hand and arm, or foot and leg, should be bandaged. Once the limb has been reduced to a reasonable size, compression hosiery can be used to maintain limb reduction. Intermittent pneumatic compression may be of use for some patients, in addition to massage and not as an alternative. The most effective type of compression is the multichamber sequential pump. The best effect is obtained by clearing fluid from the trunk before commencing treatment.

Massage is an important aspect of lymphoedema management and may be in the form of manual lymphatic drainage or simple massage. The former should be undertaken by a healthcare professional who has received training in the technique but the latter may be taught to patients or their relatives. Massage encourages the flow of lymph away from the limb. Occasionally, the swelling may have spread beyond the limb into the trunk. Massage should start on an area of the trunk free of lymphoedema before moving to a lymphoedematous area (Regnard et al., 1997). This creates a space for the lymph in the swollen limb to flow into. The massage then continues down the affected limb. The massage technique should be gentle, so that it does not stimulate blood flow into the limb and increase congestion. It may need to be a little firmer when tissue fibrosis is present. Board and Harlow (2002b) recommend that patients/relatives be advised to spend 20 minutes each day undertaking massage. Patients and relatives often find that undertaking this massage creates a sense of closeness that may be of particular benefit for those who are terminally ill.

Ko et al. (1998) monitored the effects of treatment for 299 patients over a 12-month period. They found a 59.1% size reduction in arms and 67.7% reduction in legs after initial treatment averaging 15.7 days. This was maintained in 88% of compliant patients. The non-compliant patients regained 33% of the initial reduction. McNeely et al. (2004) randomised 50 patients with lymphoedema associated with breast cancer to compression bandaging or compression bandaging plus manual lymphatic drainage. They found that all patients achieved a significant reduction in arm volume after four weeks but those with mild lymphoedema in the combination treatment group had a significantly larger reduction in limb volume. However, these numbers are small and a larger study is needed to confirm this finding.

Exercise assists in improving drainage of lymph from the limb. Muscle movement alters tissue pressure and has a massaging effect on the lymph vessels. The best effect is obtained if the exercises are carried out when the patient is wearing compression bandages or hosiery. Exercise also prevents or reduces stiffness of the joints. Passive movements should be carried out if the limb is paralysed. All patients should be encouraged to move as much as possible but lifting and carrying heavy weights should be avoided. It is important to provide encouragement to the patient to persevere with all aspects of this plan as none of these treatments is effective in isolation. Significant reduction of a swollen limb can only be achieved when all aspects of the treatment plan are implemented.

Evaluation

Reduction in limb size, improvements in skin status and greater limb mobility are all desirable outcomes that can easily be measured.

5.7 CONCLUSION

The management of chronic wounds is complex and requires skilled care that is best undertaken by a multiprofessional team. Fortunately, there is increasing access to specialist services that have made a major impact on improvement in patient care.

REFERENCES

Allen, S. (1983) Hang the patient upside down from the ceiling – it works every time. *General Practitioner*, **June 24**, 40–41.

Allman, R.M., Goode, P.S., Burst, N., Bartolucci, A.A., Thomas, D.R. (1999) Pressure ulcers, hospital complications and disease severity: impact on hospital costs and length of stay. *Advances in Wound Care*, **12** (1), 22–30.

Amlung, S.R., Miller, W.L., Bosley, L.M. (2001) The 1999 national pressure ulcer prevalence survey: a benchmarking approach. *Advances in Skin and Wound Care*, **14** (6), 297–301.

Anthony, D. (1996) Receiver operating characteristic analysis. *Nurse Researcher*, **4** (2), 75–88.

Aronovitch, S.A. (1999) Intraoperatively acquired pressure ulcer prevalence: a national study. *Journal of Wound, Ostomy and Continence Nursing*, **26** (3), 130–136.

Arthur, J., Lewis, P. (2000) When is reduced-compression bandaging safe and effective? *Journal of Wound Care*, **9** (10), 469–471.

Baker, S.R., Stacey, M.C. (1994) Epidemiology of chronic leg ulcers in Australia. *Australia and New Zealand Journal of Surgery*, **64** (4), 258–261.

Bale, S., Crook, H. (1998) The preliminary results of a comparative study on the performance characteristics of a new hydrogel versus an existing hydrogel on necrotic pressure ulcers, in (eds) Leaper, D., Cherry, G., Cockbill, S. *et al.*, *Proceedings of the EWMA/Journal of Wound Care Spring Meeting*. Macmillan Magazines Ltd, London.

Bale, S., Harding, K.G. (2003) Managing patients unable to tolerate therapeutic compression. *British Journal of Nursing*, **12** (19) (suppl), S4–S13.

Bale, S., Squires, D., Vernon, T., Walker, A., Benbow, M., Harding, K.G. (1997) A comparison of two dressings in pressure sore management. *Journal of Wound Care*, **6** (10), 463–466.

Bale, S., Banks, V., Haglestein, S., Harding, K.G. (1998) A comparison of two amorphous hydrogels in the debridement of pressure sores. *Journal of Wound Care*, **7** (2), 65–68.

Barwell, J.R., Davies, C.E., Deacon, J. *et al.* (2004) Comparison of surgery and compression with compression alone in chronic venous ulceration (ESCHAR study): randomised controlled trial. *Lancet*, **363**, 1854–1858.

Baumgarten, M., Margolis, D., Gruber-Baldini, A.L., Zimmerman, S., German, P., Hebel, J.R. (2003a) Pressure ulcers and the transition to long term care. *Advances in Skin and Wound Care*, **16** (6), 299–304.

Baumgarten, M., Margolis, D., Berlin, J.A. *et al.* (2003b) Risk factors for pressure ulcers among elderly hip fracture patients. *Wound Repair and Regeneration*, **11** (2), 96–103.

Bennett, G., Dealey, C., Posnett, J. (2004) The cost of pressure ulcers in the UK. *Age and Ageing*, **33**, 23–235.

Bergstrom, N., Braden, B., Brandt, J., Krall, K. (1985) Adequacy of descriptive scales for reporting diet intake in the institutionalised elderly. *Journal of Nutrition for the Elderly*, **6** (1), 3–16.

Bergstrom, N., Braden, B., Laguzza, A. (1987) The Braden scale for predicting pressure sore risk. *Nursing Research*, **36** (4), 205–210.

Bergstrom, N., Braden, B., Kemp, M., Champagne, M., Ruby, E. (1996) Multi-site study of incidence of pressure ulcers and the relationship between risk level, demographic characteristics, diagnoses and prescription of preventive interventions. *Journal of the American Geriatrics Society*, **44**, 22–30.

Berlowitz, D.R., Wilking, S.V.B. (1989) Risk factors for pressure sores: a comparison of cross-sectional and cohort-derived data. *Journal of the American Geriatrics Society*, **37**, 1043–1050.

Birchall, L., Clark, N., Taylor, S. (2004) Implementing the Essence of Care benchmark for pressure ulcers. *Nursing Times*, **100** (32), 63–67.

Bliss, M. (1990) Editorial – preventing pressure sores. *Lancet*, **335**, 1311–1312.

BLS (2001) *Clinical Definitions*. BLS, Sevenoaks, Kent.

Board, J., Harlow, W. (2002a) Lymphoedema 2: classification, signs, symptoms and diagnosis. *British Journal of Nursing*, **11** (6), 389–395.

Board, J., Harlow, W. (2002b) Lymphoedema 3: the available treatments for lymphoedema. *British Journal of Nursing*, **11** (7), 438–450.

Bours, G.J., Halfens, R.J., Abu-Saad, H.H., Grol, R.T. (2002) Prevalence, prevention and treatment of pressure ulcers: descriptive study in 89 institutions. *Research in Nursing and Health*, **25** (2), 99–110.

Bowering, C.K. (1998) Use of layered compression bandages in diabetic patients. Experience in patients with lower leg ulceration, peripheral oedema, and features of venous and arterial disease. *Advances in Wound Care*, **11** (3), 129–135.

Bradley, M., Cullum, N., Nelson, E.A., Petticrew, M., Sheldon, T., Torgerson, D.J. (1999) Systematic reviews of wound care management: (2) dressings and topical agents used in the healing of chronic wounds. *Health Technology Assessment*, **3** (17) Part 2, 1–174.

Brandeis, G.H., Ooi, W.L., Hossain, M., Morris, J.N., Lipsitz, L.A. (1994) A longitudinal study of risk factors associated with the formation of pressure ulcers in nursing homes. *Journal of the American Geriatrics Society*, **42**, 388–393.

Bridel, J. (1993) Assessing the risk of pressure sores. *Nursing Standard*, **7** (25), 32–35.

Briggs, M., Closs, S.J. (2003) The prevalence of leg ulceration: a review of the literature. *EWMA Journal*, **3** (2), 14–20.

Brookes, R., Thomson, J. (1997) Pressure area care and estimating the cost of pressure sores: critique 2. *Journal of Wound Care*, **6** (3), 135–137.

Buss, I.C., Halfens, R.J., Abu-Saad, H.H. (1997) The effectiveness of massage in preventing pressure sores: a literature review. *Rehabilitation Nursing*, **22** (5), 229–234.

Butcher, M. (2002) Managing mixed-aetiology leg ulcers. *Practice Nursing*, **13** (4), 161–166.

Callam, M.J., Ruckley, C.V., Harper, D.R., Dale, J.J. (1985) Chronic ulceration of the leg: extent of the problems and provision of care. *British Medical Journal*, **290**, 1855–1856.

Cameron, J. (1998) Skin care for patients with chronic leg ulcers. *Journal of Wound Care*, **7** (9), 459–462.

Clark, J. (2002) Metronidazole gel in managing malodorous fungating wounds. *British Journal of Nursing*, **11** (6) (suppl), S54–S60.

Clark, M. (1998) Repositioning to prevent pressure sores – what is the evidence? *Nursing Standard*, **13** (3), 58–64.

Clark, M. (2003) Compression bandages: principles and definitions. *EWMA Position Document: Understanding Compression Therapy*. Medical Education Partnership Ltd, London.

Clark, M., Bours, G., Defloor, T. (2003) The prevalence of pressure ulcers in Europe. *Hospital Decisions*, **Winter**, 123–127.

Colin, D., Abraham, P., Preault, L., Bregeon, C., Saumet, Jl. (1996a) Comparison of 90 degrees and 30 degrees laterally inclined positions in the prevention of pressure ulcers using transcutaneous oxygen and carbon dioxide pressures. *Advances in Wound Care*, **9** (3), 35–38.

Colin, D., Kurring, P.A., Yvon, C. (1996b) Managing sloughy pressure ulcers. *Journal of Wound Care*, **5** (10), 444–446.

Colin, D., Dizien, O., Yvon, C. (1997) The clinical investigation of a transparent semi-permeable adhesive film dressing with an extra-thin hydrocolloid in the management of stage I and II pressure sores, in (eds) Leaper, D.J., Cherry, G.W., Dealey, C., Lawrence, J.C., Turner, T.D., *Proceedings of the 6th European Conference on Advances in Wound Management*. Macmillan Magazines Ltd, London.

Collins, F. (1999) The contribution made by an armchair with integral pressure-reducing cushion in the prevention of pressure sore incidence in the elderly, acutely ill patient. *Journal of Tissue Viability*, **9** (4), 133–137.

Cooper, P., Gray, D. (2001) Comparison of two skin care regimes for incontinence. *British Journal of Nursing*, **10** (6) (suppl), S6–S20.

Cornwall, J.V., Dore, C.J., Lewis, J.D. (1986) Leg ulcers: epidemiology and aetiology. *British Medical Journal*, **73**, 693–696.

Culley, F. (1998) Nursing aspects of pressure sore prevention and therapy. *British Journal of Nursing*, **7** (15), 879–884.

Cullum, N., Nelson, E.A., Sheldon, T. (2001a) Systematic reviews of wound care management (5): pressure-relieving beds, mattreses and cushions for the prevention and treatment of pressure sores. *Health Technology Assessment*, **5** (9), 1–75.

Cullum, N., Nelson, E.A., Fletcher, A.W., Sheldon, T.A. (2001b) Compression for venous leg ulcers (Cochrane Review). *Cochrane Library, Issue 1*. Update Software Ltd, Oxford.

Danchaivijitr, S., Suthisanon, L., Jitreecheue, L., Tantiwatanapaibool, Y. (1995) Effects of education on the prevention of pressure sores. *Journal of the Medical Association of Thailand*, **78** (suppl.1), S1–S6.

David, J.A., Chapman, R.G., Chapman, E.J., Lockett, B. (1983) *An Investigation of the Current Methods Used in Nursing for the Care of Patients with Established Pressure Sores*. Nursing Practice Research Unit, Northwick Park, Middlesex.

Dealey, C. (1991a) The size of the pressure sore problem in a teaching hospital. *Journal of Advanced Nursing*, **16**, 663–670.

Dealey, C. (1991b) Causes of leg ulcers. *Nursing*, **4** (35), 23–24.

Dealey, C. (1997) *Managing Pressure Sore Prevention*, Mark Allen Publishing Ltd, Salisbury.

Dealey, C., Keogh, A. (1998) A randomised study comparing the Triple Care cleanser and cream system with soap and water for elderly incontinent patients, in (eds) Leaper, D., Dealey, C., Franks, P.J., Hofman, D., Moffatt, C.J., *Proceedings of the 7th European Conference on Advances in Wound Management*. EMAP Healthcare Ltd, London.

Dealey, C., Earwaker, T., Eden, L. (1991) Are your patients sitting comfortably? *Journal of Tissue Viability*, **1** (2), 36–39.

Deeks, J.J. (1996) Pressure sore prevention: using and evaluating risk assessment tools. *British Journal of Nursing*, **5** (5), 313–320.

Defloor, T., Schoonhoven, L. (2004) Interrater reliability of the EPUAP pressure ulcer classification system using photographs. *Journal of Clinical Nursing*, **13** (8), 952–959.

Defloor, T., de Bacquer, D., Grypdonck, M.H. (2005) The effect of various combinations of turning and pressure reducing devices on the incidence of pressure ulcers. *International Journal of Nursing Studies*, **42** (1), 37–46.

Department of Health (1993) *Pressure Sores: a key quality indicator*. Department of Health, London.

Department of Health and NHS Modernisation Agency (2003) *The Essence of Care. Patient-focused Benchmarks for clinical governance*. Department of Health, London.

Dowsett, C. (2002) Malignant fungating wounds: assessment and management. *British Journal of Community Nursing*, **7** (8), 394–400.

Effective Health Care (1995) The prevention and treatment of pressure sores. *Effective Health Care Bulletin*, **2** (1), 1–16.

Ek, A.C., Gustavssen, G., Lewis, D.H. (1987) Skin blood flow in relation to external pressure and temperature in the supine position on a standard hospital mattress. *Scandinavian Journal of Rehabilitation*, **19**, 121–126.

Ellison, D.A., Hayes, L., Lane, C., Tracey, A., McCollum, C.N. (2002) Evaluating the cost and efficacy of leg ulcer care provided in two large UK health authorities. *Journal of Wound Care*, **11** (2), 47–51.

European Pressure Ulcer Advisory Panel (1999) Pressure ulcer treatment guidelines. *EPUAP Review*, **1** (2), 31–33.

Exton-Smith, A.N., Sherwin, R.W. (1961) The prevention of pressure sores: the significance of spontaneous bodily movement. *Lancet*, **II**, 1124–1126.

Faries, P.L., Teodorescu, V.J., Morrissey, N.J., Hollier, L.H., Marin, M.L. (2004) The role of surgical revascularisation in the management of diabetic foot wounds. *American Journal of Surgery*, **187** (5) (suppl), 34S–37S.

Fentem, P.H. (1986) Elastic hosiery. *Pharmacy Update*, **5**, 200–205.

Ferrell, B.A., Josephson, K., Norvid, P., Alcorn, H. (2000) Pressure ulcers among patients admitted to home care. *Journal of the American Geriatrics Society*, **49** (5), 1042–1047.

Flanagan, M. (1997) Choosing pressure sore risk assessment tools. *Professional Nurse*, **12** (6) (suppl), 3–7.

Fowler, E. (1990) Chronic wounds: an overview, in (ed.) Krasner, D., *Chronic Wound Care: a clinical sourcebook for healthcare professionals*. Health Management Publications, King of Prussia, PA.

Gebhardt, K. (1995) What causes pressure sores? *Nursing Standard*, **9** (suppl. 31), 48–51.

Ghauri, A.S.K., Nyamekye, I., Grabs, A.J., Farndon, J.R., Whyman, M.R., Poskitt, K.R. (1998) Influence of a specialised leg ulcer service and venous surgery on the outcomes of venous leg ulcers. *European Journal of Vascular and Endovascular Surgery*, **16**, 238–244.

Girod, I., Valensi, P., Laforet, C., Moreau-Defarges, T., Guillon, P., Baron, F. (2003) An economic evaluation of the cost of diabetic foot ulcers: results of a retrospective study on 239 patients. *Diabetes and Metabolism*, **29** (3), 269–277.

Goebel, R.H., Goebel, M.R. (1999) Clinical practice guidelines for pressure ulcer prevention can prevent malpractice lawsuits in older patients. *Journal of Wound, Ostomy and Continence Nursing*, **26** (4), 175–184.

Grocott, P. (1997) Evaluation of a tool to assess the management of fungating wounds. *Journal of Wound Care*, **6** (9), 421–424.

Grocott, P. (1998) Exudate management in fungating wounds. *Journal of Wound Care*, **7** (9), 445–448.

Grocott, P. (2000) The palliative management of fungating malignant wounds. *Journal of Wound Care*, **9** (1), 4–9.

Gruen, R.L., Chang, S., MacLellan, D.G. (1996) Optimising the hospital management of leg ulcers. *Australia and New Zealand Journal of Surgery*, **66** (3), 171–174.

Guenter, P., Malyszek, R., Bliss, D.Z. *et al.* (2000) Survey of nutritional status in newly hospitalised patients with stage III or stage IV pressure ulcers. *Advances in Skin and Wound Care*, **13** (4), 164–168.

Hafner, J., Schneider, E., Burg, G., Cassina, P.C. (2000) Management of leg ulcers in patients with rheumatoid arthritis or systemic sclerosis: the importance of concomitant arterial and venous disease. *Journal of Vascular Surgery*, **32** (2), 322–329.

Haglsawa, S., Barbenel, J. (1999) The limits of pressure sore prevention. *Journal of the Royal Society of Medicine*, **92**, 576–578.

Haisfield-Wolfe, M.A., Rund, C. (1997) Malignant cutaneous wounds: a management protocol. *Ostomy and Wound Management*, **43**, 56–66.

Halfens, R.J.G., Bours, G.J.J.W., van Ast, W. (2001) Relevance of the diagnosis 'stage 1 pressure ulcer': an empirical study of the clinical course of stage 1 ulcers in acute care and long-term care hospital populations. *Journal of Clinical Nursing*, **10** (6), 748–757.

Harding, K.G. (1998) The future of wound healing, in (eds) Leaper, D.J., Harding, K.G., *Wounds: biology and management*. Oxford University Press, Oxford.

Hayes, S., Dodds, S. (2003) The identification and diagnosis of malignant leg ulcers. *Nursing Times*, **99** (31) (suppl), 8–10.

Hibbs, P. (1988) *Pressure Area Care for the City and Hackney Health Authority*. City and Hackney Health Authority, London.

Hofman, D., Ryan, T.J., Arnold, F. *et al.* (1997) Pain in venous leg ulcers. *Journal of Wound Care*, **6** (5), 222–224.

Horn, S.D., Bender, S.A., Bergstrom, N. *et al.* (2002) Description of the national pressure ulcer long-term care study. *Journal of the American Geriatrics Society*, **50**, 1816–1825.

Houwing, R., Overgoor, M., Kon, M., Jansen, G., van Asbeck, B.S., Haalboom, J.R. (2000) Pressure-induced skin lesions in pigs: reperfusion injury and the effects of vitamin E. *Journal of Wound Care*, **9** (1), 36–40.

Iglesias, C., Nelson, E.A., Cullum, N.A., Torgerson, D.J. (2004) VenUS 1: a randomised controlled trial of two types of bandage for treating venous leg ulcers. *Health Technology Assessment*, **8** (29), 1–106.

Jay, R. (1997) Other considerations in selecting a support surface. *Advanced Wound Care*, **10** (7), 37–42.

Jeffcoate, W.J., Harding, K.G. (2003) Diabetic foot ulcers. *Lancet*, **361** (9368), 1545–1551.

Jeffs, E. (1993) The effect of acute inflammatory episodes on the treatment of lymphoedema. *Journal of Tissue Viability*, **3** (2), 51–55.

Jones, J.E., Nelson, E.A. (1998) Compression hosiery in the management of venous leg ulcers. *Journal of Wound Care*, **7** (6), 293–296.

Jones, J.E., Nelson, E.A. (2001) Skin grafting for venous leg ulcers (Cochrane Review). *Cochrane Library, Issue 1*. Update Software Ltd, Oxford.

Jude, E.B., Oyibo, S.O., Millichip, M.M., Boulton, A.J.M. (2003) A survey of physicians' involvement in the management of diabetic foot ulcers in secondary health care. *Practical Diabetes International*, **20** (3), 89–92.

Kabagambe, M.K., Swain, I., Shakespeare, P. (1994) An investigation of the effects on the microcirculation of the skin (reactive hyperaemia) in spinal cord injured patients. *Journal of Tissue Viability*, **4** (4), 110–123.

Kaltenthaler, E., Whitfield, M.D., Walter, S.J., Akehurst, R.L., Paisley, S. (2001) UK, USA and Canada: how do their pressure ulcer prevalence and incidence data compare? *Journal of Wound Care*, **10** (1), 530–535.

Khoo, C., Bailey, B.N. (1990) Reconstructive surgery, in (ed.) Bader, D., *Pressure Sores – clinical practice and scientific approach*. Macmillan Press, London.

Kierney, P.C., Engrav, L.H., Isik, F.F., Esselman, P.C., Cardenas, D.D., Rand, R.P. (1998) Results of 268 pressure sores in 158 patients managed jointly by plastic surgery and rehabilitation medicine. *Plastic and Reconstructive Surgery*, **102** (3), 765–772.

Ko, D.S., Lerner, K., Klose, G., Cosimi, A.B. (1998) Effective treatment of lymphoedema of the extremities. *Archives of Surgery*, **133** (4), 452–458.

Krouskop, M. (1983) A synthesis of the factors which contribute to pressure sore formation. *Medical Hypothesis*, **11**, 255–267.

Kumar, R.N., Gupchup, G.V., Dodd, M.A. *et al.* (2004) Direct health care costs of 4 common skin ulcers in New Mexico Medicaid fee-for-service patients. *Advances in Skin and Wound Care*, **17** (3), 143–149.

Landis, E.M. (1931) Micro-injection studies of capillary blood pressure in human skin. *Heart*, **15**, 209–228.

Langer, G., Schloemer, G., Knerr, A., Kuss, O., Behrens, J. (2003) Nutritional interventions for preventing and treating pressure ulcers (Cochrane review). *The Cochrane Library, Issue 4*. John Wiley & Sons Ltd, Chichester.

Lapsley, H.M., Vogels, R. (1996) Cost and prevention of pressure ulcer in an acute teaching hospital. *International Journal for Quality in Health Care*, **8** (1), 61–66.

Lawrence, J.C., Lilly, H.A., Kidson, A. (1993) Malodour and dressings containing active charcoal, in (eds) Harding, K.G., Cherry, G., Dealey, C., Turner, T.D., *Proceedings of the 2nd European Conference on Advances in Wound Management*. Macmillan Magazines Ltd, London.

Lingren, M., Unosson, M., E.K., A.-C. (2000) Pressure sore prevalence within a public health services area. *International Journal of Nursing Practice*, **6** (6), 333–337.

Litchfield, B., Ramkissoon, S. (1996) Foot-care education in patients with diabetes. *Professional Nurse*, **11** (8), 510–512.

Loudon, I.S.L. (1982) Leg ulcers in the eighteenth and early nineteenth centuries. *Journal of the Royal College of General Practitioners*, **32**, 301–309.

Machet, L., Couhe, C., Perrinaud, A., Hoarau, C., Lorette, G., Vaillant, L. (2004) A high prevalence of sensitisation still persists in leg ulcer patients: a retrospective series of 106 patients tested between 2001 and 2002 and a meta-analysis of 1975–2003 data. *British Journal of Dermatology*, **150** (5), 929–935.

Mani, R., Vowden, K., Nelson, E.A. (2004) Intermittant pneumatic compression for treating venous leg ulcers (Cochrane review). *Cochrane Library, Issue 4*. John Wiley & Sons, Chichester.

Margolis, D.J., Berlin, J.A., Strom, B.L. (2000) Which venous leg ulcers will heal with limb compression bandages? *American Journal of Medicine*, **109**, 15–19.

Margolis, D., Knauss, J., Bilker, W., Baumgarten, M. (2003) Medical conditions as risk factors for pressure ulcers in an out-patient setting. *Age and Ageing*, **32**, 259–264.

Marston, W., Vowden, K. (2003) Compression therapy: a guide to safe practice. *EWMA Position Document: Understanding Compression Therapy*. Medical Education Partnership Ltd, London.

Mathus-Vleigen, E.M.H. (2001) Nutritional status, nutrition and pressure ulcers. *Nutrition in Clinical Practice*, **16**, 286–291.

McCafferty, E., Watret, L., Brown, C. (2000) A multidisciplinary audit of patients' seating needs. *Professional Nurse*, **15** (11), 715–718.

McKeeney, L. (2002) Legal issues for the prevention of pressure ulcers. *Journal of Community Nursing*, **16** (7), 28–30.

McNeely, M.L., Magee, D.J., Lees, A.W., Bagnall, K.M., Haykowsky, M., Hanson, J. (2004) The addition of manual lymph drainage to compression therapy for breat cancer related lymphoedema: a randomised controlled trial. *Breast Cancer Research and Treatment*, **86** (2), 95–106.

McRorie, E.R. (2000) The management and assessment of leg ulcers in rheumatoid arthritis. *Journal of Wound Care*, **9** (6), 289–292.

Meyer, F.J., McGuinness, C.L., Lagatolla, N.R.F., Eastham, D., Burnand, K.G. (2003) Randomised clinical trial of three-layer paste and four-layer bandages for venous leg ulcers. *British Journal of Surgery*, **90** (8), 934–940.

Moffatt, C.J., Franks, P.J., Doherty, D.C., Martin, R., Blewitt, R., Ross, F. (2004) Prevalence of leg ulceration in a London population. *Quarterly Journal of Medicine*, **97**, 431–437.

Mortimer, P.S. (2001) Acute inflammatory episodes, in (eds) Twycross, R., Jenns, K., Todd, J., *Lymphoedema*. Radcliffe Medical Press, Oxford.

Mustoe, T. (2004) Understanding chronic wounds: a unifying hypothesis on their pathogenesis and implications for therapy. *American Journal of Surgery*, **187** (5A), 65S–70S.

National Institute for Clinical Excellence (2003) *Clinical Guideline 7: pressure ulcer prevention*. NICE, London.

National Institute for Clinical Excellence (2004) *Clinical Guideline 10: type 2 diabetes: prevention and management of foot problems*. NICE, London.

Naylor, W. (2001) Assessment and management of pain in fungating wounds. *British Journal of Nursing*, **10** (22) (suppl), S33–S52.

Nelson, E.A., Bradley, M.D. (2003) Dressings and topical agents for arterial leg ulcers. *Cochrane Database of Systematic Reviews* (1) CD001836.

Nelson, E.A., Bell-Syer, S.E.M., Cullum, N.A. (2004) Compression for preventing recurrence of venous ulcers (Cochrane Review). *Cochrane Library, Issue 4*. John Wiley & Sons, Chichester.

Nightingale, F. (1861) *Notes on Nursing*. Appleton Century, New York.

Norton, D., Mclaren, R., Exton-Smith, A.N. (1975) *An Investigation of Geriatric Nursing Problems*. Churchill Livingstone, Edinburgh.

Nyquist, R., Hawthorn, P.J. (1987) The prevalence of pressure sores in an area health authority. *Journal of Advanced Nursing*, **12**, 183–187.

O'Brien, J.F., Grace, P.A., Perry, I.J., Burke, P.E. (2000) Prevalence and aetiology of leg ulcers in Ireland. *Irish Journal of Medical Science*, **169** (2), 110–112.

O'Dea, K. (1999) The prevalence of pressure damage in acute care hospital patients in the UK. *Journal of Wound Care*, **8** (4), 192–194.

Oien, R.F., Hakansson, A., Hansen, B.U. (2001) Leg ulcers in patients with rheumatoid arthritis – a prospective study of aetiology, wound healing and pain reduction after pinch grafting. *Rheumatology*, **40**, 816–820.

Papanikolaou, P., Clark, M., Lyne, P.A. (2002) Improving the accuracy of pressure ulcer risk calculators: some preliminary evidence. *International Journal of Nursing Studies*, **39** (2), 187–194.

Patel, G.K., Llewellyn, M., Harding, K.G. (2001) Managing gravitational eczema and allergic contact dermatitis. *British Journal of Community Nursing*, **6** (8), 394–406.

Pearson, A., Francis, K., Hodgkinson, B., Curry, G. (2000) Prevalence and treatment of pressure ulcers in northern New South Wales. *Australian Journal of Rural Health*, **8** (2), 103–110.

Pedley, G.E. (2004) Comparison of pressure ulcer grading scales: a study of clinical utility and inter-rater reliability. *International Journal of Nursing Studies*, **41**, 129–140.

Peirce, S.M., Skalak, T.C., Rodeheaver, G.T. (2000) Ischaemia-reperfusion injury in chronic pressure ulcer formation: a skin model in the rat. *Wound Repair and Regeneration*, **8** (1), 68–76.

Persoon, A., Heinen, M.M., van der Vleuten, C.J.M., de Rooij, M.J., van de Kerkhof, P.C.M., van Achterberg, T. (2004) Leg ulcers: a review of their impact on daily life. *Journal of Clinical Nursing*, **13**, 341–354.

Polignano, R., Bonadeo, P., Gasbarro, S., Allegra, C. (2004) A randomised controlled trial of four-layer compression versus Unna's boot for venous ulcers. *Journal of Wound Care*, **13** (1), 21–24.

Poore, S., Cameron, J., Cherry, G. (2002) Venous leg ulcer recurrence: prevention and healing. *Journal of Wound Care*, **11** (5), 197–199.

Preston, K.W. (1988) Positioning for comfort and pressure relief: the 30 degree alternative. *Care – Science and Practice*, **6** (4), 116–119.

Quartey-Papafio, C.M. (1999) Importance of distinguishing between cellulitis and varicose eczema. *British Medical Journal*, **318**, 1672–1673.

Ray, S.A., Minty, I., Buckenham, T.M. (1995) Clinical outcome and restenosis following PTA for ischaemic rest pain or ulceration. *British Journal of Surgery*, **82** (9), 1217–1222.

Reed, R.L., Hepburn, K., Adelson, R., Center, B., McNight, P. (2003) Low serum albumin levels, confusion, and faecal incontinence: are these risk factors for pressure ulcers in mobility impaired hospitalised adults? *Gerontology*, **49** (4), 255–259.

Regan, M.B., Byers, P.H., Mayrovitz, H.N. (1995) Efficacy of a comprehensive pressure ulcer prevention programme in an extended care facility. *Advances in Wound Care*, **8** (3), 49–55.

Regnard, C., Allport, S., Stephenson, L. (1997) ABC of palliative care: mouthcare, skin care and lymphoedema. *British Medical Journal*, **315**, 1002–1005.

Rithalia, S.V.S. (1989) Comparison of pressure distribution in wheelchair seat cushions. *Care – Science and Practice*, **7** (4), 87–89.

Royal College of Nursing (1998) *Clinical Practice Guidelines. The management of patients with venous leg ulcers.* Royal College of Nursing, London.

Royal College of Nursing (2003) *Safer Staff, Better Care: RCN manual handling training guidance and competencies.* Royal College of Nursing, London.

Ruckley, C.V., Evans, C.J., Allan, P.L., Lee, A.J., Fowkes, F., Gerald, R. (2002) Chronic venous insufficiency: clinical and duplex correlations. The Edinburgh Vein Study of venous disorders in the general population. *Journal of Vascular Surgery*, **36** (3), 52–525.

Russell, L.J., Reynolds, T.M. (2001) How accurate are pressure ulcer grades? An image-based survey of nurses' performance. *Journal of Tissue Viability*, **11** (2), 67–75.

Ryan, T.J. (1987) *The Management of Leg Ulcers*, 2nd edn. Oxford University Press, Oxford.

Sanada, H., Nagakawa, T., Yamamoto, M., Higashidani, K., Tsuru, H., Sugama, J. (1997) The role of blood flow in pressure ulcer development during surgery. *Advances in Wound Care*, **10** (6), 29–34.

Sandeman, D.D., Pym, C.A., Green, E.M. *et al.* (1991) Microvascular vasodilation in the feet of newly diagnosed non-insulin dependent diabetics. *British Medical Journal*, **302** (6785), 1122–1123.

Scanlon, E., Stubbs, N. (2004) Pressure ulcer risk assessment in patients with darkly pigmented skin. *Professional Nurse*, **19** (6), 339–341.

Schiech, L. (2002) Malignant cutaneous wounds. *Clinical Journal of Oncology Nursing*, **6** (5), 305–309.

Schoonhoven, L., Defloor, T., Grypdonck, M.H. (2002a) Incidence of pressure ulcers due to surgery. *Journal of Clinical Nursing*, **11** (4), 479–487.

Schoonhoven, L., Haalboom, J.R.E., Bousema, T. *et al.* (2002b) Prospective cohort study of routine use of risk assessment scales for prediction of pressure ulcers. *British Medical Journal*, **325** (7368), 797–801.

Schue, R.M., Langemo, D.K. (1999) Prevalence, incidence and prediction of pressure ulcers on a rehabilitation unit. *Journal of Wound, Ostomy and Continence Nursing*, **26** (3), 121–129.

Seeley, J., Jensen, J.L., Vigil, S. (1998) A 40-patient randomised clinical trial to compare the performance of Allevyn Adhesive hydrocellular dressing and a hydrocolloid in the management of pressure ulcers, in (eds) Leaper, D., Dealey, C., Franks, P.J., Hofman, D., Moffatt, C.J., *Proceedings of the 7th European Conference on Advances in Wound Management.* EMAP Healthcare Ltd, London.

Severens, J.L., Habraken, J.M., Duivenvoorden, S., Frederiks, C.M.S. (2002) The cost of illness of pressure ulcers in the Netherlands. *Advances in Skin and Wound Care*, **15** (2), 72–77.

Sieggreen, M.Y., Kline, R.A. (2004) Arterial insufficiency and ulceration: diagnosis and treatment options. *Advances in Skin and Wound Care*, **17** (5), 242–251.

Sopata, M. (1997) A comparative, prospective study of the treatment of stage II and III pressure sores in patients with advanced cancer: Aquagel versus Lyofoam A, in (eds) Leaper, D.J., Cherry, G.W., Dealey, C., Lawrence, J.C., Turner, T.D., *Proceedings of the 6th European Conference on Advances in Wound Management.* Macmillan Magazines Ltd, London.

Sorensen, J.L., Jorgensen, B., Gottrup, F. (2004) Surgical treatment of pressure ulcers. *American Journal of Surgery*, **188** (1) (suppl), 42–51.

Spittle, M., Collins, R.J., Connor, H. (2001) The incidence of pressure sores following lower limb amputations. *Practical Diabetes International*, **18** (2), 57–61.

Stacey, M., Falanga, V., Marston, W. *et al.* (2002) The use of compression therapy in the treatment of venous leg ulcers: a recommended management pathway. *EWMA Journal*, **2** (1), 9–13.

Stemmer, R. (1969) Ambulatory elasto-compressive treatment of the lower extremities particularly with elastic stockings. *Der Kassenatzt*, **9**, 1–8.

Stordeur, S., Laurent, S., D'Hoore, W. (1998) The importance of repeated risk assessment for pressure sores in cardiovascular surgery. *Journal of Cardiovascular Surgery (Torino)*, **39** (3), 343–349.

Tavakoli, K., Rutkowski, S., Cope, C. *et al.* (1999) Recurrence rates of ischial sores in para- and tetraplegics treated with hamstring flaps: an 8 year study. *British Journal of Plastic Surgery*, **52**, 476–479.

Taylor, A. (1998) The importance of tissue biopsy for non-healing leg ulcers. *Journal of Tissue Viability*, **8** (3), 32.

Tennvall, G.R., Andersson, K., Bjellerup, M., Hjelmgren, J., Oien, R. (2004) treatment of venous leg ulcers can be better and cheaper. Annual costs calculation based on an inquiry study. *Lakartidningen*, **101** (17), 1506–1513.

Teot, L., N'Guyen, C., Leglise, S., Gavroy, J.P., Handshuh, R. (1998a) Safety and efficacy of a new hydrocolloid in the treatment of stage I and II pressure sores, in (eds) Leaper, D., Cherry, G., Cockbill, S. *et al.*, *Proceedings of the EWMA/Journal of Wound Care Spring Meeting*. Macmillan Magazines Ltd, London.

Teot, L., Richard, D., Votte, A. *et al.* (1998b) Comparison of an Aquacel dressing regime and a traditional dressing regime in the management of pressure sores, in (eds) Leaper, D., Cherry, G., Cockbill, S. *et al.*, *Proceedings of the EWMA/Journal of Wound Care Spring Meeting*. Macmillan Magazines Ltd, London.

Thomas, S. (1992) *Current Practices in the Managment of Fungating Lesions and Radiation Damaged Skin*. Surgical Materials Testing Laboratory, Bridgend.

Thomas, S. (2003) The use of the Laplace equation in the calculation of sub-bandage pressure. World Wide Wounds. Available online at: www.worldwidewounds.com

Thomas, S., Banks, V., Bale, S. *et al.* (1997) A comparison of two dressings in the management of chronic wounds. *Journal of Wound Care*, **6** (8), 383–386.

Thoroddsen, A. (1999) Pressure sore prevalence: a national survey. *Journal of Clinical Nursing*, **8** (2), 170–179.

Tingle, J. (1997) Pressure sores: counting the legal cost of nursing neglect. *British Journal of Nursing*, **6** (13), 757–758.

Ukat, A., Konig, M., Vanscheidt, W., Munter, K.-C. (2003) Short-stretch versus multilayer compression for venous leg ulcers: a comparison of healing rates. *Journal of Wound Care*, **12** (4), 139–143.

Versluysen, M. (1986) How elderly patients with femoral fractures develop pressure sores in hospital. *British Medical Journal*, **292**, 1311–1313.

Voisard, J.J., Lazareth, I., Baviera, E., Priollet, P. (2001) Leg ulcers and cancer. 6 case reports. *Journal des Malades Vasculaires*, **26** (2), 85–91.

Wagner, F.W. (1981) The dysvascular foot: a system for diagnosis and treatment. *Foot Ankle*, **2**, 64.

Walsh, R. (2002) Improving diagnosis of malignant leg ulcers in the community. *British Journal of Nursing*, **11** (9), 604–613.

Walters, D.P., Gatling, W., Hill, R.D., Mullee, M.A. (1993) The prevalence of foot deformity in diabetic subjects: a population study in an English community. *Practical Diabetes*, **10** (3), 106–108.

Waterlow, J. (1985) A risk assessment card. *Nursing Times*, **81** (48), 49–55.

Waterlow, J. (1988) Prevention is cheaper than cure. *Nursing Times*, **84** (25), 69–70.

Williams, A., Venables, J. (1996) Skin care in patients with uncomplicated lymphoedema. *Journal of Wound Care*, **5** (5), 223–226.

Williams, D.F., Stotts, N.A., Nelson, K. (2000) Patients with existing pressure ulcers admitted to acute care. *Journal of Wound and Ostomy Care Nursing*, **27** (4), 216–226.

World Health Organisation (2001) Lymphatic filariasis. World Health Organisation. Available online at: www.who.int/inf-fs/en/fact102.html

Yang, D., Morrison, B.D., Vandongen, Y.K., Singh, A., Stacey, M.C. (1996) Malignancy in chronic leg ulcers. *Medical Journal of Australia*, **164** (12), 718–720.

Young, T. (2004) The 30° tilt position vs the 90° lateral and supine positions in reducing the incidence of non-blanching erythema in a hospital inpatient population: a randomised trial. *Journal of Tissue Viability*, **14** (3), 88–96.

Young, T., Williams, C., Benbow, M., Collier, M., Banks, V., Jones, H. (1997) A study of two hydrogels used in the management of pressure sores, in (eds) Leaper, D.J., Cherry, G.W., Dealey, C., Lawrence, J.C., Turner, T.D., *Proceedings of the 6th European Conference on Advances in Wound Management*. Macmillan Magazines Ltd, London.

Chapter 6
The Management of Patients with Acute Wounds

6.1 INTRODUCTION

Acute wounds can be defined as wounds of sudden onset and of short duration. They include surgical wounds and traumatic wounds such as burns. Acute wounds can occur in people of all ages and generally heal easily without complication. This section will consider the specific care needed for patients with acute wounds.

6.2 THE CARE OF SURGICAL WOUNDS

Surgical wounds are, by their very nature, premeditated wounds. This allows the surgeon to attempt to reduce any risks of complication to a minimum. However, as increasingly sophisticated surgery is performed, often on relatively elderly patients, complications are still a hazard. One aspect of nursing care is to monitor the progress of the wound, so that there is early identification of any problems.

6.2.1 Management of surgical wounds

Patient assessment

This is essential to identify any factors that might affect healing. This topic is covered in more detail in Chapter 2.

Wound assessment

This should identify the method of closure, note the use of any drains and observe for any indication of complication. Westaby (1985) described the main aim of surgical wound closure as the restoration of function and physical integrity with the minimum deformity and without infection. The method of wound closure is selected in order to achieve this aim and it will vary according to the surgery performed. There are three methods of closure: primary closure, delayed primary closure and healing by second intention.

Primary closure

Hippocrates (460–377 BC) was the first to describe this method of wound closure. He called it healing by first intention. The skin edges are held in approximation by sutures, clips, staples or tape. In these wounds the skin edges seal very quickly, first with fibrin from clot formation and then as epithelialisation occurs. Within 48 hours the wound should be totally sealed, thus preventing the ingress of bacteria.

Nursing care

The care of wounds healing by first intention is generally straightforward. A simple island dressing is commonly used to cover the wound at the end of the operation. Several studies have shown that the dressing can be removed after 24–48 hours and need not be replaced, (Chrintz et al., 1989; Cruse & Foord, 1980; Weiss, 1983). Some surgeons prefer to cover the wound with a film dressing and leave it in place until the sutures are removed. Whichever method is used, normal hygiene can be resumed and the patient may bathe or shower.

Some more recent studies have been able to add further information. Wikblad and Anderson (1995) randomised 250 heart surgery patients to an island dressing, a hydrocolloid dressing or a hydroactive dressing. They found that overall, the island dressing outperformed the other dressings in terms of being less painful to remove and causing less redness to the wound site and skin changes to surrounding skin. Significantly more wounds healed under the standard dressing than the hydroactive (57% compared with 27%). Fifty percent of the wounds in the hydrocolloid group healed, there being no significant difference with the standard dressing group. Despite requiring more dressing changes over five days, the island dressing was considerably cheaper than the comparators.

Allen (1996) also studied the care of sternal wounds following heart surgery. After an initial observation study of 100 patients to observe the impact of using gauze immediately after surgery and removing it on the first postoperative day, it was concluded that there was actually an increased risk of infection in these patients. Subsequently three dressings were trialled successively: in week 1, 73 patients received Duoderm Extra Thin™; in week 2, 75 patients had Opraflex™; and in week 3, 77 patients had Opsite Post-Op™. The author found that Opsite Post-Op™ remained in place longer than the other dressings and bathing was easier. It was also easier to remove as it did not pull on the sutures. There was no real difference in infection rates compared with the observational study.

Holm et al. (1998) compared a standard island (control) dressing with a hydrocolloid dressing on 73 patients following clean abdominal surgery, the dressings remaining in place until suture removal. Unfortunately, 29 patients withdrew from the study, leaving a relatively small number to complete the study. The incidence of wound infection was higher in the control group (5/17) compared with the hydrocolloid group (1/26). There were no other differences in respect of leakage, dressing detachment and cosmetic appearance. The authors noted that the patients seemed to find the hydrocolloid more comfortable and mobilising was easier. This finding seems to support the results from the next study to be discussed.

Briggs (1996) undertook a small study where 30 patients undergoing hysterectomy were randomised to either a dry dressing removed after 48 hours or a film dressing left in place until suture removal. She found a significant difference in pain on day 3 after the dry dressing had been removed. Those with no dressing had sufficient pain to require analgesia.

A much larger study compared three dressings used on sternotomy wounds: an island dressing, a film dressing and a thin hydrocolloid dressing (Wynne *et al.*, 2004). A total of 737 patients were randomised to one of the three dressings. The authors found no difference in the incidence of wound infection or healing rates. The island dressing was seen to be the most comfortable and cost effective of the three dressings. It seems reasonable to conclude that although there may not be a need for a dressing over a surgical incision to prevent infection, use of a dressing is more comfortable for the patient. A simple island dressing appears to be comfortable to wear and remove as well as being relatively cheap.

Surgical wounds should be monitored daily for any indication of complication.

Removal of sutures or other types of wound closure is usually carried out under medical supervision.

Delayed primary closure

This method of closure is used when there has been considerable bacterial contamination. Initially, any body cavity is closed and the remaining tissue layers are left open to allow free drainage of pus. After about five days, these layers are closed and the wound will heal as any primarily closed wound. Wound drains may be used to assist in the removal of any fluid remaining at the wound base. Cohn *et al.* (2001) demonstrated that delayed primary closure was an effective method of treatment for dirty abdominal surgical wounds compared with primary closure. There was a significantly higher incidence of infection in the primary closure group (11/23 – 48%) compared with the delayed primary closure group (3/26 – 12%).

Nursing care

The aim of management of these wounds is to allow free drainage of any pus. This may be achieved by loose packing of the cavity. As the wound will be sutured at about day 5, the promotion of granulation is not a major aim. If ribbon gauze is used, it should be kept moist and changed regularly to prevent it drying out and adhering to the wound. Alginate rope may also be used, as it is very absorbent and can be removed without pain to the patient. Once the wound is sutured, it should be treated as a wound healing by first intention.

Healing by second intention

Healing by second intention describes a wound that is left open and heals by granulation, contraction and epithelialisation. This method may be used for a variety of reasons.

- There may be considerable tissue loss, e.g. radical vulvectomy.
- The surgical incision is shallow but has a large surface area, e.g. donor sites.
- There may have been infection; for example, a ruptured appendix or an abscess may have been drained and free drainage of any pus is essential.

Nursing care

The care of varying types of surgical wounds will be described here.

● Surgical cavities ●

Surgical cavities are generally clean wounds with a healthy bed that would be expected to heal without complication. Harding (1990) suggests that surgical cavities should be boat-shaped in order to heal rapidly without premature surface healing. Simple wound measurement is usually sufficient to monitor healing rates (see Chapter 3). These wounds should also be observed for indications of infection.

Selection of a suitable dressing depends on the position of the wound and the amount of exudate. Traditionally, ribbon gauze packing, often soaked in antiseptic solutions, has been used in these wounds. Ricci *et al.* (1998) compared iodine-soaked gauze with a foam stent in patients following pilonidal sinus excision and found the foam stent to be more effective. Healing time was faster – median 33.5 days compared with 73 days. The patients with the foam stent were able to return to work after 12 days compared with 23 days. Far fewer dressing changes were required: 20 foam stents compared with 868 gauze packs. In addition, the foam stent group had pain-free dressing changes whereas the gauze group found the dressing change painful and bleeding occurred. This small study clearly demonstrates the problems found with gauze packing.

Most of the studies have been small studies like the one described above. Vermeulen *et al.* (2004) undertook a systematic review of dressings and topical agents used to manage surgical wounds healing by secondary intention. They concluded that the studies were too small to provide guidance on the treatment of choice. However, they found that foam had been most frequently studied as an alternative to gauze and that it seemed to be preferable in respect of pain reduction, patient satisfaction and nursing time. Further large studies are required to provide clear evidence as to the most effective treatment regimes.

● Skin grafts ●

Skin grafts are widely used in reconstructive surgery following trauma or burns. They may also be used to repair chronic wounds such as pressure sores or leg ulcers. Skin grafting is a technique that permits the transfer of a portion of skin from one part of the body to another. There are several ways of classifying skin grafts. They can be divided into:

- autografts – a graft of the patient's own skin
- allografts – a graft taken from another individual
- xenografts – a graft taken from another species.

Grafts can be described according to their thickness. This depends on the amount of dermis that is included in the graft. A full-thickness graft includes the epidermis and all the dermis. A partial or split-thickness graft includes the epidermis and some dermis. This type of graft can be cut to varying thickness depending on need. The graft can also be meshed in order to cover a larger surface area.

Other types of graft are flaps or pedicle grafts, pinch grafts and tissue cultures. Flaps may include other tissue besides skin and one part of the graft is still attached to original site. This provides a blood supply to the graft until a new blood supply has been established. It is particularly useful in areas where the blood supply is poor and for areas of the face. An example is a gluteal rotation flap to cover the cavity of an ischial pressure sore.

Pinch grafts are small pieces of skin that have been obtained by pinching the area with forceps or lifting with a needle and slicing off with a knife. They have been used as a method of treating leg ulcers but there is limited evidence as to their success in long-term healing of leg ulcers.

Tissue culture has been developed primarily in burns units, where repeated grafting from the same donor site may be necessary for patients with large surface area burns. A small sample of skin about 2 cm in diameter can be used to culture epithelial sheets many times this size. One of the early studies using this method was carried out by Gallico *et al.* (1984) on two children who had burn injuries affecting more than 95% of their body surface area. Tissue culture provided effective grafts for more than 50% of the body surface. When such extensive burns occur, autografting is very limited because of the lack of appropriate donor sites. Allografts are also used but they do not always take. Tissue culture can reduce the need for frequent surgery to take further grafts.

Grafts may be sutured or stapled in position or just laid in place. The graft may be left exposed or covered with a dressing to help anchor it in place. The graft must be observed carefully for any indication of infection, oedema or haematoma. It may also be necessary to immobilise the area so that the graft does not slip out of position. Tension over the graft must also be avoided as it may damage the vulnerable blood supply.

Gauze dressings and paraffin gauze have been used to cover grafts but there is no evidence to determine their effectiveness. Davey *et al.* (2003) described the use of Hyperfix™ in a paediatric burns unit over a 15-year period. It was used for over 700 grafts and found to be an effective covering, with only 18 patients (2%) requiring repeat grafts. Peanut oil was routinely applied to the strapping two hours before dressing change in order to facilitate its removal without damage to the graft.

Some small studies have been undertaken to investigate the use of a silicone net dressing. Vloemans (1994) used the silicone dressing on 45 split-thickness skin grafts and found that no grafts were lost. However, the main advantage was that dressing removal was painless, unlike the standard treatment of either a non-adherent dressing or paraffin gauze. Platt *et al.* (1996) undertook a small, randomised trial comparing the use of a silicone net dressing with paraffin gauze. There was no difference in graft take between the two groups. However, the silicone net group had significantly less pain at dressing change and the dressing was easier to remove than the paraffin gauze. Although there have been no further published studies, there is widespread use of silicone net as a fixative material.

A small study investigated the use of topical negative pressure therapy (TNP) as a fixative for split-thickness skin grafts (Moisidis *et al.*, 2004). Twenty-two patients were recruited and the donor sites divided into two halves and then each half randomised to either TNP or standard treatment of silicone net, proflavine wool and foam sponge. A narrow bridge of several layers of hydrocolloid separated the two treatments. The authors found that there was no significant difference in graft take between the two treatments but quality of the graft take was significantly better in the TNP group. However, this is a very small study and a larger study is required to determine a definitive outcome.

As the graft becomes vascularised, it turns approximately the same colour as the donor site. In Caucasians, the ideal colour is pink. It is more difficult to assess the vascularity of a graft in darker skins. Coull and Wylie (1990) suggest the use of a colour code along with an assessment chart to monitor the progress of skin flaps. Once a graft has taken, it still needs to be handled very carefully as the tissues are still fragile. It should be protected against any extremes of temperature and sunlight. Once the graft is healed, the skin should be massaged twice daily with a bland moisturising cream. This helps to improve the suppleness of the skin, as it is likely to be less well lubricated than normal.

A graft may fail to take for a variety of reasons. If there is an inadequate blood supply to the graft bed the microcirculation will fail to grow into the graft and it will necrose from lack of oxygen. Equally, haematoma formation will cause separation of the graft. If the graft slides out of position it will cause separation of some or all of the graft and lead to failure.

Infection, especially from *Pseudomonas aeruginosa* and beta-haemolytic streptococcus, will also cause failure. Infection will cause pain, odour, itching and redness around the edges of the graft and a low-grade fever (Francis, 1998). It is most likely to occur between the second and fourth postoperative days.

● *Donor sites* ●

Ideally, skin grafts are taken from a part of the body where the skin provides a good match for the recipient site. The colour, texture and hair-bearing properties of the skin have to be considered. One of the commonest areas for a donor site is the thigh, from which a large area of skin can be obtained.

Donor sites are often described as being more painful than the skin graft for which the removed skin has been used. This is probably, in part, because of the large number of exposed nerve endings. Initially, a donor site is a raw haemorrhagic area. Pressure is needed to stop the bleeding and the wound should be checked regularly in the immediate postoperative period. Analgesia is also necessary and may be needed for several days.

Traditionally, donor sites have been dressed with paraffin gauze, covered with ordinary gauze, wrapped in wool roll or gamgee and held in place with bandages (Wilkinson, 1997). The dressing is left in place for about ten days and then removed. This is often a very painful experience as the dressing has dried out and adhered to the wound. The patient may have to sit in the bath in order to soak the dressing off. Damage to the newly formed tissue can occur as the dressing is pulled away. The newly epithelialising wound may be quite sore and dessicated. Aqueous cream or a similar emollient may be applied as a moisturiser.

A systematic review by Wiechula (2003) examined the use of dressings for the management of donor sites. The outcomes of using all types of moist wound and non-moist products were compared using meta-analysis. It showed a significant benefit of moist wound products such as films, foams and hydrocolloids compared with non-moist dressings such as paraffin gauze in terms of healing, pain and wound infection. The author also compared different types of products with paraffin gauze. Hydrocolloids were significantly better in terms of healing, pain and wound infection. Films also outperformed paraffin gauze in terms of healing, pain and wound infection. There were insufficient studies of good quality to determine the relative effectiveness of alginates.

Since this review was undertaken, two studies of interest have been published. Misirlioglu *et al.* (2003) compared honey-impregnated gauze with paraffin gauze, saline soaks and a hydrocolloid in 88 patients with donor sites. They found the honey gauze performed significantly better than the paraffin gauze and the saline soaks in respect of healing, pain and wound infection. There was no difference in the results when compared with the hydrocolloid. A smaller study by Barnea *et al.* (2004) compared Acquacel™ with paraffin gauze on 23 donor sites, each dressing being randomly applied to half of the site. The Acquacel™ sites healed significantly faster and caused less pain to the patient. Dressing changes were also easier.

Donor site management seems to be one area where there is reasonably clear evidence that modern products outperform paraffin gauze. It is difficult to understand, therefore, why this outdated product is still in use.

Once the donor site has healed, the skin should be kept supple. Emollients may be of assistance and should be applied two or three times a day. The patient should be advised to avoid extremes of temperature. If it is not possible to avoid exposing the site to sunlight, sun blockers should be used to cover the area. Donor sites remain susceptible to sunburn for up to a year after healing (Fowler & Dempsey, 1998). A tubular bandage may be applied to donor sites on a lower limb to provide support and to prevent hypertrophy of the scar.

Wound drains

Wound drains are inserted to provide a channel to the body surface for fluid that might otherwise collect in the wound. The fluid may be blood, pus, serous exudate, bile or other body fluids. There are several different types of drains, which can be divided into open and closed drains. Open drains may be tubes, corrugated rubber or plastic, or soft tubes filled with ribbon gauze to provide a wicking effect. Open drains originally drained into the dressing, causing considerable discomfort to the patient. They also increased the risk of infection as the drain provided an open channel for bacteria. As a result of the classic research by Cruse and Foord (1973, 1980), which demonstrated the infection hazard posed by open drains, they are rarely used these days.

Closed drains consist of the drain, connection tubing and the collecting receptacle. They usually provide a vacuum and so have a suction effect. Chest drains are closed drains that work rather differently. The purpose of this type of system is to allow air to escape from the chest cavity and bubble into the water in the container. Closed drains are usually inserted through a stab wound adjacent to the incision.

The use of drains is essential to prevent the collection of fluid in the wound. This is more important with some types of surgery than others. Several studies have investigated the use of drains, some finding them of value and others not. Varley and Milner (1995) randomly allocated 177 patients undergoing surgery for proximal femoral fracture to receive wound drainage or no drainage. Twice as many patients (13.2%) in the undrained group developed wound infections compared to the drained group (7%). However, this difference did not reach statistical significance, possibly because the numbers of infections were small. Perkins et al. (1997) randomised 222 patients undergoing face-lift surgery to drains or no drains and found a significant reduction in the formation of seromas in the group that received drainage. There was also a reduction of haematoma formation in this group but the difference did not reach statistical significance. Holt et al. (1997) randomised 136 patients undergoing total knee arthroplasty to the use of drains or no drain. They found a significant difference between the two groups, with the undrained requiring greater dressing reinforcement and developing a greater level of ecchymosis.

Conversely, the use of drains was shown not to have any particular advantage in the following studies. Maharaj et al. (2000) randomised 440 women undergoing emergency caesarean section to either drainage or non-drainage. They found no significant difference between the two groups in terms of wound inflammation, wound infection, haematoma formation or length of stay. Purushotham et al. (2002) randomised women undergoing surgery for breast cancer to either drains or no drains and found no difference in surgical outcomes. However, they did find that the no drains group had a significantly shorter hospital stay (3.75 days versus 5.23 days). Brown and Brookfield (2004) studied the impact of drain usage in a randomised study of 83 patients undergoing extensive spinal surgery and found no difference between the two groups in a range of measures including infection rates, haematoma and length of stay.

It seems reasonable to conclude that with improving surgical techniques and materials, drains do not need to be used as frequently as they have been in the past. However, they are still of benefit in some types of surgery, especially some types of orthopaedic and plastic surgery procedures.

6.2.2 Managing complications

A variety of complications may occur following surgery. Only those related to the wound will be discussed here.

Haemorrhage

This may occur during surgery, in the immediate postoperative period and up to ten days afterwards. It is sometimes categorised as primary, intermediary and secondary haemorrhage. The main cause of both primary and intermediary haemorrhage is poor surgical technique due to failure to control bleeding during surgery or poorly tied blood vessels. As the blood pressure returns to normal levels, the clots and ties get pushed off the end of the blood vessel(s), resulting in bleeding. Secondary haemorrhage is invariably associated with infection.

Taylor *et al.* (1987) studied the effects of haemorrhage on wound strength. They found that perioperative bleeding caused a weaker suture line, which was associated with impaired fibroblast function. The researchers suggest that non-absorbable or long-lasting sutures should be used if haemorrhage occurs during surgery.

The bleeding may be brisk and rapidly seen or more insidious. Blood may be seen on the wound dressing or it may drain into a drainage bag. If the bleeding is internal, signs of shock may be the first indication of its presence. If there is only a little bleeding, the blood may ooze into the superficial tissues and show as bruising around the suture line. Slow seeping of blood may lead to haematoma formation when the blood collects in a 'dead space' around the operative site and then clots.

If there is heavy bleeding, further surgery may be needed to find and control the bleeding point. In many cases the bleeding is monitored closely to see if further clotting will resolve the problem. When a haematoma forms it is a potential breeding ground for bacteria. It is sometimes possible to remove a suture in order to evacuate the haematoma.

Infection

Despite considerable improvement in standards of asepsis, postsurgical wound infection still occurs. In a national survey undertaken in the UK, surgical wound infection was found to account for 10.7% of all hospital-acquired infections (Emmerson *et al.*, 1996). These findings are not dissimilar to those of national surveys undertaken in Switzerland, which found an infection rate of 10.1% in 1999 and 8.1% in 2002 (Sax, 2004). Measuring infection rates is one method used in evaluating standards of care for surgical audit. Recently surveys have tended to involve only those undergoing a particular type of surgery. For example, Harrington *et al.* (2004) undertook a survey of 4475 patients undergoing heart surgery in five hospitals. Of these patients, 310 (6.9%) developed 346 infections: 191 sternal infections, 89 saphenous vein site infections and 66 radial artery site infections. Using multivariate analysis, the study team also found obesity, diabetes and age to be independent predictors of surgical site infection. Herruzo *et al.* (2004) monitored trauma patients who required more than two days in hospital and found a 2% clean wound infection rate.

However, the patients in both of these studies were not followed up after discharge and therefore the total numbers of infections may be underestimated. A study by Jonkers *et al.* (2003) followed patients undergoing cardiac surgery for 90 days and divided infections into sternal wound infections (SWI) and donor site infections (DSI). They found that considerably more infections were diagnosed at 30 days compared with those identified during hospital admission: SWI rose from 4.7% to 6.8% at 30 days and DSI rose from 1.5% to 4.6% during the same period. They had risen further by 90 days to 9% (SWI) and 7.3% (DSI). The authors concluded that accurate surveillance should include follow-up after discharge.

Wilson *et al.* (1990) have produced a scoring system for infections that they found to be reproducible. The ASEPSIS wound scoring system, with the grading for the severity of infection, is shown in Figure 6.1. The authors compared this system with other methods when assessing 1029 surgical patients. Further work by Wilson *et al.* (1998) reports a comparative study of four different methods of assessing wounds for infection. Patients were assessed during their hospital stay and followed up after discharge. The authors found that the infection rate depended on the definition being used.

It is important to remember that it is not always possible to make direct comparisons between different surveys because of the varying methods of data collection. The criteria used for defining wound infection may also vary. Crowe and Cooke (1998) instigated a debate on case definitions of surgical wound infections and listed several definitions used by a variety of researchers. They hoped that the ensuing debate would result in consensus on which definition should be used for national and international surveys.

When measuring the incidence of surgical wound infections, it is essential to understand the potential causes. The causes of infection can be divided into factors related to the environment, the patient and the surgery; they are summarised in Box 6.1. The first two factors have already been discussed in Chapter 2 so only those relating to the surgery will be considered here. One of the most important aspects is the type of surgery being undertaken. Cruse and Foord (1973, 1980) categorised operations into clean, clean-contaminated, contaminated and dirty, a method that has become widely recognised and used in other studies. Box 6.2 explains these categories and shows the infection rates found by Cruse and Foord (1980). There is a quite dramatic difference in infection rates between clean and dirty surgery. The clean wound infection rate is usually used as a baseline for monitoring other factors that may affect infection rates. Kamp-Hopmans *et al.* (2003) also found different infection rates in different specialties over a five-year period, with 1.8 per 100 operations in a thoracic surgery ward, 4.6/100 operations in an orthopaedic ward, 5.3/100 in a gynaecology ward and 5.4/100 in the general surgery and vascular wards.

Probably the most important factor to consider is surgical technique. Cruse and Foord (1980) found that meticulous attention to detail was essential to keep clean wound infection rates low. Israelsson (1998) surveyed 1013 patients who underwent a midline laparotomy and found the individual surgeon's infection rates ranged from 0% to 27%. The length of surgical experience of the surgeons did not affect the complication rate in this study. Reilly (1997) audited the infection rates within a district general hospital and found a direct correlation

TABLE A

Wound characteristic	Proportion of wound affected (%)					
	0	<20	20–29	40–59	60–79	>80
Serous exudate	0	1	2	3	4	5
Erythema	0	1	2	3	4	5
Purulent exudate	0	2	4	6	8	10
Separation of deep tissues	0	2	4	6	8	10

TABLE B

Criteria for allocation of additional points to ASEPSIS Score

Criterion	Points	
Additional treatment:		
Antibiotics		10
Drainage of pus under local anaesthetic		5
Debridement of wound (general anaesthetic)		10
Serous discharge	Daily	0–5
Erythema	Daily	0–5
Purulent drainage	Daily	0–10
Separation of deep tissues	Daily	0–10
Isolation of bacteria		10
Stay as inpatient prolonged over 14 days		5

Score **Table A** daily for first week, add points from **Table B** for any criteria satisfied in first 2 months after surgery.

Category of infection: total score 0–10 = satisfactory healing; 11–20 = disturbance of healing; 21–30 = minor wound infection; 31–40 = moderate wound infection; >40 = major wound infection.

Fig. 6.1   The ASEPSIS wound score (from Wilson *et al.*, 1990, reproduced with kind permission of Academic Press Ltd).

between the grade of surgeon and infection rates. The more junior the doctor, the poorer the technique is likely to be.

Another factor that has been shown to have some relevance to the development of infection is the length of operations. Cruse and Foord (1980) found that the clean wound infection rate doubled for every hour of surgery. They suggest four possible reasons for this increase: wound cells are damaged by drying out when exposed to air; the total amount of bacterial contamination increases with time; the longer the operation, the more sutures and electrocoagulation are used; longer surgery may be associated with shock and/or blood loss, thus reducing resistance to infection. Whilst it is not possible to eliminate all these factors, the numbers of bacteria in the air can be reduced. Although air

Box 6.1   Factors increasing the incidence of surgical wound infection (based on Dealey, 1991).

Environment
Lengthy preoperative hospitalisation
High bed occupancy
Poor standards of asepsis within the theatre suite
Unsuitable layout within the theatre suite
Inadequate ventilation in the operating theatre

Patient
Age
Obesity
Malnutrition
Diabetes
Steroids
Immunosuppressive drugs
Additional lesions, e.g. pressure sore (form reservoir of bacteria)
Shaving

Wounds
Type of surgery
Length of surgery
Time of surgery
Poor surgical technique
Position of drains

Box 6.2   Classification of surgical wounds (based on Cruse & Foord, 1980).

Clean
Surgery where there was no infection seen, no break in asepsis and hollow muscular organs not entered. Could include hysterectomy, cholcystectomy or appendectomy 'in passing' if no evidence of inflammation.

Infection rate: 1.5%

Clean-contaminated
Where a hollow muscular organ was entered but only minimal spillage of contents.

Infection rate: 7.7%

Contaminated
When a hollow organ was opened with gross spillage of contents, acute inflammation without pus found, a major break in asepsis or traumatic wounds less than four hours old.

Infection rate: 15.2%

Dirty
Traumatic wounds more than four hours old. Surgery where a perforated viscus or pus is found.

Infection rate: 40%

filtration systems can be used, Cruse and Foord suggested that the same results could be obtained by taking some fairly simple measures, such as reducing conversation and the amount of movement in and out of the theatre, and excluding anyone with a skin infection.

The timing of surgery also affects infection rates. Cruse and Foord (1980) found that when clean and clean-contaminated surgery was carried out at night, there was almost double the infection rate of procedures in the day. This is most likely to be due to weariness in the surgical team leading to imperfect surgical technique.

Nursing care

Early identification of signs of infection is important (see also Chapter 3).

Dehiscence

Dehiscence means the breaking down, or splitting open, of all or part of a wound healing by first intention. Complete dehiscence may involve eviscera-tion of the gut, a condition that is commonly known as a 'burst abdomen'. If the skin remains intact when the muscle and fascia layers break down, an incisional hernia occurs which may not become obvious for some months following surgery.

Dehiscence can occur because of systemic and local factors. Several studies have looked at the effect of surgical wound closure techniques. Gislason *et al.* (1995) randomised 599 patients to three different closure types and found that there was no difference between the groups. Dehiscence occurs more frequently in those undergoing emergency surgery, those having intestinal resections with stoma formation and following wound infection. Those patients whose wounds broke down were also significantly older. Brolin (1996) found that a continuous suture was more effective for closing midline incisions following surgery for morbid obesity than an interrupted suturing technique.

Westaby (1985) considered that surgical technique may be a factor in dehis-cence. Securing sutures too tightly so that they cut into the tissues can result in dehiscence. Tight suturing also affects the vascularity of the skin edges, with areas of necrosis around the sutures. Occasionally failure of the suture mater-ial may occur although this is less common with non-absorbable sutures. Perkins (1992) suggested that dehiscence can be divided into early dehiscence, related to suture failure and/or surgical technique, and late dehiscence, which is more likely to be the result of infection.

Nursing care

If a surgical wound starts to break down, the potential cause(s) should be iden-tified and rectified where possible. The wound should be carefully assessed for indications of infection. If major dehiscence, such as a burst abdomen, occurs, the wound will require resuturing. Most wounds are treated conservatively and allowed to heal by granulation and contraction. This is particularly so when infection is present as all purulent material should be allowed free drainage.

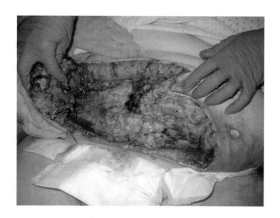

Fig. 6.2   An example of a dehiscent wound with complete breakdown of the suture line.

When this is associated with complete dehiscence of a suture line with some necrosis, as can be seen in Figure 6.2, topical negative pressure therapy may be effective in removing the wound debris and preparing the wound for late resuturing.

The wounds may be necrotic or sloughy with a heavy exudate. NICE (2001) has provided guidance on the management of these wounds. The guidance concluded that there is no clear evidence as to the most effective method of debridement or the most appropriate dressing. However, modern products were seen to be more effective than gauze in respect of pain, odour control and exudate management. As a result, the guidance recommends that selection of the method of debridement and the use of dressings should be based on patient acceptability, comfort, odour control, the type and location of the wound and total costs.

If there is only a partial dehiscence of the suture line with little exudate and necrosis then an amorphous hydrogel is appropriate. An alginate or hydrofibre is more appropriate in the presence of heavy exudate or greater dehiscence of the suture line. These dressings cause far less trauma than using traditional methods such as ribbon gauze. Once any cavity is filled with granulation tissue and there is no indication of lingering infection, foam cavity fillers may also be used.

In a few instances the exudate may be excessive and not controlled by dressings. In this situation it may be helpful to consult a colorectal nurse specialist who may suggest that an appliance similar to a drainage bag be used. It has an adhesive backing that can be cut to fit over the wound, whilst protecting the surrounding skin. The front of the appliance has a hinged lid that allows access to the wound and saves frequent removal. There is usually a tap that allows drainage. The amount of exudate can be measured accurately which is important for fluid balance. Good management of a wound following dehiscence should promote healing and permit the patient to be discharged home for care in the community.

Sinus formation

A sinus is a track to the body surface from an abscess or some material that is an irritant and becomes a focus for infection. A common irritant is suture material. Dressing material, such as ribbon gauze, may also be retained and prevent healing. Sinuses can become chronic if the causative factor is not resolved. A sinogram will show the extent of a sinus and help to identify the root problem. Surgical excision or laying open of the sinus is usually the most effective form of management. Once the focus for infection has been removed and free drainage can occur, the remaining cavity will heal by granulation and contraction.

Although wide excision is the most appropriate method of managing a sinus, it is not always possible. If the sinus is very deep the opening may be fairly narrow in relation to the sinus size. Butcher (1999) suggests that a sinus should be regularly irrigated with saline to prevent the accumulation of pus and exudate. Traditionally ribbon gauze was used in sinuses but it is painful to insert and remove and may act as a plug, preventing the drainage of exudate. The easiest dressing to apply is a hydrogel as it can easily be inserted into the sinus via the applicator. Butcher (1999) warned of the danger of maceration of the surrounding skin when using hydrogels for prolonged periods of time in the presence of heavy exudate. It is therefore advisable to use a protective skin wipe to protect the skin.

Fistula formation

A fistula is an abnormal track connecting one viscus with another viscus or a viscus with the body surface. It may develop spontaneously or following surgery. Common examples are:

- rectovaginal – connecting the rectum and vagina
- biliary – allowing leakage of bile to the surface following surgery on the gall bladder and/or bile ducts
- faecal – allowing leakage of faecal fluid through the wound, often associated with infection.

Persistent leakage of fluid indicates the possible presence of a fistula. Examination of the fluid will usually provide information to indicate the source of the fistula. Any associated infection must also be treated.

Nursing care

The management of fistulae involves care of the surrounding skin, containing and measuring the output and nutritional support. The skin can be protected by the use of ostomy pastes and protective skin wafers. Drainage bags can be applied to collect the output from the fistula. The colorectal nurse specialist may have the greatest skill in applying a suitable drainage bag over the fistula and protecting the skin.

Once the output from the fistula is contained, it can be accurately measured. This enables the correct amount of fluid to be given to replace what has been lost. Output may be considerable, sometimes a litre per day. In hospitals where there is a nutrition team, they can also be involved in the care of these patients. When it is possible, enteral feeding should be given. If the fistula is high in the gastrointestinal tract then it will be necessary to give parenteral nutrition.

Nienhuijs *et al.* (2003) reported on the management and outcomes for 17 patients with enterocutaneous fistulae. They followed the treatment described above until spontaneous healing but ten patients had skin erosion and required frequent dressing changes. Consequently topical negative pressure (TNP) was applied to these wounds. Patients were given TNP for a median of 25 days (range 14–161 days). Four patients went on to heal spontaneously after a median of 73 days, five patients had surgery to correct the fistula and one patient died, due to extensive metastasis. The four patients who healed spontaneously were discharged home with TNP therapy. Despite the high costs of using TNP, the authors calculated that the cost was cheaper than conventional treatment (€290394 versus €428311). They noted that as these figures were calculated retrospectively, they should be treated with caution. Undoubtedly, the patients in the study were very satisfied with the use of TNP and preferred it to the conventional treatment that they had been given previously.

Evaluation

Regular monitoring of surgical wounds is essential in order to identify any potential complications as early intervention may prevent further problems. Therefore good documentation is essential. Birchall and Taylor (2003) described the development of a benchmarking tool based on *The Essence of Care* (DoH, 2001). The project involved determining best practice (in the absence of any national guidelines) and improving wound assessment documents and then benchmarking practice against it. The motivation for undertaking this work was an unrelated audit that had identified that out of 40 surgical wounds, only one had a documented assessment. Projects such as this improve awareness of the need to maintain accurate records of each wound and its progress.

6.3 TRAUMATIC WOUNDS

Traumatic injuries can range from a simple cut to a major crushing injury. Major traumatic injury is beyond the remit of this book. It requires surgical intervention and specialised nursing care. Most nurses will be required to care for minor traumatic wounds from time to time. Their care will be considered here.

6.3.1 Minor traumatic wounds

Assessment

Initial assessment should identify any life-threatening problems such as airway obstruction, haemorrhage or shock. Vital signs should be recorded. Any of these problems should be addressed before treating the wound. If possible, a history should be obtained of when, where and how the injury occurred. A medical history can highlight any factors that may affect healing of the wound or the type of treatment prescribed to manage the wound.

The wound should be assessed for any bleeding. Haemorrhage may be resolved by pressure or require surgical intervention. The presence of any foreign bodies should be noted and the extent and severity of the injury. Cleansing of the wound may be necessary before a full assessment can be made. Loose particles may easily be washed off but other debris may be more difficult to remove. Bianchi (2000) reviewed the limited evidence available as to the best methods of cleansing traumatic wounds. She concluded that pain assessment and management were essential prior to the procedure, especially for children. Unfortunately, there is insufficient evidence to determine the best methods of cleansing and cleansers to use. Some accident and emergency departments use Clingfilm to cover a wound until seen by the doctor. This has the advantage of keeping the wound warm and moist and allowing easy observation.

Nursing intervention

Medical assessment and prescription may be necessary before the wound can be dressed. Whilst many nurses are competent to dress minor injuries the following guidelines should be considered. Patients should be examined by a doctor if:

- the nature and extent of the injury are uncertain.
- there is persistent bleeding.
- suturing is required.
- a foreign body is present.
- tetanus prophylaxis may be necessary.
- the injury occurred to a hospital patient.
- the nurse is uncertain of the appropriate management.
- it is required by nursing policies.

Prior to dressing, the wound should be thoroughly cleaned using saline. Any loose devitalised tissue should be removed. In some instances it may be necessary to shave the area around the wound, if there are hairs that may interfere with the healing process. An appropriate dressing can then be applied. Tetanus prophylaxis will be required if the patient has not had a complete course of tetanus toxoid or if no booster dose has been given for more than five years. Depending on the cause of the wound, the doctor may also prescribe a course of antibiotics.

If the person is not a patient in hospital, they and any carer will require information about the management of the wound. Information should also be given concerning whom to contact if any complication occurs. Potential complications such as fever, swelling around the wound, excessive pain or offensive discharge should be described to the patient. Ideally, this information should also be given in written form so that the patient has it for future reference.

Traumatic injuries occur primarily to the young and the elderly. Whilst most young people will heal easily, this is not necessarily true for the older people.

They may need to be admitted to hospital for further care. Wijetunge (1992) has provided a useful overview of a management plan for soft tissue injuries.

Evaluation

The aim of any treatment is uncomplicated healing of the wound with restoration of function and minimal scarring (Brunner & Suddarth, 1988). Patients may return to be reviewed by those who made the original assessment or they may be referred to the family practitioner. The majority of these wounds will heal without complication.

6.3.2 The management of specific types of traumatic wounds

Abrasions

An abrasion is a superficial injury where the skin is rubbed or torn and it may be extremely sore. It may occur as a result of falling on a gritty surface. Abrasions should be cleaned carefully to ensure that there are no foreign bodies embedded in the wound. In the case of extensive abrasions a general anaesthetic may be required in order to allow adequate cleansing. Failure to remove all the debris may result in unsightly 'tattooing' (Evans & Jones, 1996).

Selection of a suitable dressing depends on the extent and depth of the injury. These wounds are often very sore. Occlusive dressings have been found to reduce the pain, possibly because they keep the nerve endings from drying out. If the abrasion is superficial a film dressing or a thin hydrocolloid can be applied. Deeper wounds, with a heavier exudate, can be treated with hydrocolloids, foams or alginates.

Lacerations

A laceration is a wound that penetrates the skin and has a torn and jagged edge. They can be caused by blunt injury which produces shear forces or by a sharp object such as glass (Singer et al., 1997). The aim of treatment is to achieve uncomplicated healing with a functional and cosmetically acceptable scar.

It is important to remove all debris from the wound and any devitalised tissue. This procedure is sometimes called surgical toilet. The best way to manage these wounds is to bring the skin edges together to heal by first intention. This may be achieved by the use of sutures, adhesive strips or tissue adhesive. The choice of material depends on the position of the wound, its extent and the condition of the damaged skin. Suturing is recommended around joints or on the hand where movement is involved. Farion et al. (2004) reviewed the use of tissue adhesives for traumatic lacerations in both children and adults. They found no difference in cosmesis between adhesives and standard closures but tissue adhesives could be applied more quickly and were less painful to use. The authors of the review also noted that there was a small but significant increased rate of dehiscence with tissue adhesives compared with standard closure methods.

One of the commonest positions for a laceration is the pretibial area. Davis *et al.* (2004) undertook an audit of A&E departments in a heavily populated region of the UK and found that the mean incidence of estimated patients with pretibial laceration was 5.2/1000 A&E attendances. The extent of the injury can vary and Dunkin *et al.* (2003) proposed a method of classifying these wounds.

I   Laceration.
II   Laceration or flap with minimal haematoma and/or skin edge necrosis.
III Laceration or flap with moderate to severe haematoma and/or necrosis.
IV   Major degloving injury.

Dunkin *et al.* (2003) have also provided a useful algorithm for the management of each type of laceration. Fairly obviously, types III and IV require surgical intervention. Type I lacerations should have the skin edges opposed and then held together with short, wide adhesive strips. The wound is covered with a non-adherent dressing and a crepe bandage applied from toe to knee. It may be appropriate to place a wool bandage under the crepe bandage in order to provide additional protection. Patients should be encouraged to mobilise and to elevate their leg when sitting in order to reduce any oedema. Type II is also managed with use of adhesive strips and supportive bandages, after any haematoma has been evacuated, the non-viable wound edges trimmed and the wound edges apposed. Both these type of lacerations should heal without complication. Failure to do so indicates that the injury is more serious than originally thought (Dunkin *et al.*, 2003).

If there is any risk of infection as a result of severe contamination of the wound at the time of injury, primary closure is not appropriate. Conservative treatment with antibiotics and dressings such as an amorphous hydrogel is preferable. An iodine-impregnated low-adherent dressing may also be used for a short period of time. Once the wound is clean, skin grafting is the fastest method of wound closure.

Finger tip injuries

Crushing finger tip injuries are very common in children, mainly caused by fingers being caught in house or car doors. Buckles (1985) suggested that 14% of children below the age of 13 years suffer from this type of injury. Cockerill and Sweet (1993) described the procedure of trephining to remove a haematoma from the nail bed. They also suggest that an X-ray may be necessary to identify any fracture. Prophylactic antibiotics may be needed if a fracture is present.

The use of adhesive tapes over the finger tip can be an effective way of holding the wound edges together and then protecting the finger by applying a tubular bandage. Collier (1996) suggests that it is important to use dressings that will not stick to the wound as adherent dressings will cause pain and further trauma at dressing change. Given that many of the patients are children, this is an important consideration. Suitable dressings might be hydrocolloids or adhesive foams which can be retained without bulky dressings or strapping.

Mammalian and human bites

Patients presenting with mammalian bites account for 1% of visits to A&E departments (Medeiros & Saconato, 2004). As many as 74% of bites are from dogs; other animals causing problems include cats, rats, squirrels and, occasionally, snakes. As well as animal bites, patients also present with human bites, usually as a result of physical violence such as a punch to the mouth which causes injury to the knuckles (Higgins *et al.*, 1997).

The major problem with any type of bite injury is the risk of infection or the transmission of diseases such as HIV or hepatitis B from human bites. Higgins *et al.* (1997) stress the importance of not underestimating these wounds. After reviewing the evidence for the use of prophylactic antibiotics after mammalian bites, Medeiros and Saconato (2004) concluded that there was some evidence that they were beneficial after human bites but not after dog or cat bites. They called for further research on the subject.

Careful cleansing is essential in order to assess the extent of the injury. Saline or an antimicrobial such as povidone iodine should be used. Surgical debridement or exploration may be necessary to remove devitalised tissue, skin tags or any foreign bodies. Large cuts and facial wounds need suturing. Delayed primary closure may be used for some wounds. Chen *et al.* (2000) monitored outcome for 145 mammalian bite wounds that were treated by primary closure. They found there was an infection rate of 5.5% and considered that this was an acceptable risk for wounds where a good cosmetic result was essential. However, they also noted that appropriate selection of patients was important.

Puncture wounds should be left open because of the risk of infection. The wound should be protected. An iodine-impregnated low-adherent dressing may be suitable, unless there is a moderate to heavy exudate. Higgins *et al.* (1997) suggest that patients with human puncture wounds should be admitted for surgical exploration and irrigation. So, too, should those with bites involving joints or tendons or any indication of spreading infection. Patients with bite wounds should be followed up to ensure that there has been uncomplicated healing and the patient has regained full function of the affected area.

Skin tears

Skin tears are caused either by friction or by a combination of friction and shearing associated with thin, fragile skin. Thomas *et al.* (1999) suggest that up to 1.5 million people living in care institutions in the USA suffer a skin tear each year. A survey of 154 nursing home residents revealed that they occurred mostly on the arms in the very elderly who were frail, had limited mobility, poor appetite and ecchymosis (McGough-Csarny & Kopac, 1998). Skin tears can be classified according to severity using a classification system devised by Payne and Martin (1993), given in Table 6.1.

There is limited evidence to determine the best method for managing skin tears. Sutures are not an option as the skin is too fragile and they would cause further damage. Adhesive strips may be used for category I tears but care must be taken to ensure that they do not cause damage on removal.

Table 6.1 Skin tear classification (based on Payne & Martin, 1993).

Category	Subcategory	Definition
I	Linear type	Epidermis and dermis pulled in one layer from supporting structures, resulting in skin tear in a straight line
	Flap type	The epidermis and dermis are separated but the epidermal flap covers the dermis to within 1 mm of the wound margin
II	Scant loss of tissue	An actual loss of tissue no greater than 25% of flap size
	Large loss of tissue	Loss of tissue where more than 25% of the flap has been lost
III		Entire loss of tissue, either at the time of injury or later following necrosis of the flap

Meuleneire (2002) reported on 88 patients with category I or II (scant tissue loss) who were managed using a silicone-coated net dressing, Mepitel™. The same protocol was followed for all wounds. The flap and wound bed were irrigated and the flap gently returned to as close approximation as possible. The wound was covered with Mepitel™, a secondary low-adherent dressing applied and then a light compression bandage applied to reduce any oedema. The secondary dressing was changed daily for three or four days and then left in situ until day 7 when all dressing layers were removed. The wound was then protected using a low-adherent dressing for a further 4–5 days. A total of 83% of the wounds had healed by day 8. The remaining 17% did not heal in this time because of either bleeding or infection. The infection was a consequence of delay in initial treatment as all the infected wounds were treated six hours or more after the injury.

Edwards *et al.* (1998) undertook a pilot study to compare four dressings: a film, a thin hydrocolloid, a foam and a combination of adhesive strips and low-adherent dressing on skin tears (no indication of severity was given). Fifty-four patients were recruited to the study but 24 cases were withdrawn, 14 of these (12 film dressing and two hydrocolloid) because the wound was not progressing or it was infected. Of the 30 that completed the study, only 13 had healed by day 7 and a further 12 by day 14 while five remained unhealed. The combination dressing performed better than the other dressings as about two-thirds had healed by day 7 and the remainder by day 14. However, these numbers are very small and no real conclusions can be drawn, other than the need for further research.

6.4 THE BURN INJURY

Burns are traumatic wounds but because of the specialised care required, they need to be considered separately from other traumatic wounds. Burns are measured in terms of the percentage of total body surface area (TBSA) that is affected and they are divided into complex and non-complex burns. In the UK, there are national criteria for the referral of complex burns to a specialist burn care unit (NBCRC, 2001). They include:

- patients aged under five years or over 60 years.
- full-thickness burns involving more than 10% TBSA in adults or 5% in children less than 16 years of age.
- burns of the face, hands, perineum, feet or flexures of the body such as neck or axilla.
- circumferential deep dermal or full-thickness burns of torso, limbs or neck.
- inhalation injuries.
- suspicion of non-accidental injury.

The burn care required by these patients is beyond the remit of this book.

6.4.1 Aetiology

A burn is an injury caused by excessive heat. It primarily damages the skin, causing tissue destruction and coagulation of the blood vessels of the affected area. Burn damage consists of three areas or zones (Hettiaratchy & Dziewulski, 2004a). The central zone is the *zone of coagulation* and at this point there is coagulation of the tissue proteins and thus irreversible damage and tissue loss. The *zone of stasis* surrounds the zone of coagulation and there is decreased tissue perfusion in this zone. However, if tissue perfusion is increased promptly it is possible to prevent the tissue damage extending into this zone. The third and outer zone is the *zone of hyperaemia* and here tissue perfusion is increased. Generally this area will recover unless the burn becomes severely infected or there is prolonged hypoperfusion.

Burns can be divided into four categories depending on their cause.

- *Thermal* – caused by flame, hot water or steam, other hot liquids and hot surfaces. Smoke inhalation injuries may be associated with fire casualties.
- *Chemical* – caused by spillage of strong acids, alkalis or other corrosive substances. These are usually industrial injuries. Damage to vital organs can occur if the chemicals are absorbed into the blood supply.
- *Electrical* – caused by an electrical current passing through the body. The internal damage may be considerably greater than is obvious from the skin appearance. Such burns may also be associated with thermal injury.
- *Radiation* – due to overexposure to industrial ionising radiation or following radiotherapy treatment. (Reactions to radiotherapy are covered in more detail in section 6.5.)

Although burn injuries are usually described as accidental, it has been suggested that some individuals are more likely to suffer from them than others (Hettiaratchy & Dziewulski, 2004b).

- *Young children* – 20% of all burn injuries are in young children, predominantly boys. Most of these injuries (70%) are due to scalds.

- *Children aged 5–14 years* – 10% of burns occur in this group and may be due to illicit activity such as playing with fireworks or petrol or misuse of electrical equipment.
- *Adults of working age* – around 60% of burns occur in this group, generally as a result of flame injury. About a third of the burns in this group are due to work-related injury.
- *Elderly people* – 10% of burns occur in this group, often as a result of infirmity or disability.
- *Additional factors* – within all age groups there are other predisposing factors that can increase the risk of burn injury. They include medical conditions such as epilepsy, psychiatric illness, alcoholism and social conditions such as poor housing, including faulty wiring and overcrowding.

6.4.2 Incidence

It is estimated that around 250 000 people suffer burn injury each year in the UK (NBCRC, 2001). Out of this group, around 175 000 people attend A&E as a result of their injury and for 13 000 it is sufficiently severe as to require admission to hospital. About 1000 people, half of whom are children under 12 years, have such severe burns that they require fluid resuscitation. It should also be noted that 300 people on average will die from their burns each year.

The figures for burn injury in the UK are similar to those in other developed counties (Hettiaratchy & Dziewulski, 2004b). However, in developing countries they are likely to be much higher; for example, it is thought that 2 million of the 500 million people in India have suffered a burn injury. Mortality rates are also likely to be higher in countries with a high level of poverty. Poor housing, overcrowding and the use of open fires for cooking are likely factors in the high incidence of fires in developing countries.

Staff should be aware of the possibility of non-accidental injury to children. Gordon and Goodwin (1997) suggest that around 10% of paediatric burns are the result of child abuse. This view is supported by work by Andronicus *et al.* (1998) who reviewed 507 paediatric burn cases. They found that 8% of injuries were considered to be as a result of abuse or neglect. The staff believed that the family's social or emotional situation was likely to have been a major factor in causing the burn injury of a further 6% of children. Andronicus *et al.* (1998) provide a list of features that may indicate abuse or neglect. They include a delay between the incident and presentation, an inconsistent history of events, a history of previous accidents and presentation for treatment by someone other than the parent. Most A&E departments have specific procedures to follow if an injury is suspected to be non-accidental.

6.4.3 The severity of the injury

The skin is the organ of the body that usually suffers the greatest damage from a burn injury. Depending on the extent of the injury, several layers may be

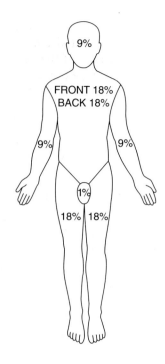

Fig. 6.3 The Rule of Nines.

affected. It is common to describe the severity of a burn according to its depth and extent. Burns are divided as follows.

- *Superficial burns* – only the upper strata of the epithelium are damaged. The stratum basale is unaffected.
- *Superficial dermal burns* – these burns extend beyond the epidermis into the top layers of the dermis. They are associated with blistering.
- *Deep dermal burn* – the burn extends into the deeper layers of the dermis and may involve hair follicles or sweat glands.
- *Full-thickness burns* – there is full destruction of the epidermis and dermis. The damage extends into the subcuticular layer and may involve muscle and bone.

The extent of the burn is determined by the measurement of the surface area of the affected part, excluding erythema. This is described in terms of a percentage of the whole body. Various methods of achieving this have been described. An *ad hoc* method is to measure the area using the palm of the hand. The palmar surface of the patient is equal to 1% of the body surface area in adults and 1.5% in children. When making the initial assessment of a burn-injured patient, it is most common to use the 'Rule of Nines' (Wallace, 1951). Figure 6.3 shows how the body is divided into sections, each measuring 9% of the whole, or multiples of 9%. The percentages for each affected area are then totalled. Thus, if one arm and the front of the trunk were affected, this would be described as 27% burns.

However, the Rule of Nines may overestimate the extent of the injury. Once the initial emergency treatment has been carried out, a reassessment of the extent of the injury is usually made. A more accurate picture can be obtained using a Lund and Browder chart (see Fig. 6.4). Lund and Browder (1944) developed a system for assessing burn injury that not only divides the body into smaller areas but also considers the age of the patient. Body proportions alter during childhood, so that the front of the head is 8.5% of the whole in a child of one year but only 4.5% of the whole in a 15 year old. Patient management may need to be adapted once this reassessment has been made.

6.4.4 Burn oedema

Almost immediately after injury, oedema starts to collect beneath the damaged tissue. This is typically maximal within 24 hours of the injury but can last for up to three or four days. As plasma continues to leak into the tissues, there is a risk of hypovolaemia developing. Without treatment, burns shock can develop and is potentially fatal. If the burn is on the face, neck or chest, the swelling from the oedema may cause obstruction of the airway. Patients with facial burns are admitted for 24 hours as a precaution. Treatment must ensure that the effects of burn oedema are minimised.

6.4.5 First aid treatment of burns

The British Burn Association has published recommendations for the first aid treatment of burns (Lawrence, 1987). Box 6.3 is based on these recommendations. The principal treatment is to remove the injured person from the source of heat and pour cold water over the affected area. Lawrence and Wilkins (1986) demonstrated that the subcutaneous temperature continues to rise after the burn injury occurs. Thus, if a burn injury at 100°C lasts for ten seconds, the affected tissue will take three minutes to return to normal body temperature. Application of cold water within ten seconds of the injury can reduce the 'burn time' to 30 seconds.

There are occasions when cold water is not readily available and other alternatives must be used. Lawrence (1996) tested a mousse containing a mixture of

---

Box 6.3 The first aid treatment of burns (based on Lawrence, 1987).

- Remove the person from the source of heat.
- Turn off the electricity in the case of electric burns.
- Apply copious amounts of water to the affected area.
- Do NOT try to remove clothing if the burns are extensive.
- Put wet compress on any exposed areas.
- Wrap Clingfilm around wet compress to hold in place.
- Seek qualified help quickly, especially if the burn is extensive.
- If no tap water, use bottled/mineral water or milk.
- Do not use solutions such as bleach, butter or oil.

CHART FOR ESTIMATING SEVERITY OF BURN WOND

NAME _____WARD_____NUMBER _____DATE ____
AGE _____ ADMISSION WEIGHT_____

LUND AND BROWDER CHARTS

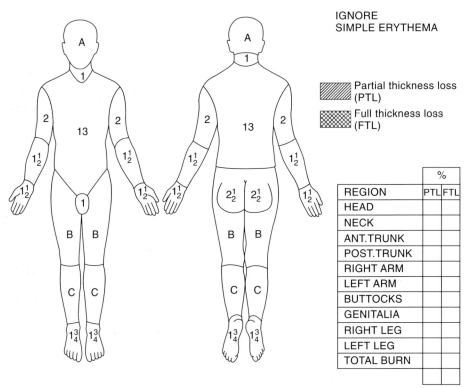

IGNORE
SIMPLE ERYTHEMA

▨ Partial thickness loss
(PTL)

▩ Full thickness loss
(FTL)

REGION	PTL	FTL
	%	
HEAD		
NECK		
ANT.TRUNK		
POST.TRUNK		
RIGHT ARM		
LEFT ARM		
BUTTOCKS		
GENITALIA		
RIGHT LEG		
LEFT LEG		
TOTAL BURN		

RELATIVE PEROENTAGE OF BODY SURFACE AREA AFFECTED BY GROWTH

AREA	AGE 0	1	5	10	15	ADULT
A=$\frac{1}{2}$ OF HEAD	$9\frac{1}{2}$	$8\frac{1}{2}$	$6\frac{1}{2}$	$5\frac{1}{2}$	$4\frac{1}{2}$	$3\frac{1}{2}$
B=$\frac{1}{2}$ OF ONE THIGH	$2\frac{3}{4}$	$3\frac{1}{4}$	4	$4\frac{1}{2}$	$4\frac{1}{2}$	$4\frac{3}{4}$
C=$\frac{1}{2}$ OF ONE THIGH	$2\frac{1}{2}$	$2\frac{1}{2}$	$2\frac{3}{4}$	3	$3\frac{1}{4}$	$3\frac{1}{2}$

Fig. 6.4   Lund & Browder chart.

paraffin oils and waxes in the laboratory and found that it gave local cooling for at least ten minutes. The same product was tested at a fire service college on 108 casualties with a variety of burns or scalds (Dunn, 1996). All subjects found immediate pain relief after application of the mousse. When the mousse fell off, a thin film remained over the burn site, obviating the need for a dressing unless there was skin loss. This product would appear to be a useful first aid treatment but further clinical evidence is required to support its use. An alternative is a cooling gel pad that can both cool the wound and relieve some of the initial wound pain (Hudspith & Rayatt, 2004).

6.4.6 The management of burn injuries

When considering the management of burns, the extent of the injury must be defined as the treatment varies drastically between complex and non-complex burns. Non-complex burns may be treated in the outpatient department but anyone with complex burns must be admitted to hospital.

Complex burns

Depending on the circumstances, it may be necessary to provide initial resuscitation before transferring a patient to a burn care unit. Gordon and Goodwin (1997) describe the importance of the primary ABCDEF assessment of the patient.

- *A = airway, B = breathing.* Check airway. Endotracheal intubation may be needed if there are deep burns to face, neck or mouth or any indication of respiratory distress.
- *C = circulation.* Check pulse. May be absent or show signs of dysrhythmias following electric burn.
- *D = disability or neurological deficit.* Identify any associated trauma. Signs of mental confusion or disorientation may be an indication of pre-existing conditions, hypoxia or unrecognised injury.
- *E = exposure and evaluation.* All jewellery or clothes should be removed from the burn-injured area because of the risk of constriction when burn oedema develops. This also allows for a rapid assessment of the full extent of the injury, using the Rule of Nines. The patient should be kept warm; a space blanket is ideal.
- *F = fluid resuscitation.* Establish an intravenous infusion – this is essential for all burns greater than 15% TBSA in adults and 10% in children. Blood samples may be taken at the same time. Catheterise the bladder if the burns are 25% or more TBSA; urinary output will indicate inadequate rehydration as well as renal function.

Analgesia may also be required, especially for those with superficial burns as they are very painful (Hettiaratchy & Papini, 2004).

It is also important to obtain a full history of cause of the injury from patient, relative or ambulance crew. This may provide information indicating potential complications such as smoke inhalation. Inhalational analgesia or systemic analgesia may be given depending on the condition of the patient.

When the patient's condition has been stabilised by the above measures, urgent transfer to the burn care unit can take place. Once in the care of a burns team, a more detailed assessment of the patient and the extent of the burn injury using a Lund and Browder chart is undertaken. Essentially, the extent of damage is assessed visually. However, Mileski *et al.* (2003) found that a Doppler flowmeter could be a useful tool to measure tissue perfusion, thus allowing easier differentiation between the different zones of the burn injury. They found that serial measurements had a positive predictive value of 81% for identifying non-healing wounds.

Non-complex burns

Managing minor burns requires assessment of both the patient and the wound, as in any other type of wound. Assessment of the patient has been discussed in Chapter 2 and wound assessment and management in Chapter 3. Specific aspects of the care of minor burns are discussed here.

Patient assessment

Burn aetiology.   Discover the cause of the injury. Non-accidental injury must be considered if the history seems inconsistent with the burn appearance. The risk of infection is always present in the burn-injured patient.

Pain.   Analgesia may be required for pain.

Nutrition.   Nutritional status should be identified. Advice on nutrition may be necessary as there will be increased nutritional demands on the body.

Sleep.   Pain or anxiety may affect sleep patterns.

Early psychological care.   Many patients will be very frightened. It is important to provide reassurance and explanation to the patient and the family.

Later psychological care.   A burn injury can be extremely disfiguring. Body image may be profoundly altered, causing distress and loss of self-esteem. Many patients may have fears of disfigurement or disability. Some may fear loss of loved ones as a result of the scarring. Specific fears should be identified and addressed.

Wound assessment

Initial assessment of a burn injury includes the extent and depth of the burn. The use of a Lund and Browder chart has already been described. The zone of hyperaemia should not be included when calculating the burn area. Identifying the depth of a burn is not always easy to do, especially as a burn injury may have varying depths. Table 6.2 shows how it is possible to differentiate between the different wound depths.

A burn injury differs from other types of wounds in several important respects (Bayley, 1990). There are frequently large areas of devitalised tissue. The wound may have a large surface area and take some time to heal. As a result, the burn wound is rapidly colonised by bacteria. There is considerable

Table 6.2   Identifying burn wound depth (from Fowler, 2003).

Depth of burn	Skin structures affected	Indicators
Superficial	Upper strata of epithelium	• Skin intact, red and very painful • Blanches under fingertip pressure • Usually no blisters but may form in the 48-hour period after injury
Superficial dermal	Epidermis and upper layers of dermis	• Blisters form immediately with a pink/red wound bed below • Wound areas may be red and moist and exuding • Easily observable brisk capillary refill • Painful and sensitive to skin changes
Deep dermal	Epidermis down to deep layers of dermis, possibly hair follicles and sweat glands	• Burn creamy/white • May have large blisters • Initially burn has little moisture • Slight pain with insensate areas not sensitive to pinprick
Full thickness	Complete destruction of epidermis and dermis; may involve muscle or tendon	• Burn appears waxy white, cherry red, grey or leathery • Little or no pain – but may be areas on the edges of the burn that are not so deep and therefore painful

risk of infection in complex burns but this is much less likely in non-complex burns. Lawrence (1989) quotes an incidence of about 1% but this may vary between centres. Nonetheless, the wound should be observed carefully for any indication of infection.

Wound management

Superficial burns may be very painful and require analgesia. Fowler (2003) suggested treating them like minor sunburn with aloe vera gel or other aftersun lotions. Aloe vera gel is soothing and feels cooling and thus helps to alleviate the pain.

Superficial dermal burns require careful cleansing with warm saline or tap water to remove all loose debris in the first instance. They have traditionally been treated with paraffin gauze dressings or silver sulphadiazine cream and covered with gauze and a bandage. Whilst healing will occur with this regime, it has several disadvantages. The dressings are bulky and hinder washing around the affected area. They may also be painful to remove, although it may not be necessary to remove the wound contact layer until the wound is healed and it separates spontaneously.

Modern products are easier to use and are also more comfortable for patients, especially when being removed. There is limited evidence to determine best practice but what evidence is available seems to favour modern products. Thomas *et al.* (1995) undertook a randomised study comparing a hydrocolloid alone, a hydrocolloid with silver sulphadiazine cream and a medicated paraffin gauze dressing in 50 patients with 54 non-complex burns. The hydrocolloid group required significantly fewer dressings than the other two groups. The hydrocolloid group also had significantly faster healing than the hydrocolloid with cream group. The researchers concluded that hydrocolloid dressings alone are useful for the management of non-complex burns.

Two studies by Subrahmanyam (1991, 1998) investigated the use of honey for partial-thickness burns compared with silver sulphadiazine. The 1991 study compared these products on 104 patients with less than 40% partial-thickness burns. Patients were randomly assigned to one of the two treatments. The author found a significantly lower infection rate in the honey group. The study in 1998 followed the same procedure as the previous study but monitored healing outcomes of 50 patients (25/group). The results showed that 84% of wounds in the honey group showed evidence of granulation and epithelialisation by day 7 compared with 72% in the silver sulphadiazine group. By day 21 all patients in the honey group ($n = 25$) and 21/25 in the silver sulphadiazine group were healed, a significant difference in favour of the honey group ($p = 0.05$).

Other dressings that can be used on minor burns include flat foam dressings, silicone net dressings and hydrogels. The foam dressings are comfortable and can be held in place with tape or a tubular net. Hydrogels can give a cooling sensation when applied, which may be comforting to the patient. Silicone net dressings are widely used as they can be left in place for 7–14 days and the secondary dressing changed when necessary.

Whatever dressing is used, the patient and wound should be reviewed at between 48–72 hours when the local oedema has subsided (Fowler, 2003). This review is especially important for patients who are being managed at home and attending the outpatient department.

Deep dermal and full-thickness burns generally require early excision of necrotic tissue and skin grafting for speedy healing.

Burns of the hands are best treated with silver sulphadiazine. Once the cream is applied, the hand should be covered with a plastic bag. This will allow free movement and help to prevent contractures. The hand should be kept elevated for the first 48–72 hours to reduce swelling (Fowler, 1996). There are several disadvantages with the use of plastic bags. They cause considerable maceration of the whole hand as large quantities of exudate accumulate in the bag. The bag becomes heavy and pulls the wrist into flexion. Once full of fluid, the bag tends to leak or tear, necessitating dressing change. Terrill *et al.* (1991) compared the use of Gore-Tex™ bags with plastic bags. Gore-Tex™ has the property of water vapour permeability. Although there was no difference in healing times, there was a considerable reduction in skin maceration and accumulation of exudate when using Gore-Tex™. Improved hand function was also noted. Witchell and

Crossman (1991) compared the use of these bags over silver sulphadiazine with paraffin gauze for children with burns of the hands. They found that use of Gore-Tex™ bags increased child activity and reduced the length of time of dressing change. More significantly, there were considerably fewer unscheduled visits to the accident and emergency department because of problems with the dressing.

Evaluation

Evaluation of the burn wound involves monitoring of the wound as it progresses towards healing and of the healed wound. Any non-complex burn that fails to heal within three weeks should be referred to a specialist unit. Once the wound is healed, special care needs to be taken of the newly formed epithelia. Bayley (1990) suggests cleansing with a mild soap and then applying water-based cream several times a day. The patient should be warned to avoid any possibility of sunburn. Fowler (2003) recommends use of total sunblock for the first year and then gradually reducing to factor 15.

Potential problems that can develop are contractures and hypertrophic scarring. Myofibroblasts contract and shorten the wound, causing the collagen fibres to become coiled. The scar develops a hard, red, raised appearance. If the burn injury is over a joint, as the myofibroblasts contract this causes flexion of the joint. Unless measures are taken to splint the joint, it will become contracted. A programme of exercise and splinting can help to counteract this problem.

Hypertrophic scarring is often managed by the use of pressure garments that the patients will have to wear for about a year. However, a randomised study by Chang *et al.* (1995) found that pressure garments made no difference to the degree of scarring. An alternative treatment, a silicone gel sheet, has been used, initially in Australia. Poston (2000) undertook a review of the use of silicone gel sheeting in the management of hypertrophic and keloid scars and concluded that it appears to improve the appearance of these scars, but there is insufficient evidence to determine its usefulness in restoring mobility and function when scarring is associated with contractures.

A few patients will develop permanent pigmentation changes. This is possibly because of damage to the melanocytes in the basal layer of the epidermis. It can present as either apigmentation or hyperpigmentation. It is not possible to predict when it will occur.

6.5 RADIATION REACTIONS

Radiation treatment or radiotherapy is the mainstay of cancer treatment. It has been estimated that nearly 20% of people in Western countries will receive radiotherapy at some point in their lives (Porock *et al.*, 1999). Radiation reaction is the reaction of the skin to the effects of radiotherapy and is limited to the treatment field or its exit point. Strictly speaking, a radiation reaction is not a wound. However, the skin reaction is akin to a superficial burn and has the potential for ulceration. There is limited research into the management of what can be a very painful problem.

6.5.1 Aetiology

Ionising radiation or radiotherapy is the mainstay of cancer treatment. Treatment is usually given in a series of doses, ranging from daily to weekly, although a small number of patients will receive just one dose. A course of treatment may last up to eight weeks. Radiation reactions are most likely to occur when the treatment field is close to the body surface, such as the head or neck, or if it includes the axillae, under the breasts, perineum or groin. The reaction is dose dependent; that is, the more frequent the treatment or the higher the dose, the more likely the reaction. A reaction may occur during a course of treatment or after it is completed. Within six weeks of completion of treatment, all but the most severe reactions have disappeared.

6.5.2 The classification of radiation reactions

The severity of radiation reactions is generally classified using the grading system developed by the Radiation Therapy Oncology Group (RTOG) (Cox *et al.*, 1995) and recommended by the College of Radiographers in the UK.

0   No change over baseline.
1   Follicular, faint or dull erythema.
2a   Tender or bright erythema with/without dry desquamation.
2b   Patchy, moist desquamation, moderate oedema.
3   Confluent wet desquamation, pitting oedema.
4   Ulceration, haemorrhage, necrosis.

It is considered that 90–95% of patients undergoing radiotherapy will have some degree of reaction (Porock *et al.*, 1999). However, in a study of 126 women treated for breast cancer, less than 10% had moist desquamation (Porock & Kristjanson, 1999). Thus it seems reasonable to assume that most patients are likely to have erythema, possibly associated with soreness and itching. In a review of the subject, Porock *et al.* (1999) noted that women being treated for breast cancer were particularly vulnerable if they smoked, were overweight and/or had large breast size or had required axillary lymphocoele drainage prior to treatment, whereas younger patients were more vulnerable than older patients in those having treatment to the sternum.

6.5.3 Preventive skin care

There is a body of evidence available to guide practice, in the form of best practice statements (NHS Quality Improvement Scotland, 2004), a summary of key research findings for breast cancer (National Breast Cancer Centre, 2004) and the clinical guidelines issued by the UK College of Radiographers (2001). Box 6.4 provides a summary of the recommended skin care. Unfortunately, despite

---

Box 6.4   Summary of recommendations for skin care during radiotherapy treatment.

- Wash treatment site daily using mild unperfumed soap.
- Avoid having a very hot shower, especially if the water jets are powerful.
- Pat area dry with soft towel, avoiding friction.
- Do not apply deodorants, perfume or aftershave to the treatment site.
- Apply a mild emollient twice daily, ensuring emollient is at room temperature.
- For men having radiotherapy to face or neck, use an electric razor rather than a wet shave.
- If the axilla is part of the treatment site, do not shave during treatment.
- If swimming, wash off chlorinated water as it is drying to skin and apply emollient.
- Wear loose clothing over treatment site to avoid friction.
- Avoid sun exposure where possible and use sunblock if it is unavoidable.

---

this guidance, there is considerable variation in the advice given to patients concerning how the skin within the treatment field should be managed whilst radiotherapy is in progress (Faithfull *et al.*, 2002).

Wells and colleagues reviewed the findings of their study of 357 patients undergoing radiotherapy and concluded that levels of skin discomfort were lower than they had expected (Wells *et al.*, 2004). They concluded that consistent advice, skin hygiene and regular assessment were major factors in reducing problems. It is interesting to postulate that a reason for previous reports of severe skin problems may have been the advice given some years ago that patients should not wash the treatment area. Happily, that advice is now seen as outdated.

6.5.4 Managing radiation reactions

The basic principles of managing radiation reactions are as follows.

RTOG score 1 and 2a

A simple moisturiser such as aqueous cream can be soothing applied to the area twice daily. If aqueous cream is not effective an alternative cream may help. There is much anecdotal evidence of the benefits of using aloe vera gel and Heggie *et al.* (2002) undertook a study of 225 patients undergoing treatment for breast cancer comparing aloe vera gel with aqueous cream. They found that aqueous cream was significantly better than aloe vera gel in reducing dry desquamation and pain. However, Wells *et al.* (2004) did not find this to be the case when comparing aqueous cream with either sucralfate cream or no cream. They concluded that patients should be given the choice to use a cream or not.

RTOG score 2b and 3

There is insufficient evidence to suggest a definitive treatment for wet desquamation. The main goal is to choose a dressing that is comfortable for the patient and promotes healing. Depending on the level of exudate, this could include hydrocolloids, hydrogels and silicone dressings (National Breast Care Centre, 2004).

RTOG score 4

There is no information in the literature about the management of this grade of radiation reaction but it would seem logical to treat them following the basic principles of wound management as described in Chapter 3.

6.5.5 Care of the patient

The most important aspect of care of any patient undergoing radiotherapy must be communication. Written information can be used to reinforce verbal explanations. This provides the patient with a permanent record that can be shared with others. Although UK radiotherapy centres provide written information for their patients, not all of this is evidence based (Faithfull *et al.*, 2002). As hospitals seek to improve the information given to patients, it is hoped that this situation will improve.

REFERENCES

Allen, P. (1996) Sternal wound dressings – a research study into risk factors. *British Journal of Theatre Nursing*, **6** (7), 38–39.

Andronicus, M., Oates, R.K., Peat, J., Spalding, S., Martin, H. (1998) Non-accidental burns in children. *Burns*, **24** (6), 552–558.

Barnea, Y., Amir, A., Leshem, D. *et al.* (2004) Clinical comparative study of Aquacel and paraffin gauze dressing for the treatment of split-skin donor site treatment. *Annals of Plastic Surgery*, **53** (2), 132–136.

Bayley, E.W. (1990) Wound healing in the patient with burns. *Nursing Clinics of North America*, **25** (1), 205–222.

Bianchi, J. (2000) The cleansing of superficial traumatic wounds. *British Journal of Nursing*, **9** (19) (suppl.), S28–S36.

Birchall, L., Taylor, S. (2003) Surgical wound benchmark tool and best practice guidelines. *British Journal of Nursing*, **12** (17), 1013–1023.

Briggs, M. (1996) Surgical wound pain: a trial of two treatments. *Journal of Wound Care*, **5** (10), 456–460.

Brolin, R.E. (1996) Prospective, randomised evaluation of midline fascial closure in gastric bariatric operations. *American Journal of Surgery*, **172**, 328–331.

Brown, M.D., Brookfield, K.F.W. (2004) A randomised study of closed wound suction drainage for extensive lumbar spine surgery. *Spine*, **29** (10), 1066–1068.

Brunner, L.S., Suddarth, D.S. (1988) *Textbook of Medical-Surgical Nursing.* J.B. Lippincott, Philadelphia, PA.

Buckles, E. (1985) Wound care in accident and emergency. *Nursing*, **2** (42) (suppl), 3–5.

Butcher, M. (1999) Management of wound sinuses. *Journal of Wound Care*, **8** (9), 451–454.

Chang, P., Laubenthal, K.N., Lewis, R.W. *et al.* (1995) A prospective randomised study of the efficacy of pressure garment therapy in patients with burns. *Journal of Burn Care Rehabilitation*, **16**, 473–475.

Chen, E., Hornig, S., Shepherd, S.M., Hollander, J.E. (2000) Primary closure of mammalian bites. *Academic Emergency Medicine*, **7** (2), 157–161.

Chrintz, H., Vibits, H., Cordtz, T.O. *et al.* (1989) Need for surgical wound dressing. *British Journal of Surgery*, **76**, 204–205.

Cockerill, J., Sweet, A. (1993) Nursing management of common accident wounds. *British Journal of Nursing*, **2** (11), 578–582.

Cohn, S.M., Gianotti, G., Ong, A.W. *et al.* (2001) Prospective randomised trial of two wound management strategies for dirty abdominal wounds. *Annals of Surgery*, **233** (3), 409–413.

College of Radiographers (2001) *Summary of Intervention for Acute Radiotherapy Induced Skin. Reaction in Cancer Patients: a clinical guideline*. College of Radiographers, London.

Collier, M. (1996) Trauma injury nursing in A&E. *Nursing Times*, **93** (20), 74–79.

Coull, A., Wylie, K. (1990) Regular monitoring: the way to ensure flap healing. *Professional Nurse*, **6** (1), 18–21.

Cox, J.D., Stetz, J., Pajak, T.F. (1995) Toxicity criteria of the Radiation Therapy Oncology Group (RTOG) and the European Organisation for Research and Treatment of Cancer (EORTC). *International Journal of Radiation Oncology, Biology and Physics*, **31**, 1341–1346.

Crowe, M.J., Cooke, E.M. (1998) Review of case definitions for nosocomial infection – towards consensus. *Journal of Hospital Infection*, **39**, 3–11.

Cruse, P.J.E., Foord, R. (1973) A five-year prospective study of 23 649 surgical wounds. *Archives of Surgery*, **107**, 206–210.

Cruse, P.J.E., Foord, R. (1980) The epidemiology of wound infection, a ten-year prospective study of 62 939 wounds. *Surgical Clinics of North America*, **60** (1), 27–40.

Davey, R.B., Sparnon, A.L., Lodge, M. (2003) Technique of split skin graft fixation using Hypafix: a 15-year review. *Australian and New Zealand Journal of Surgery*, **73** (11), 958–962.

Davis, A., Chester, D., Allison, K., Davison, P. (2004) A survey of how a region's A&E units manage pretibial lacerations. *Journal of Wound Care*, **13** (1), 5–7.

Dealey, C. (1991) Managing surgical wounds. *Nursing*, **4** (43), 29–32.

Department of Health (2001) *The Essence of Care*. Department of Health, London.

Dunkin, C.S.J., Elfleet, D., Ling, C.A., La Hause Brown, T. (2003) A step by step guide to classifying and managing pretibial injuries. *Journal of Wound Care*, **12** (3), 109–111.

Dunn, R.J. (1996) Practical application of a first-aid treatment for burns and scalds. *Journal of Wound Care*, **5** (6), 265–266.

Edwards, H., Gaskill, D., Nash, R. (1998) Treating skin tears in nursing home residents: a pilot study comparing four types of dressings. *International Journal of Nursing Practice*, **4** (1), 25–32.

Emmerson, A.M., Enstone, J.E., Griffin, M. *et al.* (1996) The second national prevalence survey of infection in hospitals – overview of the results. *Journal of Hospital Infection*, **32**, 175–190.

Evans, R.C., Jones, N.L. (1996) The management of abrasions and bruises. *Journal of Wound Care*, **5** (10), 465–468.

Faithfull, S., Hilton, M., Booth, K. (2002) Survey of information leaflets on advice for acute radiation skin reactions in UK radiotherapy centres: a rationale for a systematic review of the literature. *European Journal of Oncology Nursing*, 6 (3), 176–178.

Farion, K., Osmond, M.H., Hartling, L. *et al.* (2004) Tissue adhesives for traumatic lacerations in children and adults (Cochrane review). *The Cochrane Library, Issue 4.* John Wiley & Sons Ltd, Chichester.

Fowler, A. (1996) Superficial partial thickness burns of the hands. *Nursing Standard,* **11** (6), 56–61.

Fowler, A. (2003) The management of non-complex wounds within the community. *Nursing Times,* **99** (25) (suppl), 5–7.

Fowler, A., Dempsey, A. (1998) Split-thickness skin graft donor sites. *Journal of Wound Care,* **7** (8), 399–402.

Francis, A. (1998) Nursing management of skin graft sites. *Nursing Standard,* **12** (33), 41–44.

Gallico, G.G., O'Connor, N.E., Compton, C.C., Kehinde, O., Green, H. (1984) Permanent cover of large burn wounds with autologous cultured human epithelium. *New England Journal of Medicine,* **311**, 448–451.

Gislason, H., Gronbech, J.E., Soreide, O. (1995) Burst abdomen and incisional hernia after major gastrointestinal operations – comparison of three closure techniques. *European Journal of Surgery,* **161**, 349–354.

Gordon, M., Goodwin, C.W. (1997) Initial assessment, management and stabilisation. *Nursing Clinics of North America,* **32** (2), 237–249.

Harding, K.G. (1990) Wound care: putting theory into clinical practice, in (ed.) Krasner, D., *Chronic Wound Care.* Health Management Publications, King of Prussia, PA.

Harrington, G., Russo, P., Spelman, D. *et al.* (2004) Surgical-site infection rates and risk factor analysis in coronary artery bypass graft surgery. *Infection Control and Hospital Epidemiology,* **25** (6), 472–476.

Heggie, S., Bryant, G.P., Tripcony, L. *et al.* (2002) A phase III study on the efficacy of aloe vera gel on irradiated breast tissue. *Cancer Nursing,* **25** (6), 442–451.

Herruzo, C.R., Lopez, G.R., Diez, S.J., Lopez, A.M.J., Banegas, B.J.R. (2004) Surgical site infection of 7301 traumatologic inpatients (divided in two sub-cohorts, study and validation): modifiable determinants and potential benefit. *European Journal of Epidemiology,* **19** (2), 163–169.

Hettiaratchy, S., Dziewulski, P. (2004a) ABC of burns: pathophysiology and types of burns. *British Medical Journal,* **328**, 1427–1430.

Hettiaratchy, S., Dziewulski, P. (2004b) ABC of burns: introduction. *British Medical Journal,* **328**, 1366–1368.

Hettiaratchy, S., Papini, R. (2004) ABC of burns: initial management of a major burn: I overview. *British Medical Journal,* **328**, 1555–1557.

Higgins, M.A.G., Evans, R.C., Evans, R.J. (1997) Managing animal bite wounds. *Journal of Wound Care,* **6** (8), 377–380.

Holm, C., Pederson, J.S., Gronbaek, F., Gottrup, F. (1998) Effects of occlusive and conventional gauze dressings on incisional healing after abdominal operations. *European Journal of Surgery,* **164** (3), 179–183.

Holt, B.T., Parks, N.L., Engh, G.A., Lawrence, J.M. (1997) Comparison of closed-suction drainage and no drainage after total knee arthroplasty. *Orthopaedics,* **20** (12), 1121–1124.

Hudspith, J., Rayatt, S. (2004) ABC of burns: first aid and treatment of minor burns. *British Medical Journal,* **328**, 1487–1489.

Israelsson, L.A. (1998) The surgeon as a risk factor for complications of midline incisions. *European Journal of Surgery,* **164** (5), 353–359.

Jonkers, D., Elenbaas, T., Terporten, P., Nieman, F., Stobberingh, E. (2003) Prevalence of 90-days postoperative wound infections after cardiac surgery. *European Journal of Cardiothoracic Surgery,* **23** (1), 97–102.

Kamp-Hopmans, E.M., Blok, H.E.M., Troelstra, A. *et al.* (2003) Surveillance for hospital acquired infections on surgical wards in a Dutch university hospital. *Infection Control and Hospital Epidemiology*, **24** (8), 584–590.

Lawrence, J.C. (1987) British Burn Association recommended first aid for burns and scalds. *Burns*, **13** (2), 153.

Lawrence, J.C. (1989) Treating minor burns. *Nursing Times*, **85**, 69–73.

Lawrence, J.C. (1996) A first-aid preparation for burns and scalds. *Journal of Wound Care*, **5** (6), 262–264.

Lawrence, J.C., Wilkins, M.D. (1986) The epidemiology of burns. Burncare Symposium at Birmingham University, April.

Lund, C.C., Browder, N.C. (1944) Estimations of areas of burns. *Surgery, Gynecology and Obstetrics*, **79**, 352.

Maharaj, D., Bagratee, J.S., Moodley, J. (2000) Drainage at caesarian section – a randomised prospective study. *South African Journal of Surgery*, **38** (1), 9–12.

McGough-Csarny, J., Kopac, C.A. (1998) Objectives 1: risk factor identification. Skin tears in institutionalised elderly: an epidemiological study. *Ostomy and Wound Management*, **44** (3A) (suppl), 14S–25S.

Medeiros, I., Saconato, H. (2004) Antibiotic prophylaxis for mammalian bites (Cochrane review). *The Cochrane Library, Issue 4*. John Wiley & Sons Ltd, Chichester.

Meuleneire, F. (2002) Using a soft silicone-coated net dressing to manage skin tears. *Journal of Wound Care*, **11** (10), 365–369.

Mileski, W.J., Atiles, L., Purdue, G. *et al.* (2003) Serial measurements increase the accuracy of laser Doppler assessment of burn wounds. *Journal of Burn Care and Rehabilitation*, **24** (4), 187–191.

Misirlioglu, A., Eroglu, S., Karacaoglan, N., Akan, M., Akoz, T., Yildirim, S. (2003) Use of honey as an adjunct in the healing of split-thickness skin graft donor site. *Dermatologic Surgery*, **29** (2), 168–172.

Moisidis, E., Heath, T., Boorer, C., Ho, K., Deva, A.K. (2004) A prospective, blinded, randomised, controlled clinical trial of topical negative pressure use in skin grafting. *Plastic and Reconstructive Surgery*, **114** (4), 917–922.

National Breast Cancer Centre (2004) *Skin Care during Radiotherapy for Breast Cancer: A Summary of Key Research Findings*. National Breast Cancer Centre, Sydney, Australia.

National Burn Care Review Committee (NBCRC) (2001) *Standards and Strategy for Burn Care: a review of burn care in the British Isles*. NBCRC, London.

National Institute for Clinical Excellence (2001) *Guidance on the Use of Debriding Agents and Specialist Wound Care Clinics for Difficult to Heal Surgical Wounds*. NICE, London.

NHS Quality Improvement Scotland (2004) *Best Practice Statement: Skincare of Patients Receiving Radiotherapy*. NHS QIS, Edinburgh.

Nienhuijs, S.W., Manupassa, R., Strobbe, L.J.A., Rosman, C. (2003) Can topical negative pressure be used to control complex enterocutaneous fistulae? *Journal of Wound Care*, **12** (9), 343–345.

Payne, R.L., Martin, M.C. (1993) Defining and classifying skin tears: need for a common language. A critique and revision of the Payne–Martin classification system for skin tears. *Ostomy and Wound Management*, **39** (5), 16–26.

Perkins, P. (1992) Wound dehiscence: causes and care. *Nursing Standard*, **6** (34) (suppl), 12–14.

Perkins, S.W., Williams, J.D., Macdonald, K., Robinson, E.B. (1997) Prevention of seromas and haematomas after face-lift surgery with the use of postoperative vacuum drains. *Archives of Otolaryngology, Head and Neck Surgery*, **123** (7), 743–745.

Platt, A.J., Phipps, A., Judkins, K. (1996) A comparative study of silicone net dressing and paraffin gauze dressing in skin-grafted sites. *Burns*, **22** (7), 543–545.

Porock, D., Kristjanson, L. (1999) Skin reactions during radiotherapy for breast cancer: the use and impact of topical agents and dressings. *European Journal of Cancer Care*, **8** (3), 143–153.

Porock, D., Nikoletti, S., Kristjanson, L. (1999) Management of radiation skin reactions: literature review and clinical application. *Plastic Surgical Nursing*, **19** (4), 185–191.

Poston, J. (2000) The use of silicone gel sheeting in the management of hypertrophic and keloid scars. *Journal of Wound Care*, **9** (1), 10–16.

Purushothom, A.D., McLatchie, E., Young, D. *et al.* (2002) Randomised clinical trial of no wound drains and early discharge in the treatment of women with breast cancer. *British Journal of Surgery*, **89**, 286–292.

Reilly, J. (1997) Under surveillance. *Nursing Times*, **93** (23), 57–60.

Ricci, E., Aloesio, R., Cassino, R. *et al.* (1998) Foam dressing versus gauze soaks in the treatment of surgical wounds healing by secondary intention, in (eds) Leaper, D., Cherry, G., Cockbill, S. *et al.*, *Proceedings of the EWMA/Journal of Wound Care Spring Meeting*. Macmillan Magazines Ltd, London.

Sax, H. (2004) Nationwide surveillance of nosocomial infection in Switzerland – methods and results of the Swiss Nosocomial Infection Prevalence Studies (SNIP) in 1999 and 2002. *Therapeutische Umschau*, **61** (3), 197–203.

Singer, A.J., Hollander, J.E., Quinn, J.V. (1997) Evaluation and management of traumatic lacerations. *New England Journal of Medicine*, **337** (16), 1142–1148.

Subrahmanyam, M. (1991) Topical application of honey in treatment of burns. *British Journal of Surgery*, **78**, 497–498.

Subrahmanyam, M. (1998) A prospective randomised clinical and histological study of superficial burn wound healing with honey and silver sulphadiazine. *Burns*, **24** (2), 157–161.

Taylor, D.E.M., Whamond, J.S., Penhallow, J.E. (1987) Effects of haemorrhage on wound strength and fibroblast function. *British Journal of Surgery*, **74**, 316–319.

Terrill, P.J., Kedwards, S.M., Lawrence, J.C. (1991) The use of Gore-Tex bags for hand burns. *Burns*, **17** (2), 161–165.

Thomas, D.R., Goode, P.S., LaMaster, K., Tennyson, T., Parnell, L.K.S. (1999) A comparison of an opaque foam dressing versus a transparent film dressing in the management of skin tears in institutionalised subjects. *Ostomy and Wound Management*, **45** (6), 22–28.

Thomas, S.S., Lawrence, J.C., Thomas, A. (1995) Evaluation of hydrocolloids and topical medication in minor burns. *Journal of Wound Care*, **4** (5), 218–220.

Varley, G.W., Milner, S.A. (1995) Wound drains in proximal femoral fracture surgery: a randomised prospective trial of 177 patients. *Journal of the Royal College of Surgeons of Edinburgh*, **40**, 416–418.

Vermeulen, H., Ubbink, D., Goossens, A., de Vos, R., Legemate, D. (2004) Dressings and topical agents for surgical wounds healing by secondary intention. *Cochrane Database of Systematic Reviews* (2) CD003554.

Vloemans, A.F. (1994) Fixation of skin grafts with a new silicone rubber dressing (Mepitel). *Scandinavian Journal of Plastic and Reconstructive Surgery and Hand Surgery*, **28** (1), 75–76.

Wallace, A.B. (1951) The exposure treatment of burns. *Lancet*, **i**: 501–504.

Weiss, Y. (1983) Simplified management of operative wounds by early exposure. *International Surgery*, **68**, 237–240.

Wells, M., Macmillan, M., Raab, G. *et al.* (2004) Does aqueous or sucralfate cream affect the severity of erythematous radiation skin reactions? A randomised controlled trial. *Radiotherapy and Oncology*, **73**, 153–162.

Westaby, S. (1985) Wound closure and drainage, in (ed.) Westaby, S., *Wound Care*. William Heinemann-Medical Books Ltd, London.

Wiechula, R. (2003) The use of moist wound healing dressings in the management of split-thickness skin graft donor sites: a systematic review. *International Journal of Nursing Practice*, **9** (suppl.), S9–S17.

Wijetunge, D. (1992) An A & E approach. *Nursing Times*, **88** (46), 70–76.

Wikblad, K., Anderson, B. (1995) A comparison of three wound dressings in patients undergoing heart surgery. *Nursing Research*, **44** (5), 312–316.

Wilkinson, B. (1997) Hard graft. *Nursing Times*, **93** (16), 63–68.

Wilson, A.P.R., Weavill, C., Burridge, J., Kelsey, M.C. (1990) The use of the wound scoring method 'ASEPSIS' in postoperative wound surveillance. *Journal of Hospital Infection*, **16**, 297–300.

Wilson, A.P.R., Helder, N., Theminimulle, S.K., Scott, G.M. (1998) Comparison of wound scoring methods for use in audit. *Journal of Hospital Infection*, **39**, 119–126.

Witchell, M., Crossman, C. (1991) Dressing burns in children. *Nursing Times*, **87** (36), 63–66.

Wynne, R., Botti, M., Stedman, H., Holsworth, L. (2004) Effect of three wound dressings on infection, healing comfort and cost in patients with sternotomy wounds: a randomised trial. *Chest*, **125** (1), 43–50.

Chapter 7
Clinically Effective Wound Care

7.1 INTRODUCTION

Most nurses want to give their patients high-quality care. In the last few years there has been considerable emphasis on the importance of ensuring that clinical practice is based on research. Evidence-based care is a major component of clinical governance, the framework used by the UK Department of Health to ensure high standards of care within the NHS (DoH, 1997).

Alongside the move to identify clinically effective practice has been the development of clinical guidelines. In turn this links to clinical audit. Research is an essential component underpinning each one. This chapter will address the issues in relation to developing clinically effective practice in wound care.

7.2 EVIDENCE-BASED PRACTICE AND CLINICAL EFFECTIVENESS

Providing clinically effective evidence based care involves:

- identifying current research and 'best' practice.
- utilising appropriate national guidelines, protocols or standards where available.
- where guidelines are not available, critically appraising the available literature and evaluating its value to the proposed care setting.
- implementing guidelines or protocols, changing practice where necessary.
- undertaking clinical audits to measure outcomes and ensure patient care is clinically effective.
- sharing this knowledge with others within the clinical care setting and elsewhere.

7.3 SEARCHING AND APPRAISING THE LITERATURE

With the advent of electronic databases, literature searches have become more sophisticated. It is no longer adequate for individuals to simply use those articles that they have stored in the filing cabinet. They are likely to be out of date and coincide with the point of view of the individual. Electronic databases such as MEDLINE or CINAHL can assist in rapidly identifying relevant information

Box 7.1   Examples of different kinds of wound care journals.

General wound care journals
Advances in Skin and Wound Care
International Wound Journal
Journal of Tissue Viability
Journal of Wound Care
Ostomy and Wound Management

Journals that cover specific types of wounds
Burns
Diabetic Foot Journal
Journal of Burncare Rehabilitation
Journal of Hospital Infection
Surgery

on a specific topic. It is also important to have access to library facilities in order to retrieve the relevant journal papers.

Wound care research can be found in a wide range of journals as evidenced in the reference lists within this book. There are also a number of specialist journals that focus wholly on tissue viability or very specific types of wounds. Box 7.1 lists some examples. Hand searching these journals may also provide further information.

Other sources of information include the Cochrane Library, in particular the Cochrane Wounds Group, which is based at the University of York in the UK. The Cochrane Wounds Group is responsible for overseeing systematic reviews that follow the same specific methodology and format for presentation of the findings as any other Cochrane review on a wide range of topics relating to wounds. Another source of evidence is the Health Technology Assessment Programme in the UK. This programme has funded both primary (randomised controlled trials) and secondary (systematic reviews) research in wound care. The relevant reports are freely available on the website. It is also sometimes useful to be aware of research studies that are in progress. This information can be found on the Controlled Trials website, which also contains the meta Register of Clinical Trials. Details of all these resources can be found in Table 7.1.

Once a literature search is completed, the identified studies need to be critically appraised. All healthcare professionals should be able to critically review a piece of research in order to judge the value of a study and whether the findings have implications for their clinical practice. Unfortunately, not everyone has had training to develop this skill. In the UK, the Critical Appraisal Skills Programme (CASP) has been developed to assist large numbers of healthcare professionals in developing these skills. There are also useful proformas to guide appraisal of studies using different research methods. The broad issues

Table 7.1 Useful web-based sources of education and evidence.

Source	Type of evidence	Internet address
Cochrane Collaboration	Systematic reviews	www.cochrane.org
Cochrane Wound Group	Systematic reviews relating to wound care	www.york.ac.uk/healthsciences/gsp/themes/woundcare/Wounds
Health Technology Assessment Programme	RCTs and systematic reviews relating to wound care + wide range of other studies	www.ncchta.org.
Meta-Register of Clinical Trials	Wide range of information about current trials	www.controlled-trials.com/mrct
Critical Appraisal Skills Programme (CASP)	Details of programme for developing skills in literature searching and critical appraisal, including e-learning	www.phru.nhs.uk/casp

that the appraisal tool helps to identify for most quantitative methods such as randomised controlled trials or cohort studies are:

- is the trial valid?
- what are the results?
- will the results help locally?

whereas for an economic evaluation, the overall questions of relevance are:

- is the economic evaluation likely to be useable?
- how were the costs and consequences assessed and compared?
- will the results help in purchasing services for local people? (Milton Keynes Primary Care Trust, 2002)

The proformas are designed to guide the user through the process in a very systematic way. Further information can be found in Table 7.1.

Searching the literature is very time-consuming as there is a wealth of information available. Not everyone has the time or resources to undertake such a task in relation to all aspects of patient care. Systematic reviews of the literature can assist the healthcare professional by integrating existing information. A systematic review has been defined by Mulrow (1994) as 'the methodological and critical exploration, evaluation, collation and analysis of information from related research studies to draw conclusions about the variables and outcomes included in the studies'. Systematic reviews generally only include randomised controlled trials as they are considered to be the best research method for measuring the effectiveness of different treatments. Within the review, the results of several studies can be grouped together by means of a type of statistical analysis called meta-analysis, which can give a more conclusive result than each of the studies may do on their own (Cook *et al.*, 1997a). The websites where relevant wound care systematic reviews may be found are detailed in Table 7.1.

7.3.1 Appraising the literature on wound care

The literature pertaining to all aspects of wound care is very large, as demonstrated by the many examples that have been given in other chapters of this book. It is therefore important for the nurse to be aware of how to identify both the strengths and the weaknesses of the wound care evidence. Some of the issues are addressed here.

Study size

Early studies of modern dressings tended to compare them with gauze. As the differences between the two groups were so great, only relatively small numbers of patients were needed in a study. However, the differences are much smaller when comparing two modern products and therefore much larger numbers are needed. It may be difficult for one centre to recruit sufficient patients, so several centres may be required. This may introduce other variables if there are variations in local management patterns (Freak, 1995). High-quality research will indicate that it has sought to reduce this problem by using a power calculation to identify the required sample size and also addressing the issue of standardisation between centres.

Endpoints

Another issue to consider when appraising the wound care literature is endpoints. In other words, at what point a patient should be considered to have completed a study. Freak (1995) suggests that complete healing is not always the most suitable endpoint, although Bradley *et al.* (1999) argue that assessing the proportion of wounds healed is the most objective assessment currently available. They also propose that if reduction in wound size is used as an endpoint then both the percentage and absolute change in surface area should be measured.

Length of study

There has been considerable debate regarding the length of time that is reasonable for a trial of effectiveness of treatment, especially if time to healing is used as an endpoint. Lengthy studies are costly to undertake and there is a risk that patients may be lost to follow-up during the time of the study. Nelson (1998) suggests that healing rates for leg ulcers should be measured at intervals over time, probably more than 12 weeks. However, other authors have not always supported this view. Kantor and Margolis (2000) studied 104 venous leg ulcers and found that percentage change in area at four weeks was an indicator of healing at 24 weeks. Similarly, Sheehan *et al.* (2003), using 203 patients found the percentage change in diabetic foot ulcer area at four weeks is a robust indicator of healing at 12 weeks. There is obviously some disparity in the expected healing time between the two studies quoted, indicating the importance of not trying to extrapolate the findings directly to another wound type.

7.4 DEVELOPING CLINICAL GUIDELINES

Clinical guidelines are recommendations on the appropriate treatment and care of people with specific diseases and conditions (NICE, 2004a). They have a number of uses: to guide the care of individuals; to develop standards against which clinical practice can be measured; for education and training; and to help patients make informed choices (NICE, 2004a). Generally, guidelines consist of a series of statements around a particular topic with a rationale for each statement. The rationale relates to the evidence, usually obtained from systematic reviews, underpinning the statement. Many guidelines use a hierarchy to measure the quality of the evidence that they use and then grade the recommendation, as demonstrated in the NICE guidelines. For example, within the hierarchy of evidence, level I indicates evidence obtained from meta-analysis of randomised controlled trials or at least one randomised controlled trial; a statement based on this evidence would be graded as a grade A statement. Table 7.2 shows the grading system used in the NICE guidelines on prevention and management of foot problems in patients with type 2 diabetes (NICE, 2004b).

Preparation and publication of a guideline are not enough to ensure that it is implemented. Any national guideline tends to be written in broad terms. It needs to be adapted to include more operational detail for local use and may include policies and protocols. The implementation team should be multidisciplinary, reflecting all key personnel including representatives from purchasing authorities (Effective Health Care, 1994). Richens *et al.* (2004) undertook a review of the literature on guideline implementation and made several useful observations based on their findings.

- Guidelines and any local adaptation of guidelines should contain recommendations that are clear, specific and relevant to both practitioners and practice.
- Ownership and adoption of guidelines are more likely to occur if there is a partnership between the guideline developers, users and implementers.
- Guideline implementation can be improved by use of dedicated 'change agents' to work with individuals, teams and organisations in the clinical setting.
- The use of clinical audit is an essential aspect of guideline implementation.
- Those responsible for implementing guidelines need to be aware of organisational factors, especially linking in to the organisation's strategy and resource commitments.

7.4.1 Guidelines in wound care

There are a great number of guidelines available that relate to various aspects of wound care. A survey undertaken by the Tissue Viability Society in 2002 found that there appeared to be a major shift over a five-year period from the use of locally developed guidelines to the use of national and international

Table 7.2 Evidence grading scheme used within the NICE guideline: Type 2 Diabetes, Prevention and Management of Foot Problems (NICE, 2004)*

Recommendation grade	Evidence
A	Directly based on category I evidence
B	Directly based on: • category II evidence **or** • extrapolated recommendation from category I evidence
C	Directly based on: • category III evidence **or** • extrapolated recommendation from category I or II evidence
D	Directly based on: • category IV evidence **or** • extrapolated recommendation from category I, II or III evidence
NICE 2003	Recommendation drawn from the NICE 2003 technology appraisal of patient education models for diabetes

Evidence category	Source
I	Evidence from: • meta-analysis of randomised controlled trials **or** • at least one randomised controlled trial
II	Evidence from: • at least one controlled trial without randomisation **or** • at least one other type of quasiexperimental study
III	Evidence from non-experimental descriptive studies such as comparative studies, correlation studies and case control studies
IV	Evidence from expert committee reports or opinions and/or clinical experience of respected authorities

*(reproduced by kind permission of NICE).

guidelines (Clark, 2003). Many of these guidelines have been published in the wound care literature and others are freely available via the Internet.

At present, there is insufficient high-quality research to provide all grade A recommendations in guidelines for either pressure ulcers or leg ulcers. For example, the NICE guidelines for pressure ulcer prevention contains ten statements, of which one is grade B and the remainder grade D, demonstrating the weak evidence on which the guideline is based (NICE, 2003). Cook *et al.* (1997b) suggest that where the evidence supporting a guideline is not strong, the impact of implementation needs to be rigorously audited.

7.5 THE CLINICAL AUDIT CYCLE

Audit has been defined as:

'a clinically-led initiative which seeks to improve the quality and outcome of patient care through structured peer review whereby clinicians examine their practices and results against agreed explicit standards and modify their practice where indicated' (NHS Executive, 1998).

Burnett and Winyard (1998) suggest that clinical audit is at the heart of clinical effectiveness. Some guidelines also include an audit tool against which it is possible to measure the effectiveness of implementation. Examples can be found in the NICE guidelines on pressure ulcer prevention and the diabetic foot (NICE, 2003, 2004b).

One of the benefits of audit is that it can be used to measure the outcomes of everyday practice to provide baseline information before introducing clinical guidelines. A repeat of the audit enables the guideline team to monitor any health gains associated with the implementation of more effective practice as well as monitoring whether the guidelines are being adhered to. Clinical staff are more likely to be willing to adhere to guidelines if they can see a beneficial outcome. Providing information for staff about performance levels is an essential aspect of the audit process.

7.5.1 Auditing clinical practice

Audit provides data both for initial baseline information and to measure the outcomes of guideline implementation. In many instances this information is obtained by means of prevalence surveys and incidence monitoring. This is particularly true of pressure ulcers where there has been much debate on the most effective methods for collecting this information and on its value.

Prevalence can be defined as: 'The number of persons with a specific disease or condition as a proportion of a given population measured at a specific point in time' (Dealey, 1997), whereas incidence is defined as: 'The number of people developing a specific condition as a proportion of the local population measured over a period of time' (Dealey, 1997).

An example of a baseline pressure ulcer audit is one undertaken across France by Barrois et al. (1997). They found an overall prevalence of 8.7% as well as considerable detail about the characteristics of pressure ulcers in France. This provided a very informative baseline prior to introducing a range of prevention strategies. Incidence rates are often used to evaluate the effectiveness of prevention policies. Data collection for incidence measurement is more complicated than for prevalence surveys and subject to inaccuracies (Bridel et al., 1996). However, Dealey (1997) suggests that the main benefit of incidence rate measurement is to demonstrate improvements over time.

Lindholm et al. (1998) and Dealey (1998) undertook prevalence surveys of leg ulceration prior to instigating education and training and the implementation of management guidelines. Audit of the effectiveness of this strategy concentrated on changes in practice, nursing knowledge and healing rates (Dealey, 1998). Feedback of the results to the staff provided encouragement that adherence to the guidelines was ensuring increased healing rates. Stevens *et al.* (1997) also used healing rates to monitor the outcomes of a project establishing leg ulcer guidelines within two acute hospitals and the surrounding community. Over time they were also able to measure recurrence rates and compare them favourably with the rate from another study previously reported in the literature.

Audit of surgical wounds is usually undertaken as a surveillance of wound infection rates. This may be in the form of either prevalence or incidence. Prevalence surveys have been used in national surveys to provide a snapshot of the situation (Briggs, 1996). Incidence rates can be used to monitor the performance of individual surgeons. Frequently this type of surveillance measures the incidence of surgical wound infection (SWI) in clean surgery. Incidence may be used with case control studies or with cohort studies. Case control studies retrospectively compare a group of patients with SWI with a control group in order to determine any risk factors associated with SWI. Cohort studies are prospective and follow a group of patients over time to see who develops a SWI. Potential risk factors are determined at the beginning of the studies and then monitored for the outcome. For example, in their ten-year study, Cruse and Foord (1980) considered diabetes to be a potential risk factor and so monitored the clean wound infection rate for diabetics and found it to be considerably higher than that for non-diabetics. The findings from this type of audit can be used to improve patient care.

7.5.2 Dissemination of audit findings

As well as sharing audit results with those directly involved, it is important to discuss them with a wider audience. This may be in the form of a report for the executive board of a hospital trust or the local purchasing authority or it may be a conference presentation or a publication. There are a number of benefits.

- Internal dissemination allows other areas in the organisation to benefit from the audit findings.
- Healthcare professionals working in similar clinical areas can apply the lessons learned from the audit.
- Those involved in the audit will develop skills in writing and undertaking presentations.

7.6 CONCLUSIONS

At present, the quality of the evidence available to support clinically effective wound care is very variable. Systematic reviews can be used to determine the gaps so that future research can be directed to the area where it is most needed.

REFERENCES

Barrois, B., Allaert, F., Urbinelli, R., Colin, D. (1997) National survey in France: pressure sores in hospital institutions in 1994, in (eds) Cherry, G.W., Gottrup, F., Lawrence, J.C., Moffat, C.J., Turner, T.D., *Proceedings of the 5th European Conference on Advances in Wound Management.* Macmillan Magazines Ltd, London.

Bradley, M., Cullum, N., Sheldon, T. (1999) The debridement of chronic wounds: a systematic review. *Health Technology Assessment*, **3** (17), Part 1, 1–78.

Bridel, J., Banks, S., Mitton, C. (1996) The admission prevalence and hospital-acquired incidence of pressure sores within a large teaching hospital during April 1994 to March 1995, in (eds) Cherry, G.W., Gottrup, F., Lawrence, J.C., Moffat, C.J., Turner, T.D., *Proceedings of the 5th European Conference on Advances in Wound Management.* Macmillan Magazines Ltd, London.

Briggs, M. (1996) Epidemiological methods in the study of surgical wound infection. *Journal of Wound Care*, **5** (4), 186–191.

Burnett, A.C., Winyard, G. (1998) Clinical audit at the heart of clinical effectiveness. *Journal of Quality and Clinical Practice*, **18** (1), 3–19.

Clark, M. (2003) Barriers to the implementation of clinical guidelines. *Journal of Tissue Viability*, **13** (2), 62–72.

Cook, D.J., Mulrow, C.D., Haynes, R.B. (1997a) Systematic reviews: synthesis of best evidence for clinical decisions. *Annals of Internal Medicine*, **126** (5), 376–380.

Cook, D.J., Greengold, N.L., Ellrodt, A.G., Weingarten, S.R. (1997b) The relation between systematic reviews and practice guidelines. *Annals of Internal Medicine*, **127** (3), 210–216.

Cruse, P.J.E., Foord, R. (1980) The epidemiology of wound infection: a 10-year prospective study of 62 939 wounds. *Surgical Clinics of North America*, **60**, 27–40.

Dealey, C. (1997) *Managing Pressure Sore Prevention.* Mark Allen Publishing Ltd, Salisbury.

Dealey, C. (1998) The importance of education in effecting change in leg ulcer management, in (eds) Leaper, D., Dealey, C., Franks, P.J., Hofman, D., Moffatt, C.J., *Proceedings of the 7th European Conference on Advances in Wound Management.* EMAP Healthcare Ltd, London.

Department of Health (1997) *The New NHS: Modern, Dependable.* Department of Health, London.

Effective Health Care (1994) Implementing clinical practice guidelines. *Effective Health Care Bulletin no. 8.* University of Leeds, Leeds, pp. 1–12.

Freak, L. (1995) Evaluating clinical trials. *Journal of Wound Care*, **4** (3), 114–116.

Kantor J., Margolis D. (2000) A multicentre study of percentage change in venous leg ulcer area as a prognostic index of healing at 24 weeks. *British Journal of Dermatology*, **142**, 960–964.

Lindholm, C., Tammelin, A., Bergsten, A., Berglund, E. (1998) The Uppsala experience: implications for developing educational strategies, in (eds) Leaper, D., Dealey, C., Franks, P.J., Hofman, D., Moffatt, C.J., *Proceedings of the 7th European Conference on Advances in Wound Management.* EMAP Healthcare Ltd, London.

Milton Keynes Primary Care Trust (2002) *Critical Appraisal Skills Programme.* Milton Keynes Primary Care Trust, Milton Keynes.

Mulrow, C.D. (1994) Rationale for systematic reviews. *British Medical Journal*, **309** (6954), 597–599.

National Institute for Clinical Excellence (2003) *Clinical Guideline 7: the use of pressure-relieving devices (beds, mattresses and overlays) for the prevention of pressure ulcers in primary and secondary care.* NICE, London.

National Institute for Clinical Excellence (2004a) *About Clinical Guidelines*. Available online at: www.nice.org.uk.

National Institute for Clinical Excellence (2004b) *Clinical Guideline 10: type 2 diabetes: prevention and management of foot problems*. NICE, London.

Nelson, E.A. (1998) The evidence in support of compression bandaging. *Journal of Wound Care*, **7** (3), 148–150.

Richens, Y., Rycroft-Malone, J., Morrell, C. (2004) Getting guidelines into practice: a literature review. *Nursing Standard*, **18** (50), 33–40.

Sheehan, P., Jones, P., Caselli, A., Giurini, J.M., Veves, A. (2003) Percentage change in wound area of diabetic foot ulcers over a 4-week period is a robust predictor of complete healing in a 12 week prospective trial. *Diabetes Care*, **26** (6), 1879–1882.

Stevens, J., Franks, P.J., Harrington, M. (1997) A community/hospital leg ulcer service. *Journal of Wound Care*, **6** (2), 62–68.

8

̲̲nisation of Wound Management

8.1 INTRODUCTION

The organisation of the delivery of wound care has undergone great change in the last few years. This chapter explores some of the aspects of wound care delivery that have had a great impact on nurses and nursing, both in the hospital and in the community. Overall, these changes have ensured that patients receive more effective care.

8.2 MANAGING WOUNDS IN THE COMMUNITY

In most healthcare systems there are some restrictions on which wound management products are available in the community. In the UK, available products are listed on the Drug Tariff. Today this list is regularly reviewed and new products added to it but this was not always the case. Less than ten years ago, there were considerable restrictions on the range of products available, particularly dressings for cavity wounds and compression bandages. Dealey (1997) reported a survey undertaken by the Tissue Viability Society to gain information about how cavity wounds were managed in the community. The overall response rate was poor but the results showed that nearly one-fifth of the dressings used were obtained by illegal means such as obtaining a prescription for one product and doing a 'swap' with the pharmacist for another, more suitable product. Happily a great deal has changed since then. As well as an increase in the products available, nurses are now allowed to prescribe from a limited formulary.

8.2.1 Nurse prescribing

Nurse prescribing has followed a rocky road since Julia Cumberlege first put forward the idea in a report for the Department of Health (DHSS, 1986). The concept was seen as a way of reducing time wasting for both community nurses and general practitioners (GPs) and reducing delays in treatment. Typically a nurse would see a patient with a leg ulcer at home and decide on a particular course of treatment. The nurse would have to go to the surgery to see the GP and request a prescription for the treatment. The patient, or a representative, would then collect the prescription from the surgery. In the case of housebound, elderly patients, nurses would sometimes obtain the prescription and deliver it to the pharmacist for the patient.

Initially it was only qualified district (community) nurses and health visitors who were able to prescribe, once they had undertaken the relevant three-month training course. Since 2000, this has widened and there are now a variety of ways in which a wide range of nurses can potentially undertake prescribing using the *Nurse Prescriber's Formulary.*

- *Independent prescriber* – person who is responsible for both assessment and treatment of a range of specific conditions. This group includes doctors and dentists as well as nurses but there are obviously greater limitations to the range of conditions that nurses can treat. However, they do include skin and wound care and minor injuries.
- *Supplementary prescriber* – this type of prescribing is most frequently of benefit when caring for patients with long-term conditions. A doctor will draw up a plan of care including the range of medication that can be used and when to refer the patient back to the doctor (Dimond, 2003). The supplementary prescriber can vary the dosage, keeping within the prescribed treatment range. This type of prescribing means that supplementary prescribers can legally prescribe from a wider range of medications than can be found in the nurse's formulary and this is generally more useful within specialist multi-disciplinary teams (Hay *et al.*, 2004).
- *Patient Group Directions (PGD)* – these are documents that make it legal for specific medicines to be given to patients without an individual prescription. However, they only relate to the supply or administration of a medicine, rather than its prescription (Baird, 2003). Each PGD has to be developed locally. Although initially intended for situations such as the treatment of mass casualties, they have also been used for walk-in centres and nurse-led clinics.

Thus far, nurse prescribing would seem to be relatively successful in the UK and around 23 000 district nurses and health visitors have been trained to prescribe so far. Latter and Courtney (2004) reviewed the literature for evaluations of nurse prescribing and found that, overall, the outcome was positive with evidence of improvements in time saving and convenience. White and Biggs (2004) conducted a postal survey of health visitors and district nurses in three trusts. They found variation in the level of confidence as a prescriber and in the frequency of prescribing. There was also a strong association between prescribing more than three times a week and wound care products and elastic hosiery, indicating wound care has particularly benefited from nurses' ability to prescribe. However, as discovered by other writers (Banning, 2004; Lewis-Evans & Jester, 2004), the authors of this study found that the nurses desired greater education in applied pharmacology, both in the initial education programme and as part of their ongoing professional development.

8.2.2 Community leg ulcer clinics

Another development has been that of nurse-led leg ulcer clinics in the community. These clinics have gradually increased in number during the last ten years, encouraged by the work of Moffatt *et al.* (1992) and the development of leg ulcer courses for nurses, such as the N18 validated by the now defunct English National Board (Moffatt & Karn, 1994). Many clinics have been established under the auspices of clinical nurse specialists in tissue viability or leg ulcer nurse specialists. The rationale for establishing leg ulcer clinics is the possibility of concentrating resources and skilled nurses at the clinic to ensure that all patients have a full assessment, including a Doppler assessment, and access to appropriately applied compression bandages. However, it is the outcomes of care that are most important.

Simon *et al.* (1996) found a 38% reduction in costs after establishing leg ulcer clinics in a health authority alongside a 13-week healing rate that increased from less than 25% to 42% in the first 12 months. They compared these outcomes with a control group in a neighbouring health authority where there were no clinics and found no improvement from baseline in this group. In a later phase of this project, the project team monitored the continuing progress of the clinics as well as new clinics established in the neighbouring health authority (Ellison *et al.*, 2002). They found the new clinics showed a similar improvement in outcome but the longer established clinics did not totally maintain their initial level of improvement, most probably because of the loss of the leg ulcer nurse specialist between the two phases of the project.

Morrell *et al.* (1998) undertook a randomised, controlled trial to compare outcomes for patients randomised to a leg ulcer clinic compared with usual care at home by a district nurse. They found a trend towards greater healing in the clinic group ($p = 0.03$) and a slightly greater cost per patient compared with the controls. The authors concluded that clinics provide better outcomes than homecare. However, in a critique by Thurlby and Griffiths (2002), the authors suggest that the study was biased towards the clinic group as there was poor provision of compression bandages with less than half the homecare patients receiving them. It is also possible that the nurses were less skilled in leg ulcer care.

Despite these criticisms, there seems to be a general view that leg ulcer clinics are an effective method of proving care for patients with leg ulcers. Some patients find the social aspect important as many have poor mobility that restricts their lifestyle. A study by Liew *et al.* (2000) found an improvement in quality of life over an average of eight weeks of clinic attendance. In particular, patients had a significant reduction of pain, better sleep and greater mobility. Overall, leg ulcer clinics have more supporters than critics, although it may be that involvement of a nurse specialist is crucial in maintaining beneficial outcomes.

8.3 NURSE SPECIALISTS IN WOUND CARE

Specialist nurses in wound care have a variety of titles but the most common in the UK is clinical nurse specialist in tissue viability (TVN). They straddle both hospital and community as TVN may be found in both community and hospital trusts. It is a relatively new nursing specialty developed in the late 1980s and the numbers have grown rapidly. The precise number is difficult to determine as there is no formal register but Finnie (2004) suggests that there are now around 500 in post as well as a few nurse consultants.

Education is an essential prerequisite for the recognition of any specialty. Fletcher (1998) found that there are a variety of courses available within the UK. They comprise short courses at diploma level as well as degree and Masters level programmes. Fairbairn (2001) discussed the potential for a clinical doctorate for TVN as an alternative to undertaking a PhD following the more traditional route. He suggested that this option is more flexible, allowing the student to utilise aspects of existing work. A more recent development has been that of a competency framework devised for TVN in Scotland but it is intended for wider use (Finnie & Wilson, 2003). It involves six domains: clinical problem solving, professional practice, teamwork, reflective practice, empowerment and leadership.

Austin (2002) undertook a survey of TVN in one region of the UK and found several clearly defined aspects of the role.

- *Clinical role* – all the TVN had direct clinical contact with patients, receiving referrals predominantly from nurses.
- *Educator role* – this is an important aspect of the role. The survey found that TVN mostly taught nurses but also taught other disciplines such as doctors, allied health professionals and social workers.
- *Leadership role* – all respondents had a remit that extended across their organisation, involving advice on purchasing or commissioning resources (94%), standards or guideline development (93%), audit of care provision (83%).
- *Research role* – 57% had participated in research, predominantly product evaluations. This aspect of the role generally requires further development (Gray, 2004).
- *Management role* – respondents indicated that this involved managing a team (39%) and/or holding the service budget (42%) or influencing the budget expenditure.

Austin's survey provides a picture of TVN activity that is fairly representative. She also noted that the role is poorly understood by others. Flanagan (1996) described some of the difficulties that the TVN may face. They include unrealistic objectives or targets, role ambiguity, responsibilities across large geographical areas or multiple sites, constant pressure to reduce the cost of the tissue viability service and often having to work with insufficient resources with limited professional support. Despite the constraints, the role of the TVN still presents the post holder with considerable opportunities to enhance nursing practice and the personal satisfaction of seeing wounds healing and patients' quality of life improve.

8.4 THE MANAGEMENT OF PRESSURE-REDISTRIBUTING EQUIPMENT

As noted above, many TVN have a major role in relation to the management of equipment, especially pressure-redistributing equipment. Most trusts have some type of budget for equipment but there is considerable variety in how it is used and the ways in which distribution and maintenance are organised. Several authors have reported that *ad hoc* ordering of rental equipment or unplanned purchasing on a ward-by-ward basis is both expensive and inefficient and results in ineffective care (Birchall, 2001; Fox & Delve, 1994; Newton 2001). One alternative is an equipment store or equipment library.

8.4.1 Equipment stores

This method of control and delivery of pressure-redistributing equipment is most commonly found in the hospital setting but there are also a few within primary care trusts. Birchall (2001) described the development of an equipment store across an acute trust of 1100 beds on two sites, taking two years to become fully established. The store contained a mixture of purchased and rental equipment. The cost savings from the previous *ad hoc* rental system covered the cost of the equipment, including maintenance and repair, cost of the staff running the store, an annual foam mattress replacement programme and a five-year replacement programme for the alternating air mattresses.

Newton (2001) found similar problems in her trust. In particular, there were problems with staff attitudes as they were careless with equipment, unwilling to share equipment with other wards, kept patients on dynamic systems for longer than necessary and tended to order rental equipment as an easy option, rather than seeking out trust-owned equipment. As a result, rental expenditure was spiralling out of control. After implementing an equipment library, Newton found a marked change in staff attitudes and a more appropriate and cost-effective use of equipment.

Both Birchall (2001) and Newton (2001) implemented improved education programmes for staff that covered not only the appropriate use of equipment but also how to set it up. The use of a central database is also an essential aspect of this type of service as it enables the store staff to determine the whereabouts of every piece of equipment, making it easier to monitor usage.

8.4.2 Total bed management

An alternative to the establishment of an equipment store is the use of total bed management (TBM). This concept means that a trust and a contractor enter into partnership, with the contractor supplying the trust with all its tissue viability, manual handling and bed therapy needs (Preece, 1999). Obviously, this type of contract means that the equipment is supplied at a reduced cost. Preece (1999) described similar problems as those described above. In addition, there was also a major problem with existing bed frame stock as 492 bed frames failed at least one of five assessment criteria; also 389 of them were a manual handling risk. An audit of the foam mattresses showed that 75% needed replacement. There was also an excessive use of low air loss systems. The implementation of TBM enabled the trust to replace the worn-out bed frames with electric bed frames, which they found reduced both the manual handling risks and also the need for low air loss beds. The foam mattresses were replaced with high-specification foam mattresses and a suitable range of other pressure-redistributing equipment was included in the contract.

8.5 WOUND-HEALING CENTRES

Wound care falls into the remit of a great many specialist areas: vascular surgery, dermatology, diabetology, plastic surgery, geriatrics and so on. This has resulted in considerable fragmentation of services and lack of ownership in many areas. Bennett (2000) suggested that unless wound care is able to establish its own unique national profile, it is in danger of being subsumed into other specialties such as those listed above. There is also little awareness of the benefits of providing a multiprofessional specialist centre for non-healing wounds. The one exception seems to be diabetic foot ulcers as the NICE guidelines state that patients should have access to a multidisciplinary footcare team (NICE, 2004); even then, it only refers to the one wound type. There are a number of centres of excellence caring for one wound type, such as leg ulcers or diabetic foot ulcers, but very few that provide care for wounds of all aetiologies.

Four wound-healing centres will be discussed: two in the UK and two in Denmark. All of these centres are based within the national healthcare systems of the two countries and there is no charge associated with attendance. This is in contrast with the wound-healing centres in the USA that are commercially run.

Despite the fact that nurses have led much of the work in improving wound care provision, it is doctors who have pioneered the concept of wound-healing centres. In the case of the two centres in the UK, one centre was established by a general practitioner, although it is based in a department of surgery in a university hospital, and the other by a geriatrician (Bennett, 2000; Harding, 2001) and in Denmark, the two wound-healing centres were established by a surgeon (Gottrup, 2004). Although the centres all function differently, they have a number of common features:

- The staff working in wound-healing centres include physicians from different specialisms, as well as a variety of other healthcare professionals, including nurses. The range of professionals varies from centre to centre.
- They are based within teaching hospitals and provide education programmes of varying types.
- They treat both inpatients and outpatients, referred from both the primary and secondary healthcare sectors, although the number of inpatient beds may be limited.
- All the wound-healing centres are involved in research programmes.

Beyond this common ground, the centres all function differently, due to the circumstances in which they were developed. The centres in Denmark have been fully integrated into the national health service, allowing for country-wide referrals. Gottrup (2004) suggests that for Denmark, with its 5.2 million inhabitants, only one or two clinics are necessary. Obviously, larger or more densely populated countries would require more centres to provide the same levels of care provision.

Wound-healing centres have a great deal to offer in terms of specialised care for problem wounds, educational opportunities to increase the numbers of clinical staff with specialist knowledge and an important research function to assist in developing the evidence base for this important subject.

8.6 CONCLUSIONS

Wound care is increasingly being recognised as an important aspect of nursing care and it is becoming ever more sophisticated. Despite this, there are still areas of poor practice and patients who receive less than optimum care. It is hoped that these variations in practice will decrease as more evidence and more guidelines become available to guide the practitioner.

REFERENCES

Austin, L. (2002) A survey of tissue viability nurses' role and background in one region. *Journal of Wound Care*, **11** (9), 347–350.

Baird, A. (2003) Nurse prescribing – how did we get here? *Journal of Community Nursing*, **17** (4), 4–10.

Banning, M. (2004) Nurse prescribing, nurse education and related research in the United Kingdom: a review of the literature. *Nurse Education Today*, **24**, 420–427.

Bennett, G. (2000) Is there a role for the multidisciplinary approach within tissue viability in the next millennium? *Journal of Tissue Viability*, **10** (2), 43–44.

Birchall, L. (2001) Centralising supply of a trust's pressure-relieving equipment. *Journal of Wound Care*, **10** (6), 214–219.

Dealey, C. (1997) A survey of the management of cavity wounds in the community. *Journal of Tissue Viability*, **7** (3), 75–76.

Department of Health and Social Security (1986) *Neighbourhood Nursing – a focus for care. Report of the Community Nursing Review.* HMSO, London.

Dimond, B. (2003) The introduction of nurse prescribing 2: final Crown Report. *British Journal of Nursing*, **12** (16), 980–983.

Ellison, D.A., Hayes, L., Lane, C., Tracey, A., McCollum, C.N. (2002) Evaluating the cost and efficacy of leg ulcer care provided in two large UK health authorities. *Journal of Wound Care*, **11** (2), 47–51.

Fairbairn, G. (2001) The role of a clinical doctorate in the advancement of practice. *British Journal of Nursing*, **10** (15) (suppl), S4–S5.

Finnie, A. (2004) We must act to move tissue viability forward. *British Journal of Nursing*, **13** (6) (suppl), S3.

Finnie, A., Wilson, A. (2003) Development of a tissue viability nursing competency framework. *British Journal of Nursing*, **12** (6) (suppl), S38–S44.

Flanagan, M. (1996) The role of the clinical nurse specialist in tissue viability. *British Journal of Nursing*, **5** (11), 676–681.

Fletcher, J. (1998) A survey of courses available that are relevant to the field of tissue viability, in (eds) Leaper, D., Dealey, C., Franks, P.J., Hofman, D., Moffatt, C., *Proceedings of the 7th European Conference on Advances in Wound Management*. EMAP Healthcare Ltd, London.

Fox, P., Delve, M. (1994) Equipped to care. *Nursing Times*, **90** (30), 46–47.

Gottrup, F. (2004) A specialised wound-healing centre concept: importance of a multidisciplinary department structure and surgical treatment facilities in the treatment of chronic wounds. *American Journal of Surgery*, **187** (5) (suppl), 38S–43S.

Gray, D. (2004) Specialists must accept challenge of improving clinical outcomes. *British Journal of Nursing*, **13** (6) (suppl), S4.

Harding, K.G. (2001) Meet the innovators in wound care. *Journal of Wound Care*, **10** (5), 180.

Hay, A., Bradley, E., Nolan, P. (2004) Supplementary nurse prescribing. *Nursing Standard*, **18** (4), 33–39.

Latter, S., Courtenay, M. (2004) Effectiveness of nurse prescribing: a review of the literature. *Journal of Clinical Nursing*, **13** (1), 26–32.

Lewis-Evans, A.B., Jester, R. (2004) Nurse prescribers' experiences of prescribing. *Journal of Clinical Nursing*, **13** (7), 796–805.

Liew, I.H., Law, K.A., Sinha, S.N. (2000) Do leg ulcer clinics improve patients' quality of life? *Journal of Wound Care*, **9** (9), 423–426.

Moffatt, C.J., Karn, A. (1994) Answering the call for more education. Development of an ENB course in leg ulcer management. *Professional Nurse*, **9** (10), 708–712.

Moffatt, C.J., Franks, P.J., Oldroyd, M. *et al.* (1992) Community clinics for leg ulcers and impact on healing. *British Medical Journal*, **305**, 1389–1392.

Morrell, C.J., Walters, S.J., Dixon, S. *et al.* (1998) Cost effectiveness of community leg ulcer clinics: randomised controlled trial. *British Medical Journal*, **316**, 1487–1491.

National Institute for Clinical Excellence (2004) *Clinical Guideline 10: type 2 diabetes: prevention and management of foot problems*. NICE, London.

Newton, H. (2001) Developing an equipment library: the solution to increasing demand. *British Journal of Nursing*, **10** (22) (suppl), S59–S64.

Preece, J. (1999) Total bed management: the way forward in pressure sore prevention. *British Journal of Nursing*, **8** (22), 1524–1529.

Simon, D.A., Freak, L., Kinsella, J. *et al.* (1996) Community leg ulcer clinics: a comparative study in two health authorities. *British Medical Journal*, **312**, 1648–1651.

Thurlby, K., Griffiths, P. (2002) Community leg ulcer clinics vs home visits: which is more effective? *British Journal of Community Nursing*, **7** (5), 260–264.

White, A., Biggs, K. (2004) Benefits and challenges of nurse prescribing. *Journal of Advanced Nursing*, **45** (6), 559–567.

Index

Page numbers in *italics* refer to figures or tables.